**Perspectives in
Personality Research**

DISCARD

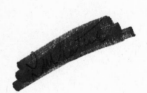

Perspectives in Personality Research

Edited by HENRY P. DAVID, Ph.D.

and

J. C. BRENGELMANN, M.D., Ph.D.

under the auspices of the

INTERNATIONAL UNION OF SCIENTIFIC PSYCHOLOGY

SPRINGER Publishing Company, Inc., New York

Type set at The Polyglot Press, New York

Printed in U.S.A.

BY NOBLE OFFSET PRINTERS, INC.

Contributors

ARTHUR M. ADLERSTEIN, Ph.D.
Neurological Research Center, Children's Hospital, Philadelphia, Pennsylvania, United States

IRVING E. ALEXANDER, Ph.D.
Training Branch, National Institute of Mental Health, Bethesda, Maryland, United States

LEONARDO ANCONA, Ph.D.
Professor of Psychology, Catholic University, Milan, Italy

GERALD S. BLUM, Ph.D.
Professor of Psychology, University of Michigan, Ann Arbor, Michigan, United States

J. C. BRENGELMANN, M.D., Ph.D.
Institute of Psychiatry, Maudsley Hospital, London, England

HENRY P. DAVID, Ph.D.
Chief Psychologist and Psychology Consultant, N. J. State Department of Institutions and Agencies, Trenton, New Jersey, United States

NORMAN L. FARBEROW, Ph.D.
Central Research Unit, Veterans Administration Center, Los Angeles, California, United States

FRANZ G. FROM, Ph.D.
Professor of Psychology, University of Copenhagen, Denmark

E. P. HOLLANDER, Ph.D.
Associate Professor of Psychology, Washington University, St. Louis, Missouri, United States

BÄRBEL INHELDER, Ph.D.
Professor of Child Psychology, Institute J. J. Rousseau, University of Geneva, Switzerland

OTTO KLINEBERG, M.D., Ph.D.
Secretary-General, International Union of Scientific Psychology; Professor of Psychology, Columbia University, New York, New York, United States

A. R. LURIA, M.D., Ph.D.
Professor of Psychology, University of Moscow; Director, Research Section, Institute of Defectology, Academy of Pedagogical Science, Moscow, Union of Soviet Socialist Republics

ROBERT B. MacLEOD, Ph.D.
Professor of Psychology, Cornell University, Ithaca, New York, United States

NOËL MAILLOUX, Ph.D.
Treasurer, International Union of Scientific Psychology; Professor of Psychology, University of Montreal, Quebec, Canada

RICHARD MEILI, Ph.D.
Professor of Psychology, University of Bern, Switzerland

DANIEL R. MILLER, Ph.D.
Associate Professor of Psychology, University of Michigan, Ann Arbor, Michigan, United States

LOIS B. MURPHY, Ph.D.
Research Psychologist, Menninger Foundation, Topeka, Kansas, United States

HENRY A. MURRAY, M.D., Ph.D.
Professor of Psychology, Harvard University, Cambridge, Massachusetts, United States

GERALD NOELTING, Ph.D.
Research Associate in Child Psychology, Institute J. J. Rousseau, University of Geneva, Switzerland

JOSEPH NUTTIN, Ph.D.
Professor of Psychology, University of Louvain, Belgium

WILLIAM RABINOWITZ, Ph.D.
Assistant Professor, Division of Research and Evaluation, Division of Teacher Education, Board of Higher Education, New York, New York, United States

EDWIN S. SHNEIDMAN, Ph.D.
Central Research Unit, Veterans Administration Center, Los Angeles, California, United States

AASE GRUDA SKARD, D.H.L.
Associate Professor of Psychology, University of Oslo, Norway

RONALD TAFT, Ph.D.
Reader in Psychology, University of Western Australia, Perth, Australia

RENATO TAGIURI, Ph.D.
Associate Professor, Harvard University, Graduate School of Business Administration, Boston, Massachusetts, United States

HANS THOMAE, Ph.D.
Professor of Psychology, University of Erlangen, Germany

SILVAN S. TOMKINS, Ph.D.
Professor of Psychology, Princeton University, Princeton, New Jersey, United States

Foreword

THREE YEARS AGO, when *Perspectives in Personality Theory* appeared under the editorship of Henry P. David and Helmut von Bracken, with contributions by twenty-two psychologists from nine different countries, I described it as "a real landmark in international cooperation among psychologists." All of us connected with the International Union of Scientific Psychology were delighted with this tangible expression of increased communication among psychologists, who too often remain content to read the writings of their own countrymen in their own language. Our pleasure was increased with the publication of the volume in German as well, thus widening even more the circle of international contact. The favorable reception accorded the first *Perspectives* was convincing proof that such publications met a real need in the psychological community, and the hope was expressed on many sides that what had succeeded so well would establish a precedent for the future. After all, psychologists are not usually content with just a single case!

It is therefore with even greater pleasure and pride that, in the name of the International Union of Scientific Psychology, I write these few words of introduction to the second volume. *Perspectives in Personality Research,* again edited by Henry P. David, this time in cooperation with J. C. Brengelmann, contains contributions from twenty-seven psychologists from eleven countries, an even wider range than that represented by its predecessor. We are indeed, in the happy phrase used by Joseph Nuttin as the title of his chapter, going "beyond provincialism." The distinguished scholars who have collaborated in this important undertaking have placed all of us in their debt, and our very special thanks go to the two editors who were responsible for the volume as a whole.

The International Union of Scientific Psychology, like *Perspectives,* is becoming more international. It now consists of twenty-six national societies, those of Australia, Belgium, Brazil, Canada, Cuba, Denmark, Egypt, Finland, France, German Federal Republic, Great Britain, Holland, Israel, Italy, Japan, New Zealand, Norway, Poland, Spain, Sweden, Switzerland, Turkey, United States, Uruguay, U.S.S.R., and Yugoslavia. Associated organizations include the International Association of Applied Psychology, the Inter-American Society of Psychology, and the Society of French-Speaking Psychologists. It has consultative status with UNESCO, from which it receives a generous annual subvention, and for which it carries out specific tasks under contract. It is now engaged in conducting an extensive cross-national study of the development of national stereotypes in young children of different ages. It is also closely associated with the International Union of Biological Sciences (affiliated with the International Council of Scientific Unions), and the International Committee of Social Science Documentation.

The Union was founded in 1951 on the occasion of the International Congress in Stockholm, with Henri Piéron of France as the first president, and H. S. Langfeld of the United States as secretary-general. In 1954 when the Congress took place in Montreal, Canada, Jean Piaget of Switzerland was elected president, and three years later, in Brussels, he was succeeded by Albert Michotte of Belgium. The first *Perspectives* resulted primarily from papers and discussions presented on the occasion of the Montreal Congress, and the second volume is similarly related to the Congress which took place in Brussels. There is no guarantee that this pattern will continue indefinitely, but we are grateful for what we have already received. The editors and authors have made a contribution, in the truest and most literal sense, to international understanding.

Otto Klineberg
Columbia University
Secretary General
International Union of Scientific Psychology

Editors' Note

WITH THE PUBLICATION OF *Perspectives in Personality Theory* in 1957, an idea conceived at the 1954 Montreal International Congress of Psychology had become reality. Colleagues from many lands had jointly demonstrated the international scope of their science and profession, and the International Union of Scientific Psychology was receiving modest royalties.

When a second volume was suggested at the 1957 Brussels Congress, and the editors were again urged to serve, von Bracken recommended Brengelmann as co-editor. Having previously presented the varied directions of personality theory, it now seemed appropriate to consider how theories are translated into empirical research.

Once more colleagues from many lands readily responded to our request to expand their Congress papers into reports of ongoing research. An equally gratifying response came from additional contributors invited to discuss their latest (1959) work. All of the material was then organized into appropriate sections with integrated commentaries and surveys of current personality research by distinguished psychologists. We are pleased that *Perspectives in Personality Research* will be published in time for the 1960 Bonn International Congress.

As before, there is much to acknowledge: the steadfast support of our colleagues, especially Robert MacLeod, Henry Murray, and Silvan Tomkins; the encouragement of the International Union and its Secretary-General, Otto Klineberg; the editorial counsel of David McClelland and Arthur Rosenthal; the secretarial assistance of the New Jersey State Department of Institutions and Agencies and the Maudsley Hospital; and, again, the understanding patience of our wives.

Trenton, New Jersey
London, England
January, 1960

H. P. D.
J. C. B.

Contents

PART ONE

Overview

Henry A. Murray

I

Historical Trends in Personality Research

INTRODUCTION

SCIENCE-MAKING relevant to a better understanding of human states, activities, and achievements is proceeding in different languages and terminologies at widely-separated places in both hemispheres at such a healthy rate and in such multifarious ways and directions that no single array of papers of the sort that we have here could possibly be representative of all its diversities of being and becoming; nor could any psychologist keep abreast of it on all fronts without abandoning his own researches. Allow me, then, to start with a disclaimer of the Olympian connotations of the assigned heading, "Overview," as well as of the above title for my prelude to this second triennial concert of eminent performers.

After re-reading Gordon Allport's knowledgeable overview of the preceding (first) volume of *Perspectives*,[1] my tentative conclusion was that he had already said well as much as I could say about trends in the sphere of personology, as much as could reasonably be said without a far more analytical, comprehensive, and chronological survey of the field. Indeed, he had succeeded, it seemed to me, in writing an excellent preface to both *Perspectives*. What was left? It is true that Allport's focus of attention was theoretical trends, rather than research trends, in Europe and America; but, since research and theory, at their best, are functionally intermeshed, each being both the

3

determinant and consequence of the other, Allport's review necessarily took note of the main currents of investigation as they are ordinarily defined and named today. It is also true that Allport chose to emphasize contrasts of orientation—especially between Germany and the United States—rather than similarities and convergences; but, in so doing, he omitted very little that is pertinent to our topic. In short, he competently covered a good deal of the ground that otherwise would have fallen to my lot, and the reader of this second volume should therefore have the advantage of a brief summary as reminder of his chief points.

SUMMARY OF ALLPORT'S DISTINGUISHING MARKS OF ANGLO-AMERICAN AND CONTINENTAL THEORIES

Allport's first conclusion, supported by the judgment of several other contributors to the first volume, was that the preoccupations of theorists in Great Britain and in the United States have been more similar than dissimilar. "The same kind of theories—psychoanalytic, factorial, positivistic, projective, and interpersonal—prevail in the two countries." But when he compared these shared Anglo-American trends to those which were most conspicuous on the Continent, dissimilarities became more apparent than similarities. "With some trepidation"—yet, in my scales, with considerable acumen—Allport proposed the following "distinguishing marks of Anglo-American and Continental theories respectively":

Philosophical assumptions: The Lockean tradition is dominant in England and America; the Leibnitzian and Kantian on the Continent. Anglo-American theorists are more apt to conceive of personalities as reactive (rather than internally aroused and proactive) and also as readily modified by environmental influences (rather than as basically and enduringly structured by genetical determinants).

The whole and its parts: Holistic (global, synthetic) conceptions, with fewer differentiations of various components of personality, are more prevalent on the Continent. Typology, existential psychology, and *Verstehen* psychology are cited as illustrations of this outlook.

Points of view: There is less meliorism and optimism, more fatalism and pessimism on the Continent.

Social interaction: There is less attention to the formulation of interpersonal transactions on the Continent.

Brain models: Anglo-American psychologists are currently more interested in theoretical models derived from neuro-physiology and cybernetics, as well as in physiological determinants generally.

Methodology and creativity: A far greater attachment to positivistic tenets, both in thought and practice, is characteristic of British and American psychologists. In the judgment of theorists of this persuasion, some of the dominant trends on the Continent—phenomenology, existential psychology, stratification theory—yield little that is clearly communicable, precise, and susceptible of verification. And yet there is the undeniable fact that Europe has been the breeding ground of all, or almost all, fundamentally new and important ideas. Besides the all-pervasive influence of Freud, Allport mentions the typologies of Jung, Kretchmer and Spranger, the psychometric and psychodiagnostic methods of Binet, Jung, and Rorschach, the formative labors of the Würzburg school as basis for studies of attitudes, Lewin as generator of various lines of theory and research, the philosophy of existentialism, the pioneering work of Janet, Pavlov, Stern, Adler, and Piaget. (To this list of originators, some of us might be inclined to add the names of Köhler, Wertheimer, Koffka, and Goldstein; the Bühlers, Luria, Werner, and Mareno; Melanie Klein, Rank, Alexander, Horney, Fromm, Else Frankel-Brunswik, and Erikson; Marx, Durkheim, Weber, and Pareto; Boas, Malinowski, and Sapir; Bergson, Heidegger, Carnap, and many more. Among great British sources of ideas and methods, there is Darwin, of course, and Tyler, Fraser, Sherrington, McDougall, Galton, Karl Pearson, Spearman, Fisher, and a host of others.) "Where would we be without them?"

COMMENTARY

Although pure positivism seems to be dying of inanition, positivistic measures of scientific worth—as best exemplified in physics—are assuredly accorded a far higher status in the value systems of many British and American psychologists than they are in the value systems of our Continental colleagues, and I agree with Allport that the consequences of these two contrasting estimates constitute the clearest difference between the nature of their respective contributions. The picture in the United States is not clear-cut, because so many European "ideamen" have emigrated to this country and leavened in diverse ways the course of psychological thought and action. What America has done is to provide congenial pots for the melting, marriage, and systematic integration of the transported ideas, as well as the necessary technical resources, inventiveness, and ingenuity for the testing, correction, and revision of these ideas according to increasingly rigorous criteria.

This positivistic trend was initiated, in large measure, by the ideal formula, created in the mind of Pavlov and established by his experiments, which was seized by that persuasive, one-tracked, charismatic, timely publicist, James B. Watson, labeled "behaviorism," and sold to all but a few American psychologists as the only model on which to build a veritable science. With this sword he murdered, on his right hand, the meandering introspectionism of Titchener, and, on his left, the nativistic drive theory of McDougall; and ever since that triumph, Watsonian behaviorism has constituted the fixed image of American psychology—shallow, mechanistic, Philistine, soulless—in the minds of a large number of Continental, including Soviet, thinkers. Although Watson failed to stem the tide of Freudian ideas and although, in due course, the method of introspectionism and the concept of purposive disposition were each (with a new look) officially resurrected, so indelible has proved the imprint of Watson's message that even today Americans must honor him with a semantic gesture by speaking of the "behavioral sciences," although "behavior" now embraces everything that Watson excluded from the realm of science, everything, in fact, that can be studied.

After the definite separation of psychology from academic departments of traditional philosophy—a strategic turning-point —a number of veteran experimentalists raised their sights from biology and physiology toward the far more perfected physical sciences with their mathematics, symbolic logic, operational definitions, systems of postulates and theorems; and nowadays it is the mounting ambition of these theorists to build, so far as possible, a psychology in the image of physics. Since the advance toward this ideal is facilitated by studying the most consistent organisms in stable, rigidly-constrained situations, psychologists with this extravagant ambition have (with certain recent exceptions) almost invariably restricted their fields of concern to the behavior of lower organisms or to the simplest perceptual or physiological processes of human beings. Although thereby divorcing themselves, strictly speaking, from the sphere of personology, these experimentalists have been notably influential, first, by providing the general outlines of a sophisticated learning theory, and second, by holding up their scientific standards which, though forever unattainable by anyone who is genuinely interested in human nature, nevertheless induce the personologist to work toward more explicit and verifiable propositions, greater numbers of subjects, more rigidly controlled experiments, instrumental recordings, and the mechanical and statistical manipulation of his data. The general effect of this ideal has been to put excellence of means (and scientific prestige) ahead of importance of ends (significance of obtained knowledge). To this twist may be ascribed, in part, the technical fecundity but conceptual parasitism of American psychology.

I would guess that this popular, militant, philosophical, positivistic, behavioristic movement is enough to account for all of Allport's above-listed characteristics of American trends (exemplified to a less extent by British trends). With this ultra-scientific orientation and with Pavlov as grandfather figure, the activist American psychologist—an empirical, inductive, thinking extravert, in contrast, say, to the more numerous rationalistic, deductive, thinking introverts of Germany, the Netherlands, and Switzerland—is predisposed toward controlled experimentation and hence to initiate action himself by stimulating his subjects (animal or human) and thereby making them *reactors* (rather than proactors). Following Pavlov, one of the more frequent aims of an American psychologist will be to discover how to

change or condition (train or socialize) the reactions of his subjects by rewards and punishments, and hence he necessarily will
stress *modifiability* through *environmental influences,* even
though he may end as Pavlov did, by discriminating different
constitutional types of subjects. Since it is not possible to elicit
and record more than a very few *parts* of a subject's personality
in any one session or in any series of sessions of the same kind,
an experimentalist will rarely, if ever, obtain enough data to
justify his speaking of a "whole personality" in any meaningful
sense. The study of *social interactions* is merely an extension of
the experimental method to include human beings as stimuli,
instead of restricting psychology to knowledge about responses
to physical things or to written words and pictures. From physics
was derived the hope of constructing integrated theoretical
systems such as Hull's and topological field theories such as
Lewin's, and, more recently, theoretical *models* based on cybernetics and information theory.

This covers in a rough way Allport's chief classes of distinctive marks of Anglo-American theories as compared to Continental theories. No doubt some burden of determination must
be assigned to temperamental and characterological differences.
British and American psychologists, let us say, are more apt to
be extraceptors, starting from what they see on the periphery,
and either staying there or working in; whereas many Continental (though relatively few Norwegian and French) psychologists
are intraceptors, starting from what they feel and think, and
either staying there or working out. The difference may also be
connected with the fact that traditional philosophy and psychology have not been so sharply divided on the Continent, and
students who elect the latter are more likely to be part-philos-
ophers than part-biologists. There is relatively little animal
experimentation, Pavlovian psychology, or statistical confirmation of propositions in Germany; the greater emphasis is on the
rational evaluations, aspirations, subjective experiences, and
basic styles of superior men or at least of mature and educated
persons in their more conscious, exalted or despairing, moments.

The *Verstehen* school of psychology, for example, assumes
the possibility of an intuitive grasp of "events as fraught with

significance in relation to a totality" (Allport quoting Spranger); and there is no doubt that many people have intuitive experiences of this nature. But the question is, to what extent they are delusory. Have a number of *Verstehen* psychologists, as well as psychologists of other persuasions, independently observed, or been presented with a report of, the same series of events in which a given subject participated, and have they all "grasped" them in the same way and apperceived them as "fraught" with the same "significance" in relation to the same "totality"? If so, we can speak of high inter-judge reliability and declare that, according to this criterion, we have something public and objective which belongs in the domain of science. But, if not, then each apperception is private and must be understood partially in terms of the personality of the apperceptor. This, however, calls for another group of apperceptors, and so on in an infinite regression. Here, following Allport, I have been thinking back three or four decades to an earlier Germany, the birthplace of academic psychology. My comments are not at all applicable or less applicable to the Soviet Union, Norway, Denmark, Belgium, France, and Switzerland.

Having chosen to identify *differences* of trends, rather than dominant trends, in Europe and America, Allport necessarily called attention to what was unique, distinctive, or exceptional in each country. As already noted, for example, what stands out in the United States—like the head of an acromegalic—are the theories and objective standards of experimental animal psychologists who have denounced reports of subjective processes simply because the entities they study do not speak a language they can understand. With this as reference point, what stands out on the Continent, then, is its polar opposite, existential psychology, developed by those who are more interested in the interior environments and experiences of human beings than they are in the muscular responses of lower organisms. Here one is comparing Continental personologists to American biologists rather than to American personologists. Furthermore, by stressing in this way the more striking contrasts and minimizing the similarities, one is likely to disregard preoccupations flourishing on both sides of the Atlantic and end with a somewhat misleading picture. As Allport pointed out, there are numerous exceptions and overlaps among the differences he enumerated.

We grant that all psychology in the United States has been influenced to some extent by the standards of positivism, and that behavioristic learning theory, in one form or another, is an integral part of most developmental personality theories; but this is nowhere near the whole story in the sphere of personology. The widespread use of paper-and-pencil tests, questionnaires, and inventories, supplemented by factor analysis, is a rather distinctive Anglo-American occupation, which can only pretend to be positivistic. Psychoanalytic theory, which is far more comprehensive and pervasive than either of these two concerns in both England and the United States, includes minute explorations of interior states and processes, via projective tests or more directly in interviews. Field theory is also prevalent in the two countries; and last, but certainly not least, are role theory, social systems theory, and culture theory. All these may be relatively more favored in Great Britain and the United States; but they are also found pretty nearly everywhere in Europe, in the Scandinavian countries, the Netherlands, Switzerland, France, and Belgium, witness the fertile Ombredane and the accomplished personality theorist, Nuttin.

DIFFICULTIES IN PLACING AND CLASSIFYING TRENDS

Do we estimate the strength of a certain trend in each country by the absolute number or by the percentage of psychologists who sustain it? In the United States there is more of almost everything because there are many more psychologists. In twenty years the existential psychologists in this country may outnumber those in Europe. Again, do we use as our criterion the country of origin or the country where the trend is most widely supported? Roughly speaking, all trends have originated in Europe, and yet all trends (with a few exceptions) are more widely supported in the United States. The conception of "personality-as-a-whole" is properly attributed by Allport to the Continent; but since the emigration to this country of the leading Gestalt psychologists of Germany, the publication of the holistic conceptions of the biologists, Ritter and Childs in America and E. S. Russell in England, and the derivation of systems theory from the more developed sciences, the whole-part concept has been taken for granted in the United States and has been more elaborately developed here than it appears to have been in Europe.

And then, what shall we say about psychoanalytic theory, which Allport includes as one of the shared Anglo-American currents, but not as one which distinguishes them from those on the Continent? Psychoanalysis is a medical psychology that is entirely Continental in origin; but yet it has not permeated university circles on the Continent, or even in England, to the extent that it has in the United States. In this country, I would say, it is the most popular theory in the field of personality, inspiring and shaping a multiplicity of productive researches. If we omit it as a characteristic of personological developments in England and America because it had its genesis in Austria or because it is also prevalent in several European countries, we may be leaving out the hero of the drama. On the other hand, if we include it as a dominant influence, it is harder to hold to the proposition that Anglo-American theories do not give sufficient weight to constitutional factors (e.g. stages of psychosexual development), to basic character structure (e.g. constellation of infantile complexes), to stratifications of the personality (e.g. id, ego, superego), or to internally generated activity (e.g. libido, wish).

The biggest obstacle, however, to a revealing discussion of scientific inclinations is the names that have been given to them. It was said above, for example, that British and American psychologists have been concerned with the "same kind of *theories* —psychoanalytic, factorial, positivistic, projective, and interpersonal." Now, psychoanalysis is a complex theoretical system which is intended for representations (both differentiated and integrated) of "entire" personalities. Projective tests, on the other hand, are techniques for obtaining imaginations, imaginations which are open to interpretation in the light of any theory. Factor analysis is a method of processing data, the result of which may be used in various ways with the minimum of theoretical assumptions. Positivism is a scientific philosophy which is largely concerned with rules and procedure and criteria of meaning and validity. "Interpersonal" refers to events in which the chief participants are human, events which are susceptible of formulation and interpretation in terms of any adequate theory of personality. One finds comparable medleys and confusions of terms pretty nearly everywhere: different kinds of things classed together, different words for the same kind of thing, and over and over again the name of a theory or movement which combines diverse components, some of which are integral to theories or movements with other names.

How, for example, shall we deal with the copious, variable, still-evolving phenomenological-existential movement in Europe? It seems to incorporate a general assumption relative to the participation, even in the most "objective" observations, of the scientist's unconscious mental sets and suppositions, an assumption which is shared by physicists as well as by a large number of psychologists. And, then, existential phenomenologists appear to be particularly concerned with regions and modes of investigation (e.g. *covert* psychic experiences as much as overt acts, *total* experiences rather than isolated parts of experiences, *stages of processes* as much as their final products, *qualities* as much as quantities, etc.) which are also stressed by quite a few psychologists who are nominally affiliated with other movements or who do not choose to think and work within the confines of any single creed. Take, say, the following three, often-quoted existential principles: first, that one must not abstract the person from his world; second, that every person apperceives and feels his world in a way that is unique—though similar, in certain respects, to the ways of other persons of the same type; and third, that the psychologist by various means (assisted by the process of empathic identification) must attempt to apperceive each subject's world as the subject does himself. These principles are basic to the concept of "beta situation" as I have defined it, and of the "behavioral environment" as defined by Koffka and Lewin, and basic to the rationale of numerous projection tests, such as Van Lennep's, as well as to an understanding of the "transference situation" in psychoanalysis. But besides these and other significant counter-positivistic, counter-introspectionistic (in the old sense), and counter-rationalistic orientations and principles, existential psychology seems to focus very largely on a doctrine (only one of several applicable diagnoses) relative to the plight of modern men: men estranged from faith, love, and the regnant values of their society, victims of a profound, essential anxiety, men desperately facing death and nothingness. Must a psychologist limit himself to one or two sources of widespread distress?

One difficulty, especially for an American psychologist, is that this important, infectious existential movement has come out of a complex of philosophies from which it has borrowed unfamiliar terms and expressions, and one suspects at times that, like mysticism, it is necessarily outside the furthest extensions of science, however defined, and that what it knows is essentially incommunicable, except possibly through poetry, art, or religious symbolism. Here, of course, I am merely exposing the ignorance and blockheadedness which, in this special sphere of thought, Continentals rather ascribe to English-speaking philosophers and psychologists. As van Kaam has pointed out, Buytendijk has his Dutch publications translated into French and German, but not into English. What I have said about phenomenology and existential psychology, however, applies to every composite of diverse elements which has been given a name. Once named, it achieves identity as a trend, and we soon find ourselves coping with a galaxy of names, rising and declining in popularity, signifying different sorts of things—much, little, or practically nothing. Trends that are not named are not likely to be mentioned.

WOULD WE BENEFIT BY KNOWLEDGE OF THE MAGNITUDE OF TRENDS?

The title of this chapter suggests that my assignment calls, first, for a discrimination of different scientific movements such as those that I have listed (in conformity with Allport though with more emphasis on research); second, for a rough annual estimate of mass, say of the number of publications exemplifying

each movement in each successive year since its inception or
since some arbitrarily selected date; and third, for a figure,
based on these data, indicating the rate of expansion or con-
traction of each trend through time. Readers of this volume
might reasonably expect this much of a social scientist, especially if they did not look too closely at the difficulty of properly
classifying trends and the labor of counting the scientific works
which manifest and sustain each of the defined classes. I once
expected this much of myself, but I was eventually deterred from
the endeavor, partly by the difficulty and the labor of doing a
really thorough job in the way I judged it should be done, and
partly—if I were to settle for less than this—by Montaigne's
crucial question, *cui bono*?

By reading, traveling, and attending meetings most of us
have a general impression of past and present currents of psychological interest and productivity; and if this impression is
felt to be too fuzzy there are numerous masterly articles in the
literature—especially for Americans in each excellent *Annual
Review of Psychology*—which will do away with some of the
vagueness of our knowledge. Is anything valuable to be gained
by making our impressions more precise? Might not mere
estimates (without evaluations) of quantities of work prove
more misleading than instructive? Indeed, might not increased
publicity as to which bandwagons are leading the procession
do more harm than good?

In this fashion I rationalized myself out of the difficulties of
constructing a comprehensive classification of trends and out of
the toil of counting their supporters. It seemed that on the
majority of us the effect, if any, of learning that there is a rising
movement among our colleagues in a certain scientific direction
would be to incline us toward that direction. Joining this trend,
we would be likely to enjoy a greater amount of companionship,
mutual aid and stimulation, intellectual and economic security,
and, to boot, professional recognition in the nearer future. If
this gregarious disposition, this dependent need for acceptance
and social identity—so prevalent in the United States—is veri-
tably one of the impediments to fundamental, radical creativity,
should it be stimulated more than it is already? Contrariwise, on

a certain number of us—those who must be different or unique at all costs, who would rather be wrong alone, or with a few choice spirits, than right with the confident and vociferous majority—on these the effect, if any, of definite information regarding dominant concerns would be to bend them in the opposite direction, to end, possibly, in some isolated *cul-de-sac*.

What I am suggesting is that every psychologist probably knows as much about the magnitude of different current interests as is good for the best health of his own researches; which, please note, is very different from saying that he knows all he needs to know about the current investigations of his colleagues. The report of an experiment which may be of signal relevance to his own work may be either one of numerous representatives of a massive, on-going movement, such as developmental studies, in which it will merely add one to the tally for that trend, or it will not be counted at all, because the trend it represents (say, reactions to sensory deprivation) is either unique or exemplified by too few publications to be included in any general survey. Anyhow, whether included or not included, there will be no mention of the significant details of the experiment. And then, is it not the new and promising direction that is illustrated by a lone experimenter which should be heralded? By the time its current has gathered momentum and become a sizable river of cognitive energy, it will be obvious to everyone, and its fountain-head may already have started to dry up, a fact which the figures will obscure. We psychologists, like other mortals, have our fixations and vested interests in trends, departure from which is not easy, and we are not immune from the tendency to re-double our efforts, as Santayana put it, when we have lost sight of our aim, or when our aim has become trivial. Here, the commonplace point which democrats and social scientists on both sides of the Atlantic are conditioned to overlook is that a large quantity, even an increasing quantity, of research is no guaranty of quality or ultimate importance. A mountain of scientific work may give forth, with much labor, what on close inspection proves to be nothing but a mouse.

In contrast to all these considerations, however, I would like to suggest that if we had a comprehensive and fitting classification of elementary trends, and were able to trace their evolutions and inter-marriages over a sufficient number of years, including tentative, retrospective evaluation of their several contributions to the science of human nature—if we were capable of this, not only would the above-mentioned possibility of hindering contemporary developments be eliminated, but we would learn more than we know now about how creativity has operated in our discipline down the years, and we might envisage better paths ahead of us in the future. We would find that a movement which declines and falls may rise again with renewed vigor in combination with some other movement, and we might also see which veins of thought are near exhaustion and what possibilities have yet to be explored.

What I am proposing here is an extensive, analytic and synthetic history of the career of basic ideas relevant to our understanding of personality, a book to be written in the future by somebody, not myself, with sufficient competence and energy. Since the author of this hypothetical book is an unknown, I shall call him X. Eventually, I suspect, there will be an actual X who will be wise enough to discard almost everything that I have to say in the next section. For the time being, however, X is a purely imaginary person who, though ideal in certain ways, necessarily suffers from some of the prejudices and limitations of his maker.

PROLEGOMENON FOR A HISTORY OF TRENDS

The trends exemplified by the work of every psychologist are, in certain general respects, like those exemplified by *all* other psychologists; and, in certain less general respects, like those exemplified by *some* other psychologists (of this or that class—nation, school, or specialty); and, in certain particular respects, like those exemplified by *no* other psychologist.

All of us, I assume, are trying in one way or another to add to the common fund of relatively valid knowledge as to the manifestations in environments of human nature (of all human natures, of some similar human natures, or of unique human natures), and/or to perfect modes of eliciting, recording, ordering, and understanding these manifestations in situations. Or, to put it another way, there is one notable, massive trend of thought, action, observation, and evaluation toward the construction of a better theoretical system of concepts and propositions, in terms of which the subjective and objective manifestations of psychic events may be analytically and synthetically observed, recorded, formulated, explained, predicted (under specified conditions), and, if possible, produced (within specified limits under specified conditions). Although this *ultima Thule* of the science of human nature must be placed beyond the ever-receding horizon of a questionable future, it is the target, nonetheless, of countless approximating efforts.

But since, as we all realize, personality is an exceedingly complex, continuing, yet changing, system of manifold part-systems and sub-systems operating from birth to death in diverse, successive situations with diverse outcomes and consequences, no single psychologist or small group of psychologists would even dream of studying all parts of all types of personalities under all kinds of circumstances at all ages. Inevitably we find a large variety of trends which may be grossly differentiated in terms of 1) *class of events studied* (regional trend), that is, differentiated in terms of which aspect or aspects (states, functions, achievements) of personality are being studied, separately or interdependently, in relation to which class or classes of entities or situations. We find trends which may be differentiated in terms of 2) *class of subjects studied* (population trend), that is, in terms of subjects of which race, age, sex, society, status, vocation, etc., or subjects with what degree of health, wealth, knowledge, or ability, or with what pathological diagnosis, or belonging to what somatic or psychological type, are being studied, separately or comparatively.

Since most, if not all, psychologists, in their observations, speculations, experimental designs, and manipulations, are guided, implicitly or explicitly, by one or another theoretical construct, assumption, or hypothesis, each of them is likely to contribute—by way of illustration, validation or invalidation, reconstruction, or creation—to one of a third class of trends:

3)*class of concepts, theories, or theoretical systems tested or developed* (theoretical trend), that is, a trend which is defined in terms of what kind of already proposed concept, postulate, or model is being tested, corrected, or revised, or what kind of new variable, perceptible or hypothetical, has been distinguished, defined, and classified, or what type of new proposition has been stated, or what kind of new combination or new system of variables and propositions has been constructed. Another major division of interests would surely be 4) *class of techniques used or developed* (technical trend). What kind of means does the psychologist employ to obtain the information he is seeking? What procedure does he design? What type of test or instrument does he invent or improve? And then, 5) *class of data-organizing methods used or developed* (data-ordering trend): the psychologist may present a simple, chronological account of what he has seen or heard, or he may classify, count, tabulate, represent on a graph, correlate statistically, or factor-analyze his data in one or another way. Last, but more fundamental than any of these divisions, would be trends classified in terms of 6) *class of basic (philosophical) assumptions or evaluations exemplified* (basic assumption trend) by a psychologist's theories or researches.

I surmise that our ideal, mythic author, X, will distinguish large categories of this sort, though his divisions may be somewhat different, and his classes will certainly be more fully and explicitly defined. In all likelihood he will want to add another category, 7) *class of final intentions* (intention trend), in order to distinguish—besides knowledge for its own sake—various kinds of applications of this knowledge, such as diagnosis, therapy, selection of personnel, vocational guidance, education, and so forth. The highly articulate X will come out with better names for some of these categories. "Regional trend" and "population trend," as used here, may confuse some readers. "Region" points to the psychologist's field (area, domain) of observation and reflection, commonly consisting of a subject in a specified environment manifesting certain kinds of states and activities (e.g. needs, perceptions, locomotions, manipulations, etc.). "Population," in this context, means nature of population of subjects studied (e.g. children, Polynesians, endomorphs, schizophrenics, etc.).

The perspicacious X will point out, with unexcelled clarity, how a single experimenter could advance seven classes of trends at once. For instance, he might increase our knowledge of the imagination (class 1, regional trend) as well as of the personalities of primitive peoples (class 2, population trend) by comparing the styles and products of story-composing processes of whites and Negroes in the Belgian Congo. In this investigation he might use a special type of "imaginal eductor" that he invented and record the subjects' spontaneous responses on tape (class 4, technical trends). He might employ a phenomenological frame of reference in discriminating styles of composition and several modified Jungian concepts in dealing with the thematic content (class 3, theoretical trends). Returning to his laboratory, he might use a computing machine to intercorrelate his protocol variables (class 5, data-ordering trend), and discover that a certain combination of these variables was a sufficiently valid indicator of good adjustment to white standards, and hence could be of service to personnel selection agencies (class 7, intention trend). I shall let you decide which philosophical position (class 6) is indicated by these labors.

The discerning X will also demonstrate lucidly, with numerous apt illustrations, the interdependence of these major trend categories: how technique is determined in part by the selected region of concern (processes to be studied) and in part by the hypothesis to be tested, and vice versa; how a certain theory may determine what population is chosen for investigation, and how the evaluation of the findings of an investigation may result in a revision of the initial theory; and how everything is largely dependent on the final intention of the psychologist, whether it be pure knowledge, therapy, or propaganda. We shall be shown, for example, that the adoption of a strict, positivistic position (trend 6), will exclude the study of free verbal expressions (trend 1)—since so many of these are susceptible to critically-different interpretations—and will thereby limit the scope of theory (trend 3) and the range of permitted techniques (trend 4). All of this, of course, is common knowledge. But there are unrecorded, instructive details in the history of the mental interactions between assumptions, intentions, theories, regions, populations, and techniques, which X will not fail to describe in a way that will be helpful to his colleagues.

Of comparable interest should be X's revealing story of the temporal procession of studied regions, designed techniques, and formulated theories. Here, instead of the mutual influence of *different* classes of trends (e.g. regions, techniques, theories, etc.), the topic will be the dependence of each novel scientific achievement on preceding achievements of the *same* class. A new psychological theory, for example, may be derived by analogy from physics, chemistry, or biology. From these sciences have come concepts such as that of energy, force, vector, affinity, attraction and repulsion, positive and negative valence, field, region, boundary, system, level, organism and environment, part-whole, self-preservative, herd-preservative, and race-preservative instincts, structure and function, differentiation and integration, hierarchical organization, dynamic equilibrium, homeostasis, adjustment, competition, survival of the fittest, evolution, law of entropy, open system, and so forth. See MacLeod's illuminating comments in this volume on Newtonian (physical) structuralism and Aristotelian (biological) functionalism in psychology. Other concepts and theories have come as explicit, abstract formulations, either of common sense (implicit theories) or of aphorisms (the wisdom of the ages), or of new facts discovered through diffuse explorations or focused experiments, or of signal experiences in which the psychologist himself was emotionally involved (e.g. Freud's self-analysis). Further concepts and theories have been the resultant of a generalization, extension, differentiation, or modification of an existing psychological theory, of an opposition to some existing theory, or of a synthesis of two or more theories. In addition to such sources and modes of theoretical composition, the all-embracing X will surely take account of their principal culturological, sociological, and personological determinants (e.g. the influence of Marxism, of capitalism, of war, of social disintegration, of the psychologist's temperament or his imbedded values). And X will deal, in a like manner, with the history of instruments and methods, of regions and populations studied, of basic assumptions and avowed intentions.

Of one thing we can be reasonably certain: The astute X will not often be confused by names—names for philosophical positions, concepts, theories, techniques, schools of psychology, and so forth. He will not assume, for example, that entities with different names are necessarily different, or that entities with the same names are similar, or that the nature of an entity (object, process, relation, theory, method) corresponds to the dictionary meaning of the word by which it is denoted. He will not take for granted, let us say, either that a so-called "projective test" is actually a *test* (of anything that can be specified before the administration of this procedure), or that the responses it educes are, for the most part, actual *projections* (according to any dynamic definition of this word). Furthermore, X will rarely see fit to traffic with unspecified terms (e.g. interview, as a method) or terms which refer to complex wholes (e.g. psychoanalysis, as theory). He will almost invariably analyze the objects of his discourse into their component parts, qualities, properties. He will realize, say, that there are several essentially different sorts of interviews as well as different classes of interviewers, and also realize that psychoanalysis is a more or less integrated system of numerous component concepts and theories, some of which are low or declining, and some of which are high or rising in the estimation of psychologists. In short, X's ambitious endeavor will be to identify the basic, elementary ideas involved in each class of trends (regional, theoretical, technical, etc.), to show how these have been combined, separated, and re-combined historically, and then to point to possible promising combinations which have yet to be explored.

REGIONAL TRENDS

I imagine that before starting his exposition of regional trends, the systematic X will first, for his own guidance, distinguish (a) every analytically-separable psychological state (e.g. sleep, state of anxiety, state of want), and process (e.g.

explanation, evaluation, actional decision, exposition, locomotion, donation) which has been or might be studied, and then list (b) every association of these variables whose mutual relationships have been or might be demonstrated (e.g. state of hunger and perception, state of mental fatigue and memory, activated need achievement and story composition). Next, with such variables and relationships in mind, X may be disposed to construct (c) a classification of external situations (in terms, say, of touch, sight, sound, or sight and sound, of discrete sensations, of words and sentences, of objects or composites, inanimate or animate, actual or represented, pictured, stationary or moving, mute, sounding, or speaking, of contrived—artificial or realistic—or "real" occasions from which the subject remains detached as a mere witness or in which he is involved as a participating actor and/or observer, and so forth). After this, I would suppose, X will list (d) the different, possible combinations, tried and untried, of the various, defined psychological states and processes, on the one hand, and the classes of confronting situations, on the other (e.g. interpretation of an actual, stationary, symbolic object or of the representation of a person's path of locomotion, explanation of a person's reaction to a situation as described in tape-recorded sentences, emotional reactions to a contrived, mechanically-produced, stressful situation, verbal reactions to criticism in a contrived, realistic, dyad discussion). Finally (to be used when relevant), X will distinguish (e) different kinds and degrees of immediate effects or outcomes of such activities (e.g. degrees of success or failure, kinds of error or distortion) and of later consequences of these activities and effects (e.g. degrees of positive or negative evaluation by others, depression or elation, gain or loss of confidence, better or worse performance, learning).

Drawing from his immense cranial library of knowledge, X will trace the history of these trends in academic and medical psychology, recording the emergence of successive regions of concern, starting with sensation, perception, memory, and other elementary cognitive processes. This first phase was largely guided by a philosophical orientation, concerned with questions such as, what can we know about the external world? and by what means? and with what degree of certainty? Some supposed that at best, the mind was analogous to a photographic plate, free from modifying dispositions, either acquired or innate. The next distinct phase, coming out of an indifference to, if not utter contempt for, traditional philosophical problems and speculations, consisted of an attempt to elevate the status of psychology by reducing it to the conceptual level of biology or physiology. Here the successive regions of attention were: overt physiological (glandular, emotional-autonomic, and effective-muscular) reactions to controlled stimulation, conditioned reflexes, and means-end motor learning resulting from hunger, sex, and other drives. Both of these major regional trends were personologically peripheral and superficial. It was French, and later Austrian, medical psychology—oriented by the wish to discover the hidden determinants of neurotic illness—which provided the depth dimension for an adequate theory of personality. A new set of cathected regions emerged from these labors: the phenomena of hypnotism, unconscious psychic processes, underlying compelling emotions and needs (anxiety, love, hate, sex, need for superiority and prestige), dreams, fantasies, word-associations, and defense mechanisms. Contemporary with this large aggregate of concerns was an expanding measurement and assessment trend, the successive regions being: general mental intelligence, special aptitudes and abilities, avowals of interests and of cultural evaluations (sentiments, attitudes), and self-estimates pertinent to various personality traits, including needful dispositions.

The history of these developments, being well-known to psychologists, will be covered in a short space, even counting X's penetrating discussion of the probable determinants of choice of each new region of investigation. Less elementary will be X's account of subsequent studies of the mutual dependence of certain dispositional states and certain mental products: of needs, evaluations, and emotions, for instance, as determinants of word-associations, perceptions, apperceptions (inferences), and story compositions, as well as of different cognitions and beliefs as determinants of emotions and evaluations. The operation of a counteractive endopsychic need (denial) in influencing fantasy productions is beautifully demonstrated in Miller's first-rate chapter. The effect or lack of effect on (a) the emotional reactivity of subjects to the highly-charged topic of death, of (b) an avowed, relevant, religious belief (e.g. immortality) constitutes the region of the well-controlled investigation by Alexander and Adlerstein. All substantial researches of this sort contribute to the great task of formulating the interdependence of various variables and sub-systems of personality.

Full of suggestiveness, I suspect, will be X's chronicle of the different, progressively-more-complicated combinations of (a) psychological processes and (b) confronting situations: First, say, studies of visual perceptions of the qualities of stationary, inanimate objects; then of moving pictures of expressive human beings in action; and, finally, studies of visual and auditory perceptions (inferences, interpretations, explanations, predictions) of sound films of conversing persons, as well as of persons in the flesh with whom the experimental subjects have interacted. Here surely are evidences of trends of change from static configurations in space to dynamic patterns in time as regions for experimentation, and from sheer visual perceptions to complex apperceptions based on both visual and auditory cues, from artificial to realistic situations, and from detached to involved subjects. Comparable trends of change will become apparent when X reviews the story of memory research, reaching from memories of discrete, printed, nonsense syllables to memories of stressful conversations in which the subject himself participated. Both of these topics—perception and memory—will be discussed later in connection with an appropriately large section of this volume dealing with "person perception."

The book of our ideal author, X, will be especially interesting, I would guess, when he starts pointing to emergent regions of investigation and regions which are still awaiting the invasion of a venturous explorer. I am not in a position to say what these will be. But as illustration of an emergent region we have the unforeseen phenomena, associated with the perception, recognition, and reproduction of figures, as revealed by the delicate and ingenious techniques of Brengelmann (e.g. stages in the actual-genetic process of perception, as well as other extremely significant micro-analyses of relatively simple functions). As another illustration of an emergent region, I might call attention to Luria's brilliant study of the maturation of the capacity for deliberate, voluntary movements, more particularly his report of the differential effects in a young child (a) of being told to make a specific movement at a given signal and (b) of telling himself to make this movement. Piaget started a great trend of longitudinal researches in the regions of perception and cognition in young children, a trend which is represented in this volume by Inhelder's and Noelting's short discussion of experiments to reveal successive stages of reasoning ability in children. But only Soviet psychologists, so far as I know, have performed multifarious, comparable studies in the region of conscious planning, initiation, and control of effective muscular and social actions. Not related to these, we have Lois Murphy's long series of investigations devoted to children's "coping methods and styles," all-too-briefly abstracted in this volume.

Among other regional trends which today are relatively new and promising X might mention studies of (a) various effects of sub-liminal stimulation, (b) reactions of various sorts of different kinds of stress, including sensory deprivation, (c) general dispositional sets (response sets) in experimental subjects, (d) phenomenology of various mental processes—perception, evaluation, description, explanation, prediction, fictional composition—with special emphasis on styles, or modes, of performance, (e) processes, ("defense mechanisms" and others) operating in the service of favorable evaluations of self by self and by others, (f) the interdependence of sthenic and asthenic emotions, apperceptions and evaluations of self and alter, occurring during and after participation in an argumentative dyadic or polyadic (small group) proceeding, (g) emotional and imaginal reactions to music, poetry, and other forms of art, (h) time-sense and time-perspective (past, present, and future), and feelings and conceptions relative to the passage of time and occurrence of death, (i) creativity, its component processes, its styles and products, the characteristics of creative personalities, et cetera, et cetera. Among several unexplored regions, X might possibly include the phenomenology and the determinants of ordination (planning), one of the most universal and consequential of mental operations, though as yet scarcely mentioned in the textbooks, except occasionally in connection with the psychology of decision-making.

EXPERIMENTATION AND THE REGION OF PERSONALITY

So far my rambling comments have been confined pretty much to the fringe of personality research, concerning, for the most part, the kinds of events, or regions (different combinations of classes of external situations and classes of reactive processes, and classes of outcomes), that are studied by experimentalists. Here the psychologist's ideal target might be a general proposition which is applicable to almost all normal personalities within a given age range, an ideal that is not infrequently approximated when attention is restricted to associations among relatively simple psychophysiological processes (sensory, sensory-autonomic, sensory-motor, motor) in connection with relatively simple configurations or arrays of stimuli. But even in such elementary experiments and even with animals—as Pavlov and others have demonstrated—marked individual and typological differences are often found, which call for some intervening personological variable, compound of variables, or model. In personality research, the simplest hypothesis to be tested is not unlikely to be one which states that the reaction, let us say, to situation A will be R1 in personalities of class X1, and R2 (the exact opposite) in personalities of class X2. Although one test is often considered sufficient to distinguish personalities of the two classes (X1 and X2), the standards of less debonair and slapdash personologists are rarely met so easily. Anyhow, our consideration of experimental regions has brought us to the mysteries and riddles of personality, a huge, embracing region of part-regions, super-regions and sub-regions.

Experiments are of course invaluable and necessary to the development of a science of human nature, but they yield, at best, relatively precise and reliable answers to definitely stated questions. Yet if all personologists were to confine themselves to experimentation—each necessarily in one or in a few regions—no sufficiently comprehensive formulation of a single personality, and hence of a type of personality or of an abstract of most personalities, would ever be attained. Experimentation is almost inevitably limited by scientific standards, time, and circumstance to the observation and measurement of a few (rather than many), restricted (rather than unrestricted) reactions (rather than proactions) to a few (rather than many), artificial (rather than "real") situations, at a particular temporal point or over a single period (rather than at different points or over several successive periods) of a subject's on-going changing personality. And even when the experimenter sees fit to inquire about his subject's covert (imperceptible, inner) states and processes during the experiment, his data is almost inevitably limited to those aspects of the experience which the subject is both able to recall and willing to communicate. Experimentalists are apt to forget what varieties of "guinea-pig" roles may be adopted by their subjects and to what extent.

Besides devotion to experimentation, the marks of a serious, full-fledged personologist—if X agrees with me—are: (a) a sturdy interest in many different regions (part-systems) of personality, during (b) successive periods in the life-span (on the assumption that the history of the personality *is* the personality—a cross-section being a convenient, though often highly artificial, abstraction from temporal events), and, since personality changes through time, (c) a pre-occupation with transformations (progressive and regressive) of personality, and hence (d) the practice of obtaining detailed, chronological reports of numerous concrete events (illustrative of the operation of significant dispositions and abilities) in which the subject participated in the course of his past and recent life, and, since such reports are almost invariably vague and distorted, in one way or another, (e) the practice of exposing, by various procedures (e.g. questionnaires, aptitude and situational tests), numerous parts of the subject's current personality and comparing these findings with the autobiographical data, and also (f) an incessant interest in the repressed and concealed, yet operating, parts of the personality, and hence (g) the practice of obtaining, by various indirect means (e.g. eliciting free-associations, fantasies, and story compositions), the processes and productions from which hypothetical inferences can be made relative to childhood and adolescent dispositions and events which the subject is unable or too reluctant to report, and, then, (h) the practice of conducting "open-ended" interviews, subtly guided towards certain apparently critical, yet ambiguous and baffling, areas of experiences revealed by the outlined procedures. In brief, a confirmed personologist is apt to be a glutton for multifarious, concrete facts, as detailed and precise as he can get them (usually more than he can use), since only from the chronology of "real" events, failures and successes, recurrent and exceptional (representative of the personality at its "best" and at its "worst") can one derive a sufficiently plausible reconstruction of the evolution of an adult personality.

In the above account of the "real," rather than the artificial, events of personological concern, I could not help mentioning assessment methods (technical trends)—interviewing, especially —being the only means of obtaining certain necessary kinds of information. Every person, for example, has had and continues to have a number of wholly or largely private and secret experiences—covert fantasies, hopes, aspirations, dreads, envies, hatreds, ignoble temptations, transgressions, humiliations, sexual practices, and so forth—knowledge of which may provide the key to some of his otherwise inexplicable attitudes or actions; and there never will be any other way of acquiring actual facts (rather than hints and clues) about these veiled parts (not to speak of the repressed parts) of personality except through the avowals of the subject himself.

Consideration of this topic could bring us to the intriguing problems of so-called "person-perception," with the psychologist himself as chief "perceptor," deciding, from moment to moment, on the basis of his feelings and his inferences (derived from everything he sees and hears) what he should say next and how, and then correctly or incorrectly apperceiving the effects on the subject of what he has just said, et cetera. Viewed in this light, "person-perception" (considered in Part III of this volume) is synonymous with personality assessment (considered in Part IV), except that the former is generally carried out without the use of instruments and the latter is sometimes carried out without even looking at the subject. I shall return to this matter later. It is mentioned here merely as a pointer to a possible, much-needed, future technical trend (about which, with a little luck, X may have something to report), namely, the training of person-ologists themselves as instruments of precision, through partici-pation in experiments in the perception and interpretation of other people's transient manifestations of psychic states, proc-esses, and styles, including suppositions, or inferences, respecting the existence of established (recurrently active) dispositions or complexes, and including, possibly, explanations and predictions —not to speak of the perception and interpretation of the signs of somatotype, age, race, nationality, socio-economic status, vocation, knowledge, intelligence, special abilities, and so forth.

But to return to the important, generally inaccessible, secret experiences of subjects, it can be confidently predicted that the even-handed X will give due credit to the medical and clinical psychologists, especially the psychoanalysts, for devising gentle and unhurtful methods of exposure (technical trend). He will no doubt devote an ample chapter to a chronicle of their dis-coveries and another chapter to the writing of case-histories (the-oretical and technical trends), indicating what regions must be explored by what available methods, and what criteria must be met before a formulation of a subject's personality can be con-sidered satisfactory. Formulations presented by psychoanalysts are characteristically most illuminating, though almost inevitably onesided, because these are primarily devoted to representations of repressed determinants of neurotic illness and of mechanisms of defense, and because only couch and transference personalities are directly observable in the orthodox psychonalytical pro-cedure. For a more balanced, comprehensive picture, other re-gions must be examined by appropriate techniques. Indeed, as I see it—and I pray that the fastidious X will agree with me on this point—only by comparing and evaluating the findings from a multiplicity of different methods can a *team* of per-sonologists arrive at a sufficient degree of certainty respecting those past experiences and those current dispositions and abilities upon which a plausible reconstruction of any personality must be founded.

So far as I can judge, present academic trends—determined partly by the high status of positivistic standards, partly by the current rage for little, neat experiments (at any cost), partly by existing requirements for a Ph.D. degree, and partly by lack of sufficient personnel, time, and cash—are indicative of an abandonment, in many quarters, of the endeavor to explore, measure, explain, and represent the various, interdependent component parts and systems of individual personalities, each as an on-going participant in various transactions with things, people, and ideas. I trust that by the time our awaited author X embarks on his momentous enterprise, this trend of change will be reversed, and there will be numerous, now unsuspected relations to be reported (theoretical trend).

No doubt, the so-called "longitudinal" way of studying personalities is ideal, starting in infancy with periodic observations of the subjects, combined with interrogations of the parents, continuing these examinations at less frequent intervals through childhood, and ending with follow-up assessments in later years to confirm or prove predictions made at different points in the course of infancy and childhood. A number of extended investigations of this type have been conducted in the past and some are still in progress. But for various reasons (Skard mentions several major difficulties) the trend of change seems to be moving toward more restricted programs of research. Illustrative of the best of these are the interesting investigations which several of the authors of the volume have conducted: notably Thomae in Germany, Lois Murphy in America, Inhelder and Noelting in Switzerland, Luria in the Soviet Union, and Skard in Norway, a fragment of each of which is outlined in the pages that lie ahead of you. In her Introduction and Commentary, Skard presents for our benefit some of the fruits of her long succession of intimate experiences with growing children and of the enlightened attempts to discriminate some of the determinants of change. Here I should not omit (though they are not summarized in this book) the illuminating, longitudinal experiments performed in Switzerland by Meili, author of the Commentary on Assessment. And, as so clearly shown in Shneidman and Farberow's chapter on suicide, it is equally important to consider socio-economic determinants of individual behavior.

This looks like the appropriate place for a few words about the tangled subject-matter of *person perception,* a department requiring a high degree of "snafu" tolerance, since the two designating terms—perception and empathy—have become incorrigible rovers, refusing to stay put. First, we were persuaded by Köhler and others that all of us are capable of "perceiving" and identifying feelings and emotions in another person, just as we perceive the movements of his facial muscles, despite the fact that we often disagree radically among ourselves and with the perceived subject about the former but not about the latter —bear me out in this, Mona Lisa—and the fact that an emotion can be feigned by a talented actor, if not by any one of us, and the fact that it is not possible to give an adequate operational definition (in terms of dependable, perceptible cues) of any feeling or emotion except a few in their fleeting moments of intensity. From "perceiving" emotions we progressed to the point where we could all "perceive" intentions, needs, and motives, oblivious of the years of sweat and sorrow psychologists have devoted to the seemingly simple enterprise of defining a motivation or even of demonstrating that "purpose" was a necessary and distinguishable concept for psychology. How gratifying it would be for positivists, what high inter-judge reliabilities we would get if we could all "perceive" a person's conscious intention registered on his forehead, and just below it his unconscious, underlying need! But the Napoleonic word "perception" could not be stopped at this border. It pushed on, and pretty soon we were "perceiving" that somebody we saw for the first time was an habitually tactful and punctilious, politically conservative, introverted, upperclass barrister, with a father complex, who was on his way to a psychotic episode. Then, there were still more fields to conquer as psychologists conducting "person-perception" experiments began to provide autobiographical data and test-findings to be "perceived." Enough said to explain my general agreement with Taft's dissatisfaction relative to pan-perceptionism expressed in

his systematic survey and, unhappily, my disagreement with
MacLeod on this semantic issue.

It is useful to have two terms (for me, they are perception and
apperception), partly because there are typological differences
between those who, in their descriptions, limit themselves literally
to the perceptible qualities of other persons (the sheer facts) and
those who give you a host of inferences about imperceptible
states, processes, and dispositions (these I term *perspections*—
to "look through" the surface manifestations), and also, very
often, placements (in this or that status, type, category), explanations and predictions. In my language, apperception includes at
least these four distinguishable processes: (immediate) perspection, placement, explanation, and prediction (anticipation).

All this becomes clear enough in the rich and informative
protocols derived from From's most original experiments, particularly the second. In my opinion, what he shows, besides many
other things, is that the total covert *experience* of a perceptor
of a subject's physical movements, acts, and words includes a
galaxy of *imaginations* pertaining to the subject's momentary
inner states and subsequent acts, as well as muscular tensions,
somatic sensations, feelings, and evaluations, placements, explanations of various sorts, and further predictions, not to speak
of impulses and decisions to intervene or actual, overt expressions
of approval or disapproval. It is not possible to describe the
perceptor's experience without using additional words, without
indicating that the perceptor is also an imaginer, perspector,
interpreter, evaluator, predictor, ordinator, and so forth. "He
reached in his pocket for a match" would be (in my terminology) a "perspection" of the alter's intention; but "he took a
match out of his pocket" (when he did no such thing) would be
what? an actual perception? an imaginal anticipation recalled as
an actual perception? or a hallucination? I trust that the accomplished X will be capable of settling these various semantic
issues, and that, between our day and his day, many experimenters will have followed Tagiuri's inviting lead, and with
comparable clarity and style, defined more of the cues which
help us to perspect correctly the psychic states and traits in other
people. I venture to predict that experiments in person-appercep-

tion will be performed in conjunction with studies of the assessment process and that the offspring of their union will be outstanding.

The only substantive contribution to the present volume which is devoted to an analysis of situations involving adult personalities is the finely-wrought and perspicacious chapter by Mailloux and Ancona. The authors present brief, pertinent case reports supportive of their contention that any one of the classical psychopathological syndromes (e.g. phobic, obsessive-compulsive, paranoid) may be provoked not only by a moral conflict of a sexual or social nature, but also by a moral conflict of a religious nature, occasioned, say, by a waning of genuine involvement, and belief. Loss of faith, its distressful concomitants and consequences, is a not uncommon variety of human experience, which the majority of psychologists either disregard entirely (never mentioning it in their textbooks), or, if they be clinicians, set aside as something which does not require study in its own right, on the assumption that *all* the determinants of a patient's suffering are operating on a deeper, unconscious level, dating, possibly, from an over-dependent, yet highly ambivalent, father-son relationship in childhood. The widely acknowledged fact that the persistence of a convincing, superpersonal "ideology" (religion, philosophy of life, or set of cultural values and ideals) is conducive, in many people, to psychic health, unity, serenity, and joy, and that the loss of it may be shattering, is all too often overlooked by psychoanalytically oriented psychiatrists and clinical psychologists, despite their own experience of being encouraged and sustained in their endeavors by a belief in the essential validity and efficacy of Freud's theories and procedures, as well as by a more embracing belief in the value of science and scientific psychotherapy. In a sense, psychoanalysis is their religion, although for them moral commitment is likely to be less binding than it is for devout Christians. A better analogy would be the attachment of fully indoctrinated Communists to *their* system of beliefs. In any case, it seems to me, the evidence is favorable to Mailloux's and Ancona's thesis that conflicts on this superordinate level may be protracted and intense in some people, productive of pathological symptoms, and hence deserving of being considered on their own terms. But must we necessarily agree with the authors' implicit assumption that Catholicism is the sole occupant of the superordinate region of personality?

POPULATION TRENDS

Academic psychology, which subsisted for many years on a meager diet of responses from educated, European, male adults, has been substantially invigorated by the initiation and growth of a succession of other population trends, exemplified by the study of animals, of females, infants, children, and adolescents, of neurotics and psychotics, of subjects of different societies and cultures, of different somatotypes, psychological types, degrees of intelligence, social classes, and vocations, and now of an emergent trend, marked by studies of aging men and women. What other possibilities are left for the conscientious X to record or to foresee?

TECHNICAL TRENDS

I will now ask you to imagine a large section of X's encyclopedic book devoted to an analysis of all known procedures into their component parts and to an account of the different combinations of these components as they have occurred in the history of psychology. Besides (a) different kinds of objects or materials presented—which could be subsumed under (situational) regions—there are (b) different modes and conditions of presentation (e.g. tachistoscope), (c) different kinds of directions given (e.g. "Speak the first word that comes to mind"), and (d) different kinds of recording techniques (e.g. tape, moving-picture, camera, electrocardiograph). Some of these have already been mentioned in connection with the survey of regions; some are set forth and judiciously weighed in David's and Rabinowitz's review of brief projective methods; some are well described in other chapters too numerous to mention; but the majority I shall entrust to the analytic and synthetic powers of the indefatigable X. My pet hope, as confessed earlier, is that he will lay sufficient stress on ways of studying the not-yet-defined "whole" person as well as on a trend which, in his day, will be moving toward the systematic training of psychologists as instruments of exact perception and adequate interpretation.

By the time X's book is underway, computing machines should have produced a very consequential revolution, having made possible, on the one hand, the precise determination of numerous interrelationships of clinically estimated variables within a single personality, and having encouraged, on the other hand, the construction of a galaxy of new questionnaires leading to the identification of basic factors and of empirical scales to measure them. There is no telling how far from actuality we may be getting in a few years as a result of the propagation of more and more wholly abstract, paper-and-pencil personalities. In any event, this section of X's book will be useful in so far as it elucidates the processes and determinants of technical invention and suggests to workers in one region methods that have proved their worth in others.

THEORETICAL TRENDS

Allusions to some of the items that belong under this heading are dispersed over the length of this chapter. A number of today's more favored concepts and theories were named in my commentary on Allport's introduction to the first volume of *Perspectives*. Later, various psychological constructs derived from the more basic sciences were listed, most of which are involved in endeavors to compose a system-of-system's frame of reference. Other conceptions were included, implicitly or explicitly, in my survey of regional trends exemplified by researches reported in this book. The findings of several authors—Brengelmann, From, Luria, and Mailloux and Ancona, for example—seem to point to some required conceptual or theoretical revision or innovation. Still more pertinent at this point is the one chapter of this collection which is primarily devoted to theory construction: Blum's definition of a brave and promising model (out of parts of psychoanalytic theory and information theory) in terms of which predictions respecting certain classes of responses to his Blacky Test can be made and tested. His first trials were encouraging and it looks as if modified forms of the model would be applicable to other situations.

Also relevant to the present topic is Hollander's critique of the concept of conformity as a personological variable, a critique which, in most respects, is applicable across the board of conceptualized *general* dispositions, and, pushed a little further, might cancel the hope of ever arriving at a sufficient formulation of a personality. Crucial here is the everlasting generality *vs.* specificity issue. How often has *any* needful, directional disposition been repeatedly observed or measured in enough *different kinds* of situations to justify our speaking of a diffuse, free-floating, *general* disposition—a disposition to achieve results, to compete, to gain attention or approval, to direct others, to comply, to resist, to empathize, to emulate, to withdraw, to avoid, to construct, et cetera? But if we adopt the opposite, extreme position and cleave to the particularities of events (which are always unique) we shall come out, at best, with a list of scores on particular tests taken under particular conditions and/or a biography or case history composed of a number of particular endeavors and experiences, with no justification for conceiving of the existence of more general and enduring dispositions. A mid-position—which I favor and which Hollander might be willing to accept—requires a classification of types of situations (A, B, C, D, etc.), in terms of which dispositional specifications can be given. One might say, for instance, that subject S is consciously or unconsciously disposed to conform to the patterns of behavior or to the consensual expectations of others in situations of type C (e.g. characterized by the presence of "authority figures") less readily, less exactly, and/or less frequently than most subjects of his age; but that he conforms more readily, more exactly, and/or more frequently than most subjects in situations of type G (e.g. informal peer group), et cetera. Of course, to predict behavior in any particular situation, a number of other specifications would be required. In any case, a personologist seldom, if ever, arrives at anything more than a plausible and probabilistic formulation of potential, semi-general and semi-specific, interdependent dispositions and abilities, which will serve as *one* basis for predictions of behavior in the future.

What the profound X will have to say about theoretical evolutions related to personality research is beyond me. I would suppose that the present puritan trend towards cleanliness of language and immaculate conceptions, with physics as fashion-plate, will continue for a while with fresh flowerings of snobbery. But sooner or later with a little luck, we should grow wise enough to bend down to the humbling proposal that psychology, infant among the sciences, might advisably return to short pants, and begin again, nearer to the beginning, in contact with the naturalistic facts, instead of dressing up in the too-big authority of its father's embarrassingly long trousers. Of course, if the majority of personologists—in accord with present experiential (phenomenological, existential) trends—do return to the naturalistic facts, they will be greatly advantaged by the purifying mentations of today's more fastidious theorists and in retrospect will gratefully bless them for their illuminating treatises, most particularly for their demonstrations (instead of mere hunches) as to why, *in the sphere of personology,* perfection of diction and of definition is highly correlated with paralysis and barrenness.

The heart of X's massive work will undoubtedly be found in the several chapters he devotes to the classification and chronology of theoretical trends. In accord with the bent ascribed to him, what he will do first, I guess, is to analyze each theory into its basic components, or ideational genes, and then, going back to the genesis of each, trace the careers, the marriages and divorces, the decompositions and recompositions of these genes, showing how they became incorporated in the theoretical systems that are now in process of evolution.

Mr. X may choose to divide theories and hypotheses according to their chief focus of concern, such as propositions respecting (a) the microdevelopment of one, or the succession or interdependence (co-variation) of two or more, reported, covert, psychic states, processes, or products; (b) one or more momentary, situational or relational-situational determinants or

modifiers of covert or overt dispositional processes or effects;
(c) one or more momentary, physiological, pharmacological or
pathological determinants or modifiers; (d) one or more immediately antecedent experiences as determinants or modifiers; (e)
one or more hypothetical establishments of personality (e.g. persisting dispositions and aims, integrates and patterns of dispositions, systems of patterns; cathected images, configurations,
concepts, postulates, or formulations; regions, places, and bound-
aries, e.g. id-ego) or one or more of their hypothetical properties as determinants or modifiers; (f) genetical-maturational
(e.g. inheritance, sex, age) determinants or modifiers of one or
more establishments of personality; (g) one or more extraordinary or recurrent experiences or enterprises (e.g. accidents, successes or failures of endeavors, social treatments, the acquisition
of knowledge through listening and reading) as determinants
or modifiers of one or more establishments of personality; (h)
one or more established, territorial and social positions and
relations (e.g. family position, group memberships, roles, friend-
ships, marriage) as determinants or modifiers of one or more
establishments of personality; (i) some type of mental illness
as determinant or modifier of one or more establishments of
personality; and so forth.

Whether or not Mr. X happens to be interested in the personalities of the different theorists, he might choose to characterize their formulations in terms of such familiar ratios of
emphasis as: overt, perceptible/covert, imperceptible, experiential variables; conscious, covert/unconscious, covert variables;
empirical, phenomenological/hypothetical, theoretical variables;
analytic/synthetic variables; energic, dynamic/static, structural;
independent/relational variables; conceptions or flexible, chang-
ing/fixed, permanent variables; temporal, successional, historic/
stationary, cross-sectional, unhistoric; conceptions of flexible,
changing/fixed, permanent variables; psychophysiological/psy-
chosociological variables; modal, stylistic expressional/purposive,
directional terminal variables; proximal, purposive/distal, purposive variables, and so forth.

But now, having occupied more than my allotted space, I
must leave in your hands all further speculations as to how our

future author will deal with the complex thought-stuff that marks the history of our science. My sole, confident prediction is that his bents of interest and evaluation will bear no resemblance to mine. May he have a galaxy of clarifying and generative new theories to report!

References

1. Allport, G. W. European and American theories of personality. In David, H. P. and von Bracken, H. (Eds.), *Perspectives in personality theory*. New York: Basic Books, 1957, 3-24.

PART TWO

Explorations in Behavior

II

Studies of
Denial in Fantasy

INTRODUCTION

OF ALL THE PSYCHOANALYTIC CONCEPTS, none have won such widespread acceptance as the mechanisms of defense. At the present time, a case study without an analysis of the patient's defenses is almost inconceivable. It is a rare textbook in introductory psychology, principles of psychiatry, or casework which omits references to defenses. The hero of many a current novel is a pawn of the forces described in *The Ego and the Mechanisms of Defense*,[8] and words like repression, projection, and denial have become part of the intelligent layman's vocabulary.

The importance of defense mechanisms is not difficult to appreciate when we consider the many topics which they help clarify. There are the symptoms of patients and the process of therapy, as well as the many daily experiences of normal adults. Defensive distortion has been invoked to explain such varied topics as dreams, slips of the tongue, content of artistic production, and conceptions of character.

Actually the understanding of defenses is very incomplete. They are very helpful in explaining the phenomena just listed, but just how they affect perception is not at all clear. In view of their promise, they cry out for empirical work and theoretical elaboration. In this chapter, I shall describe three investigations of a particular mechanism, denial in fantasy. In describing them, I shall try to highlight two issues, the problem of defining psychoanalytic concepts in operational terms and the promising extensions of current theory which can be made by controlled empirical investigations.

DESIGNING STUDIES OF DEFENSE

Status of the concept of defense: While there is a common acceptance of the theoretical importance of defensive distortion, the various mechanisms have been the subject of surprisingly few theoretical publications by psychoanalysts.[14, 20, 25] Psychologists[2, 17, 23] have demonstrated considerable interest in certain aspects of the topic but have not made much of an attempt to integrate them with defenses described in the psychoanalytic literature. Unlike such topics as psychosexual development or the techniques of therapy, the defense mechanisms have not been elaborated in terms of an organized body of theory. Only a beginning has been made, thus far, in defining principles which explain the operation and interrelations of different mechanisms.

Various psychoanalytic authorities do not agree in their lists of basic defenses.[6, 8, 19] They do agree, however, in their definitions of many mechanisms. Clinicians have little difficulty in identifying defenses such as projection or turning on the self. And most observers would concur, for example, that a patient has repressed a forbidden impulse if he cannot recall it but refers to it in a disguised form when recounting a dream.

It is not always possible to agree on a defense. It may be very difficult to judge the mechanisms of a man who has been unintentionally hurt by a friend and then goes out of his way to do the friend a favor. The man's well-meant efforts may represent reversal, denial, or a deliberate attempt to overcome his anger. Similar problems may arise when we consider some unconsciously motivated automobile accidents. They can represent the undoing of aggressive impulses, turning on the self, indirect attempts to hurt the original object, all three, or even other mechanisms.

Before we can identify different defenses with some reliability, we must first define criteria. These have not yet been proposed. This lack of theoretical development is somewhat surprising when we realize that the concept of defense is one of the cornerstones of the psychoanalytic system. One of Freud's first papers was called "The defence neuro-psychoses."[9] Sprinkled through many others are discussions and instructive examples of defensive distortion. Unfortunately, he had to delay a systematic examination of the mechanisms until he could first explore other topics connected with the resolution of conflict. Only in his final publication did he return to the mechanisms of defense; even then he did not focus on the topic.

Methodological problems: Suppose we wish to expand our knowledge of defenses. How do we begin? By collecting more descriptive information where we lack facts. Then we have to study how defenses affect perception and how they are learned. In research of this sort, controlled experiments should provide valuable supplementary material to the clinician's observations.

The investigator who proposes to study topics such as defense mechanisms faces the unique problem of measuring psychoanalytic concepts objectively without violating their original meanings. Such concepts were originally developed by clinicians to account for the symptoms of personality disorders. Compared to the experimenter, the clinician is less concerned with exact meanings. He is not disturbed by general definitions of terms. When he uses them, he implements his definitions by illustrative cases. His publications often convey his meanings only implicitly. He can usually state them explicitly, but he does this primarily when he is training new clinicians or when he is discussing cases with colleagues. The investigator who has not been clinically trained thus takes the risk that he may not understand the principles which he intends to study.

It is possible to take the position, and some psychologists do, that any concepts which are stated as generally as some of the psychoanalytic ones are not worth the investment of time required to develop a more precise translation. People with this point of view often agree that some of these topics are worth investigating, but when they investigate they feel free to select definitions on the basis of their susceptibility to precise definition rather than their fidelity to the psychoanalysts' intentions. This position has some serious drawbacks. Psychoanalysts probably know more about the concept of defense than anyone else; they first proposed it and have observed its manifestations in clinical situations for more than fifty years. If we hope to study the same phenomenon, it pays to define our terms as similarly as we can to the original conceptions and to take advantage of the psychoanalysts' finding. Only if our definitions are congruent with theirs can we gain this advantage.

Even if the investigator does understand a psychoanalytic concept, he invites a second pitfall when he attempts to define the concept by means of his techniques of measurement. The typical experimenter tries to standardize his instruments, to use control groups, and to evaluate the significance of his results by means of statistical procedures. There are some obvious advantages in these methods. They maximize the reliability of results; they enable the investigator to collect data from many subjects in a relatively short time; and they entail techniques which can be used by other investigators with relatively little training. But these advantages are lost if the instruments sacrifice the meaning of the original concepts. To avoid this is often difficult, especially when the concepts refer to transitory states like defenses, which require special precipitating conditions, and which are sometimes hard to recognize even when they occur.

These problems concerning the understanding and translation of psychoanalytic concepts had to be faced before the studies which follow could be conducted. As members of a continuing project, we first devoted a cooperative effort to careful coverage and thorough discussion of the psychoanalytic literature relevant to our topics. Next, we discussed our interpretations and instruments with a number of psychoanalysts. Finally, we made deductions from our interpretations about the conditions which would reinforce different defenses. In the next section, I shall summarize the concepts and principles which guided us in planning our studies of denial. Following that, I shall describe the results of our research and their implications for the learning of defenses.

IMAGERY, FANTASY, AND STAGES OF PERCEPTUAL DEVELOPMENT

While there are few theoretical discussions of denial, the clinical literature is replete with many interesting examples. These plus the discussions by Sigmund Freud,[9-13] Anna Freud,[8] Rapaport[21] and, particularly, Ferenczi[7] provided the bases for our speculations.

In formulating hypotheses about denial, we took a developmental approach. We started with the commonly accepted assumption that people are born with the capacity to recapitulate perceptual events. Even in the infant, such events leave a "trace" which permits them to be re-experienced. To illustrate the significance of this point, let us picture the first time that an infant becomes hungry, cries, and is fed. According to the assumption about traces, the next time he becomes hungry he can have images of being fed. Since he has no inborn conception of reality, there is no reason to believe that he can tell these need-induced images from his picture of the actual event. The distinction between the memory and the true occurrence must be learned. In time, the normal infant comes to discriminate between the different properties of the internally induced, or fantasied, images of the real event. There are at least three major differences between them. Compared to the fantasied event, the actual one is experienced more vividly. It also has a property of disappearing and of reappearing when one's eyes are closed and then opened. Finally, the sensations resulting from the actual feeding produce greater pleasure than the infant can obtain from the fantasied event. It is this greater pleasure which gradually motivates a child to favor the image of the real event when he relates to people.

Images of actual occurrences as well as internally induced images remain part of every person's repertory because both are reinforced. Every child gets some consolation from fantasies of being fed when no food is present, or from fantasies of being loved when his mother is unloving. Hence the capacity to generate such images as a means of fulfilling frustrated wishes remains a part of his potential reactions.

As a child matures, he uses fantasy for increasingly constructive purposes. When the four-year old plays games about school, he acts the roles of pupil and teacher. Under conditions which he controls, he can try out different kinds of behavior without having to worry about the consequences. This activity prepares him for school and helps him to master the insecurity aroused by the anticipation of being away from his mother.

As a boy approaches manhood his fantasies do not diminish; they are applied to new ends. When the normal man finds that he lacks access to a goal, he, too, develops fantasies. Some are only remotely related to the unaccessible goal, others more closely. Unlike the young child, the adult judges his images in terms of their relevance to his purposes. He selects the ones which may solve his problem and rejects the irrelevant ones. Fantasy is thus a necessary ingredient of thinking and of artistic creation. It may also provide a primary ingredient of some relatively mature defenses.

Instead of implementing his goals by means of his fantasy, an adult can use it as a substitute for action. By this means, he replaces frightening or depressing occurrences by pleasant daydreams. Instead of being humiliated by his financial failures, the man who denies them in fantasy can luxuriate in the imaginary success which he enjoys as an industrial tycoon. Instead of acknowledging his rejection by the opposite sex, he can picture himself as a handsome youth besieged by beautiful women.

Why should a person substitute a daydream for the greater gratification of striving to solve a problem? The answer to this question is basic to most of our predictions. The greater the gratification provided by a group of actual experiences, the stronger should be one's tendency to manipulate real objects rather than to retreat into fantasy. If a child's relationship with his mother has been generally gratifying—if she has usually fed him on timé and loved him—he should seek out still other experiences with people. He need not be overwhelmed by certain inevitable frustrations since he has learned to expect eventual gratification if he continues to strive. His memories of past gratifications motivate him not to avoid problems but to find their practical solutions.

We expect very different behavior if a child's relationships with people have not been generally gratifying. If actual occurrences provide him with less gratification than do his wishfulfilling images, he may become inclined to retreat into his world of fantasy whenever he is faced with an emergency. Even if he has not learned to favor this defense in early life, he may be forced to resort to it in later years if, say, he is treated very harshly by people whose respect he needs or if he suffers humiliating failures.

EMPIRICAL STUDIES

Problems: On the basis of conjectures listed above, members of our project investigated five general topics pertaining to denial. 1) We studied the extent to which denial is a product of hardship. Since people in the working class suffer more hardships than people in the middle class, we anticipated that the former would resort to the defense more frequently. It also seemed probable that denial would be employed more by subjects whose parents favored harsh rather than mild methods of child rearing. 2) We investigated variations of denial in different ages. We assumed that it is a primitive defense, is available very early in life and is relinquished earlier than most other mechanisms. From this, we deduced that younger children should exceed older ones in denial of anxiety. 3) One reason for relinquishing denial may be its inefficiency as a method of solving problems. Although awareness of a conflict may be obliterated, the conflict itself often persists and may even become aggravated because it is ignored. In view of this observation, we anticipated that denial might be related to sociometric ratings. Our remaining topics were exploratory, namely 4) The difference in rates of denial

by boys and girls, and 5) The extent to which denial can be
deliberately taught to children by their parents.

METHODS

Story Completion Test and denial of failure: To elicit defenses,
we administered projective tests consisting of incomplete stories.
In the first study,* conducted by Betty J. Beardslee,[1] each story
depicted a serious failure. One theme, for example, was about a
high school boy who wanted to be a concert violinist. After devot-
ing much effort to his music, his teacher said that "the hero" did
not have much promise and that he was being dropped from the
orchestra so he could catch up with his neglected academic
courses.

Subjects were instructed to finish each story. In the analysis
of results, endings were coded for amounts of denial in fantasy
and of realistic solutions. Denial was tabulated when a theme
violated the limiting conditions of the story or included events
which were so improbable as to distort the initial facts. In one
such ending, a subject wrote that the hero, who had just been
informed of his questionable musical ability, gave a concert in
Carnegie Hall the following week.

Endings coded as realistic or non-defensive took a number
of forms. In some themes, the hero accepted the situation and
tried not to be too concerned. In others, he analyzed the situation and decided on a practical course of action, or he substituted a less attractive activity that was similar to the original.
In one instance of practical action, the hero decided that the
teacher was mistaken and went to a professional music school
which provided intensive training. In a theme about substitution,
he concluded that his teacher was right, gave up music as a
vocation, and opened a music store so as to maintain contact
with the musical profession.

Experimentally induced failure: In the initial study, the subjects first completed three stories and then took a group of tests

────────────
* This research was part of Project M-564 which was supported by the
U.S. Public Health Service.

which were so designed that they could not be passed by any-one. To create an experience of failure, Beardslee first asked each subject about his vocational aspirations. Then she said the tests would reveal his qualifications for the job which he pre-ferred most. After failing the tests, he completed three other stories.

Actual failure was created on the assumption that there would be no need to defend oneself unless faced with a real problem. In analyzing the results, we used the initial endings as a baseline. The score for each subject was the difference between the frequency of denial in his initial and in his final set of story endings.

Story Completion Test and denial of anger: In a second study,* conducted by Virginia Douglas,[5] each story described a situation in which the hero was unintentionally frustrated by the well-meaning efforts of a friendly adult. The cause of con-flict was thus shifted from failure to unacceptable anger. One story, for example, described the events which occurred when the aunt of a boy named Harry came to stay with him because his mother was going away on a long trip. The aunt had always pampered Harry and he liked her very much. For a long time, Harry had saved his money to buy a ticket for the biggest foot-ball game of the year. He and his best friend had been lucky enough to get the last two available tickets. The day of the game, the aunt, noticing that Harry had not straightened up his room, cleaned it for him and burned the trash. On his way to the game, he went to his room and was happy that it was so neat and clean. He looked for his ticket in his desk but it was not there. He frantically looked in all the other possible places, but to no avail. He tried to find his aunt but she had gone visiting. When the clock told him that the game was almost over, he gave up. He had missed the game. As he sat there, his aunt came in and told him about burning the papers. Harry then realized that his aunt had unintentionally destroyed his football ticket.

The coding of denial was the same as in the Beardslee study.

---

* This research was part of the Flint Youth Study, Project 3M-9109 (c), which was supported by the U.S. Public Health Service.

One ending, which was interpreted as describing a denial of
anger, indicated that the ticket "wasn't burned up and it was
raining so that the game was called off and he got a raincheck
and he got to go another time." This ending disregarded two
basic facts presented in the plot: the ticket was destroyed, and
the game did take place. In a more realistic conclusion, the hero
used his charm to convince his aunt that she should buy him
tickets for another game. Instead of following the scoring practice of the first study, Douglas used the sum of all references to
denial and not a discrepancy between scores before and after
denial.

Denial of anger and objective endings: In the third investigation,* conducted by Arthur Kovacs,[16] subjects were given
story beginnings, each of which was followed by seven possible
endings. From the seven, all depicting frustrations of boys by
well-meaning adults, three were to be chosen in their order of
probable occurrence. In a typical story, a boy had set his heart
on a dog. After he had saved enough money to buy one, his
parents took him to a kennel. There he saw the dog of his dreams,
but his parents explained that it was too big for their apartment.
The hero did not like any of the other dogs and the one he
wanted was purchased by another boy.

Each of the possible endings described a reaction which
would result from the use of a particular defense. The hero could
do such things as blame himself for upsetting his parents, project his anger to them, or reverse his resentment.

RESULTS

Denial of anger and hardship: In summarizing the results, I
shall report them in order of the five topics listed in the previous
section. The first postulated a relationship between denial and
hardship. To test the initial hypothesis, Beardslee compared the
incidence of denial in boys from the middle and working classes.

* This research is part of a project sponsored by the Ford Foundation
on the basis of contract 50732.

In the initial study, the 115 subjects were white males in the seventh or eighth grade and of above borderline intelligence.

Social class: Sociological descriptions[4,22] indicate that working class children have a much harder time than their middle class peers. Some sons of blue collar workers suffer from poor heating, crowded homes, and inadequate food. Often the mother works, and her son is unsupervised for part of the day; in such situations he may be hurt or exploited by strangers. He may live in a part of town where schools and recreational facilities are barely adequate, or he may acquire values which make him ashamed of doing well in school. As a result, he cannot get the training necessary for advancement in the economic system.

Before the amounts of denial in the two classes are discussed, it is first necessary to report an unanticipated relationship. Denial of both anger and failure varied significantly with verbal intelligence, as measured on Thurstone's Verbal subtest of his Primary Mental Abilities.[27]

The predicted difference in denial between boys in the two classes was not supported by the data. The difference was significant, however, among children in the lower half of the distribution of verbal intelligence. In this population, boys from working class families had the higher rate of denial. The difference between classes was not significant for children in the higher half of the intelligence distribution. Apparently, if a boy is above a certain level of intelligence, he seems to rise above the handicaps of his background.

Child rearing: Another form of hardship investigated by Beardslee was the type resulting from certain parental practices. We gained our information about social status and methods of child rearing by interviewing the mothers. They provided information about three practices: the extent to which requests for obedience were explained, type of discipline, and frequency of reward.

It was anticipated that arbitrary requests for obedience would be associated with a greater increase in denial than explained requests. If a child is expected to obey requests when he does not understand the reasons for them, he may find it difficult to comply. He may even learn to avoid taking any initiative for

fear of doing wrong. An analysis of the data supported the prediction. Requests for obedience were significantly related to
denial. Arbitrary requests were associated with denial of failure;
explained requests were associated with lack of denial.

Discipline, too, was significantly associated with denial. Each
mother was classified according to the type of discipline she favored. One was psychological, including such methods as appeals
to guilt, deprivation of privileges, and distractions. A second type
of discipline was corporal, and a third was a mixture of corporal
and psychological. We initially considered the corporal method
the harshest. Contrary to our anticipation, corporal and psychological discipline were both associated with denial. Only the
more flexible, mixed type of discipline was associated with lack
of denial.

In classifying mothers with respect to reward, we assigned
them either to a group who provided incentives more than twice
a week or to a group using less frequent rewards. The association between reward and denial was in the predicted direction
but not quite significant.

Reward did interact significantly with discipline and denial.
With frequent reward, denial tended to decrease or remain the
same, regardless of the type of punishment. With infrequent
reward, denial tended to increase except when discipline was
mixed; then the incidence of denial tended to decrease. Type of
reward also interacted significantly with obedience and denial.
The harsher the combination of obedience requests and reward,
the greater was the frequency with which failure was denied. In
other words, arbitrary requests and infrequent reward were associated with most denial.

Denial and age: In the second study, Douglas tested the relationship to denial of age, sociometric status, and sex. Her subjects were 115 white boys and girls in the elementary and high
school of the University of Michigan. Almost all the subjects
were above average in intelligence and from middle class families. In analyzing age differences (topic 2), she compared three
groups. The children in one were in the second and third grades,
and the ages varied between 7 and 9 years. In the second group,
the children were in the fifth and sixth grades, and the ages

varied between 10 and 13 years. In the third group, the children were in the ninth and tenth grades, and the ages varied between 15 and 17 years.

We anticipated that the older the group, the more they should have relinquished denial in favor of more efficient methods of resolving conflict. It was not possible to foretell, however, whether each age group would differ significantly from the two others. As anticipated, there was a decrease in denial with an increase in age. Since there were six stories, it would have been difficult to make more than six references to denial. The mean for the first two grades was 2.4, the mean for the intermediate grades was 1.8, and the mean for the upper grades was .63. Non-defensive problem solving increased progressively with age. The means were 1.29 for the first two grades, 1.56 for the second two, and 2.58 for the final two. On both responses to conflict the oldest group differed significantly from the two others.

Denial and choice by peers: In the second study an exploratory analysis was made of the relationships between defense and sociometric status (topic 3). Denial should make it difficult for a child to get along in a social group. The more he ignores actual events, the greater should be his difficulty with other children. To determine the quality of relationships among peers, we asked the children in each class to rate each other on a four-point scale. The distribution was divided at the median so that a subject was classified as being either high or low.

Being liked was not significantly related to denial in the youngest or in the intermediate groups. Possibly, these results reflect the instability of the social choices of younger children. Only in grades 9 and 10 was there a significant and inverse association between denial and being liked. On the average, a child who was inclined to deny his anger in fantasy was among those least liked by his peers.

Sex differences: In another analysis, Douglas obtained sex differences in frequency of denial (topic 4). The comparison was based on a hunch rather than on any theoretical principles. When we asked people to predict the result, they usually guessed that girls would relinquish the defense earlier than boy. Often it was assumed that girls are more mature than boys either because of biological reasons or social pressures. The data revealed a significant difference between the sexes, but only in the first two grades. Boys exceeded girls in rate of denial. In the intermediate and older groups, the differences were negligible.

Kovacs also obtained sex differences in the denial of anger. His subjects were 125 boys and girls between 9 and 14 years of age. They were obtained from camps operated by various churches and local associations. Compared to the samples of the first two investigations, this third sample was much more heterogeneous. It included white and Negro children of all intelligence levels, from the middle and working classes, from different parts of the United States and Europe, and from broken and intact families. In contrast to the results of the second study, older boys and girls differed very significantly in rate of denial. Also contrary to the previous results was the finding that girls denied anger more than boys. While the populations of the second and third investigations were not comparable in every detail, it seemed warranted, for purposes of exploration, to assume homogeneity and then to account for the disparity in results. To throw light on the possible causes of the change in trend, sex differences were analyzed within the middle and working classes. Among children from the working class, females significantly exceeded males in the denial of anger; among children from the middle class, males exceeded females. The latter finding is compatible with Douglas', since most of her subjects had fathers in white collar occupations.

The indoctrination of denial: The greater frequency of denial in the population of the third study may have occurred because many of the subjects attended fundamentalist churches. We developed an interest in religious training because the dogma of certain churches practically requires the frequent use of certain defense mechanisms. An acceptance of the Calvinist doctrine of predestination, for example, should result in a tendency to turn one's unacceptable aggression against oneself. An acceptance of the dogma of many fundamentalist churches should reinforce denial. It even seemed possible that defenses compatible with dogma might be deliberately reinforced by parents (topic 5).

Our interest in the deliberate teaching of denial was initially kindled by the results of an earlier pre-test. To determine parental attitudes toward denial, we asked each of a group of mothers how she would feel if her son did a lot of daydreaming. The number of subjects was small, but the responses differed in terms of social class. Most wives of white collar workers indicated that they would regard daydreaming with alarm. Many thought they would distract their children by challenging them with special tasks—anything to stop the practice. Most wives of manual laborers had a very different reaction. While a few of the mothers were negative about daydreaming, most of them said that it is a help in getting over one's disappointments.

We next decided to study a combination of social class and degree of religious fundamentalism. Kovacs obtained another sample of 48 subjects and compared the rate of denial by children in fundamentalist Methodist and Presbyterian churches with the combined rate of denial by children in liberal and moderate groups of the same denominations. The difference between the two groups was very significant. As anticipated, the fundamentalists showed a much greater tendency to deny anger than the liberals and moderates. Unfortunately, the number of subjects did not permit a simultaneous analysis of church, class, and denial. From the trends, it seemed probable that it was the fundamentalists from the working class who denied the most but that fundamentalism would be related to denial if socioeconomic status were held constant.

Even if fundamentalists are more inclined to deny anger, this does not mean that the defense is necessarily a product of parental indoctrination. As one approach to this hypothesis, we asked parents in the three kinds of churches to fill out an attitude scale, part of which referred to denial. In a representative item, parents were asked to affirm or deny the statement: "Thinking and dreaming about pleasant things helps when you are in trouble." Compared to the parents in liberal and moderate churches, those in fundamentalist churches were more inclined to choose items which signified positive evaluation of denial. Among the middle class, but not the working class, fundamentalists, the positive evaluation by the parents was significantly related to the frequency with which their children chose the defense. It would have been desirable to analyze the interaction among class, religion, attitude, and defense, but this was not possible because of the small number of cases.

DISCUSSION

The measurement of denial: In view of the different methods of scoring denial, we may well question the comparability of the three studies. One score of denial was a discrepancy between an initial set of stories and a final set which was completed after an experience of failure. The second score was the sum of references to denial in all the story endings. The third score was the sum of references to denial chosen from alternatives which we provided. There were differences not only in methods but also in the problems of the stories. In one study, the themes described intolerable failures; in the other studies, the themes referred to conflicts about anger.

The changes in method reflected attempts to test alternative techniques of investigating defenses. How confident can we be that the three techniques measured the same defense? Even if they did, have we any evidence that the three kinds of scores are valid indicators of denial?

To answer the first question, both the writing of endings and the objective choice of alternatives were obtained from subjects in the third study. The relationship between the two measures of denial was very significant. Less direct evidence of validity is provided by the fact that different measures of denial were related to the same antecedent variable in two different studies. In the first and third investigations, the different measures of denial were significantly associated with social class. In the second and third investigations, there were significant inverse relationships between denial and realistic problem solving.

We can also invoke construct validity[3] in support of the different measures. In the first study, for example, a consideration of denial led us to predict that it would be associated with such independent variables as social class, harshness of discipline, extent to which requests for obedience were explained, and amount of reward. The fact that all the predicted relationships were significant lends support to the assumption that the projective technique must have measured denial or some significantly associated variable.

To validate the objective test of denial, we constructed two independent criteria. One was a self-rating on socially desirable traits, and the other was a rating of one's parents on a similar kind of scale. Both of these variables were significantly and positively associated with the objective index of denial. Frequent denial was associated with improbably high ratings of self and of one's parents.

Denial as a learned response: Basic to all the predictions was the assumption that defensive distortion is learned and that it changes with experience. The results tend to support this assumption. The significant variations of denial with different child rearing practices, and the fact that the relative preference for the defense by boys and girls differed in the two social classes, both these findings indicate that frequency of denial varies with specific experiences.

The social consequences of denial: We made two other assumptions about denial. We pictured it as a relatively simple defense which is available early. We also postulated that it is socially handicapping in later years because its obliteration of awareness precludes constructive action. Compatible with the first premise is the high incidence of denial in the youngest group. Compatible with the second is the decreasing incidence of denial with increasing age. The decrease seems to represent a response to two kinds of pressures, both of which are revealed in our results. For fear of the difficulties created by the defense, many mothers try to keep their children from daydreaming. In addition, children who are inclined to deny their problems are often rejected by their peers. Since these pressures are most common in the non-fundamentalist, middle class groups, this may contribute to their comparative lack of denial.

Inadequate mastery of other defenses: Finally we assumed that a child relinquishes denial only when he has developed other, more complex, techniques of resolving conflict. These alternatives have to be learned. In some cases the process is lengthy and intricate. To attain facility in turning his aggression on himself, for example, a child must first learn many other lessons. He must develop a body image, the concepts of self and non-self, and an awareness of the characteristics of other people. He must also recognize forbidden acts, and internalize prohibitions so that their violation creates guilt. Finally, he must acquire the concept of blaming. In contrast to this lengthy training process for turning aggression against oneself is the minimal experience needed for defensive use of denial. All it requires is the direct inhibition of a cue affecting awareness.

If harsh parental techniques or a child's own deficiencies prevent him from mastering the more complex defenses, he has no recourse but to fall back on simpler mechanisms. According to our findings, parental methods which delay the learning of more mature techniques are lack of reward, excessive punitiveness, arbitrary requests for obedience, and deliberate reinforcement of denial. Average, or less than average, intelligence may also interfere with acquisition of complex skills.

Defenses and realistic problem solving: In much of the literature about defenses, their difference from thinking is stressed; yet it is their similarity which stands out when one reads the subjects' stories. Thinking and denial are alternative methods of solving a problem. According to psychoanalytic theory, all such reactions are initiated when a person faces a barrier to a goal. In the clinical literature, the typical example of such a barrier is the moral standard which proscribes certain kinds of behavior; the goal usually cited is need gratification. When the moral standard prohibits the direct satisfaction of a need, the person must find a substitute act which expresses the need but does not violate the moral standard. This can be done by deliberate, rational techniques or by various defensive distortions.

When viewed in terms of their common functions, the various problem solving techniques can be compared with respect to such characteristics as degree of distortion and efficiency. Rational problem solving results in least distortion, and promotes the most adequate satisfaction of needs in line with social pressures. The use of some defenses, such as turning against the self or reversal, results in minor distortions. In self-attack, only the awareness of the original object is changed; in reversal only the awareness of the act is changed. Like more rational methods, such defenses implement one's adjustment to social pressures and facilitate the control of direct aggression. Because the facts are distorted, control is usually more rigid than that which occurs as a result of realistic problem solving. Defenses such as denial in fantasy create considerable distortion, and are least adequate socially. Control is unpredictable and action can seldom be deliberate.

Social position and denial: Among our best indicators of a person's probable tendency to deny his problems are such social indices as age, sex, social class, and religion. These variables point to the most fundamental social forces affecting the individual in every society.[18] Certain psychoses, which, according to psychoanalytic theory, are determined, in part, by a tendency to favor denial, vary with age, sex, social class and religion.[15, 22] Such findings gave us confidence that these indices might also forecast rate of denial in normals with social positions that are similar to those of psychotics. The results of our studies support the postulated relationships between the social indices and the defense.

Interactions: Without taking interactions among social variables into account, we might misinterpret some of the findings. Sex differences illustrate this possible pitfall. We would be oversimplifying the results if we thought in terms of the general rate of denial by all girls, because the rate differs with age, social class, and religion. While denial is punished in the middle class, this punishment is only common in non-fundamentalist groups. Even they do not become very coercive until the children reach a certain age. The girls then begin to give up denial more than boys. The results are quite different for boys and girls who come from working class families. Unless we take the patterns of different social pressures into account simultaneously, we get a picture which is incomplete and possibly erroneous.

Significance of social position: Why study social indices at all? We could confine our antecedent variables to methods of child rearing, differences in values, accessibility of certain kinds of friends, and the like. One reason for beginning with the society has already been mentioned. Social positions point to some of the potent, general, and enduring forces to which an individual has to adjust. Social positions may thus enable us to determine the major sources of conflict, of variations in moral standards, and of different kinds of defenses and expressive styles in a particular society.

A second asset of social indices stems from the fact that the learning of many aspects of personality cannot be ethically duplicated under the artificial conditions of the laboratory. Our theory indicates, for instance, that traumatized children should exceed others in rate of denial. It would be unthinkable to actually traumatize a group of children, nor is such a step necessary. It is, unfortunately, all too easy to find children who have been subjected to exceptionally traumatic experiences, particularly if we select subjects from different social classes.

A third benefit may be gained from the study of social antecedents. They facilitate the task of obtaining broad ranges of certain variables. The investigator who restricts his populations to college sophomores or to the children of professors runs the risk of erroneously rejecting some hypotheses because of the narrow range of scores on some variables. He can often avoid this pitfall by the simple precaution of selecting subjects with an eye to social variables which may affect the range of scores.

SUMMARY

An exploration of the problems involved in doing empirical work with psychoanalytic concepts was followed by a group of principles concerning the meaning and origins of the defense mechanism of denial. These principles provided the hypotheses for three studies. According to the results of these studies, the tendency to favor denial is related inversely to verbal intelligence, age, liking by peers, and realistic problem solving. Denial is directly related to social class within the group who were in the lower half of the distribution of intelligence, and to the degree of fundamentalism of the subjects' churches. Denial was most frequent when children had been subjected by their parents to arbitrary rather than explained requests for obedience, and to corporal discipline or psychological rather than mixed types of punishment. Use of denial varied with sex, but the trends differed in terms of social class. In the middle class, boys exceeded girls; this trend was reversed in the working class. The findings also indicated that denial may be deliberately indoctrinated by parents in the working class and in fundamentalist churches.

References

1. Beardslee, Betty J. The learning of two mechanisms of defense. Unpubl. Ph. D. dissertation. Univ. of Michigan, 1955.

2. Bruner, J. S. and Postman, L. Emotional selectivity in perception and reaction. *J. Personal.*, 1947, 16, 69-77.

3. Cronbach, L. J. and Meehl, P. E. Construct validity in psychological tests. *Psychol. Bull.*, 1955, 52, 281-302.

4. Davis, W. A. and Dollard, J. *Children of bondage*; the personality development of Negro youth in the urban South. Washington, D. C.: American Council on Education, 1940.

5. Douglas, Virginia I. A developmental study of two families of defense. Unpubl. Paper.

6. Fenichel, O. *The psychoanalytic theory of neurosis*. New York: Norton, 1945.

7. Ferenczi, S. Stages in the development of a sense of reality. *Contributions to psychoanalysis*. London: Hogarth, 1952.

8. Freud, Anna. *The ego and the mechanisms of defence*. London: Hogarth, 1948.

9. Freud, S. The defence neuro-psychoses. *Collected papers.* Vol. 1. London: Hogarth, 1949.

10. Freud, S. Instincts and their vicissitudes. *Collected papers*. Vol. 4. London: Hogarth, 1949.

11. Freud, S. Negation. *Collected papers*. Vol. 5. London: Hogarth, 1949.

12. Freud, S. Analysis terminable and interminable. *Collected papers*. Vol. 5. London: Hogarth, 1949.

13. Freud, S. Splitting of the ego in the defensive process. *Collected papers.* Vol. 5. London: Hogarth, 1949.

14. Gero, G. The concept of defence. *Psychoanal. Quart.*, 1951, 20, 565-578.

15. Hollingshead, A. B. and Redlich, F. C. Social stratification and psychiatric disorders. *Amer. Sociol. Rev.*, 1953, 18, 163-169.

16. Kovacs, A. L. Religion and the mechanism of denial. Unpubl. Paper.

17. Lazarus, R. S., Eriksen, C.W., and Fonda, C. P. Personality dynamics and auditory perceptual recognition. *J. Personal.*, 1951, 19, 471-482.

18. Linton, R. *Culture and mental disorders.* Springfield, Ill.: Thomas, 1956.

19. Monroe, Ruth L. *Schools of psychoanalytic thought.* New York: Dryden, 1955.

20. Novey, S. Utilization of social institutions as a defence technique in the neuroses. *Int. J. Psychoanal.*, 1954, 35, 82-91.

21. Rapaport, D. *Organization and pathology of thought.* New York: Columbia Univ. Press, 1951.

22. Rose, A. M. *Mental health and mental disorder;* a sociological approach. New York: Norton, 1955.

23. Rosenzweig, S. and Sarason, S. An experimental study of the triadic hypothesis reaction to frustration, ego-defense, and hypnotizability I. Correlational approach. *Charact. & Pers.*, 1942, 11, 1-20.

24. Ruesch, J. Social technique, social status, and social changes in illness. In Kluckhohn, C. and Murray, H. A. (Eds.), *Personality in nature, society, and culture.* New York: Knopf, 1949.

25. Sperling, S. J. On denial and the essential nature of defence. *Int. J. Psychoanal.*, 1958, 39, 25-38.

26. Sterba, R. F. Oral invasion and self defence. *Int. J. Psychoanal.*, 1957, 38, 204-208.

27. Thurstone, L. L. *Primary mental abilities.* Chicago: Univ. of Chicago Press, 1938.

Irving E. Alexander
with
Arthur M. Adlerstein

III

Studies in the Psychology of Death *

INTRODUCTION

EACH MAN LEARNS EARLY in life that some day he must die. What role does this information play in his development? How does it affect his aims, his wishes, his behavior? At the present time our best sources of information on these questions are outside the field of psychology—in literature, philosophy, religion, and medicine. While such sources have yielded rich insights about the meaning that death has for human beings, there has been little attempt to apply scientific procedures to select among these ideas. Perhaps it is time for this further step to be taken. It is the purpose of this chapter to describe some primitive attempts, utilizing the more traditional techniques and methods of our science, to study some aspects of man's reaction to death.

First let us glance briefly at the state of our knowledge about death as it exists in the psychological literature.

THE THEORISTS

The most fruitful sources of theory are to be found in "depth" psychology and in "existential" philosophy, more specifically, the

* The studies reported herein were supported in part by grants from The National Institute of Mental Health.

work of Freud, Jung, and Heidegger. In the early theory of psychoanalysis death was assigned a relatively minor role. Fear of death was discussed as a derivation of Oedipal and pre-Oedipal stages.[17] Two antecedent conditions were postulated, either of which could serve as a basis for this fear: separation anxiety or castration anxiety.

The appearance of the book *Beyond the pleasure principle*[18] in 1920 ushered in Freud's later views on death. He postulated a death instinct in man that operated on a biological level. Its only representation in the ego was in the aggressive impulse. The ego could not conceive of its own death. The proposal of a death instinct solved the problem of aggression in psychoanalytic theory. No longer did one have to puzzle whether the aggressive act belonged to the ego instincts or to the libidinal instincts or to both. A new dichotomy was created, Eros and Thanatos, in basic opposition to one another. In this final version death became a cornerstone of Freudian doctrine.

The problem of death interested and challenged Freud personally throughout his life. One cannot come away from a reading of the three volume Jones biography[25] without this conviction. In 1906 and again in 1918 Freud predicted that those years would be his last (Vol. 2). The numerous examples of his repeated reference to death even before the long struggle with cancer makes one feel that this was a person who lived constantly in the shadow of death (Vol. 3, p. 279). His later views on this subject generated little enthusiasm in psychoanalytic ranks. In fact some writers began to seek the roots of these ideas in Freud's personal life as though this would explain away the unacceptable doctrine. Wittels[52] postulated that Freud's concern with the death instinct came shortly after the unexpected death of his daughter, Sophie, and could be traced to this event. Jones (Vol. 3) points out in answer that Freud's speculations preceded that event, thus providing no basis for the hypothesis of personal involvement. It must be clearly recognized that acceptance of the death instinct as having some personal meaning in Freud's life by no means precludes a judgment of its value as an explanatory concept. For this purpose other more desirable criteria are available. If one wishes, however, to speculate about events in Freud's life that may have been associated with his introduction of a biological drive to return to an inanimate state, one should not overlook that the appearance of this doctrine coincided with what Jones refers to as a precancerous stage of cancer, a time when Freud was suffering pain from a recurrent swelling of the palate. It was the later stages of this illness that ultimately caused his death.

Never in his writings did Freud tie together the two aspects of death that he theorized about independently. Fear of death was entirely a libidinal matter with no stated connection to the death instinct.

In Jung's theory, death also plays a prominent role.[29] He sees it as the central problem of the second half of life. Just as sexuality is the dominant force in the first half of life so do the ensuing aspects of decline face man with his ultimate fate and his attitude towards it. The process of individuation, described by Jung,[28] leads to a completion of the personality, and, as a consequence, a solution of the death problem. Death emerges as a psychological problem only in the second half of life except in pathological instances.

Existentialist views about death are varied although most see it as an important human problem. Heidegger assigns death a central role in his philosophy.[6] He postulates that the idea of our eventual nothingness is always with us, in each moment of time, providing a background upon which both existence and time can be made meaningful. Death is also seen as an ever-present source of tension and anxiety in the organism. While Heidegger was not especially concerned with individual psychological problems, one might extend these ideas into the realm of individual psychology by hypothesizing that thoughts of death and their attendant anxiety are always present somewhere in man's psychic life, sometimes close to consciousness, sometimes more distant. Stated in this way one can recognize the basic opposition to Freud's view, where death anxiety results from particular antecedent conditions.

Other theorists have recognized the importance of death and have utilized the concept in various ways. Adler, in Bottomé's biography,[7] refers to a critical incident in his early life that led him toward a career in medicine. While stricken with pneumonia at age five, all hope for his survival was abandoned by the attending physician. The fear generated by the doctor's announcement led him to a firm resolution, when he recovered, to study medicine. In this way he felt he would be better able to defend against the danger of death. Here is an instance in which the pursuits of a lifetime were initiated by a frightening brush with death. It is not without meaning that the guiding theme of Adler's therapy was "courage," the ability to face what life held in store.

Fromm[19] also writes about the problem of death. He claims that man's awareness of his own end is an inherent property of mind. The anxiety that this dichotomy of life and death induces can only be alleviated by a recognition of one's position of "aloneness" in the universe. Man must also recognize that he alone is responsible for giving meaning to life by what he does. The similarity of these views to those of Sartre is striking.

Zilboorg's[54] approach has within it some aspects of Heidegger's views and also some of Freud's. He talks of the universality of the death fear within the framework of a Freudian topography of mind. He postulates that the fear of death is a very powerful factor in man's mental functioning and that this fear is always with us. The fear of death is related to the instinct of self-preservation; the fear being the affective aspect of the instinct. Zilboorg contends that the fear of death is necessarily repressed so that the ego can carry out its assigned function of dealing with the affairs of every day life.

A final view worth mentioning, one that is little known, is that of G. Stanley Hall[22] who early in this century called attention to the importance of the death concept for psychology. Hall stated that underlying all fears and phobic reactions is the fear of death and that this basic fear is of no less importance to the psychology of the individual than the well-recognized drives of hunger and love which are said to "rule the world." A more detailed discussion of some of these positions may be found in Eissler.[15]

Even within this small group who gave a place to death in their writings, wide differences in opinion exist. Some see it as a pervasive factor strongly influencing man's behavior; others see it as more restricted to certain phases of life or else differentially influential as a function of particular kinds of infantile experiences.

EMPIRICAL STUDIES

Empirical data on reactions to death are rather scarce. Some early work[21] was done in Hall's laboratory where responses to a questionnaire on fear revealed that the fear of death appeared in approximately 5 percent of the total fears reported by a group of pupils and students ranging in age from 5 to 22. Scott[43] carried this work further to include a much wider range of ages. He concluded that death is an important element in man's consciousness. A hypothetical course of concern was charted for the life span. Peaks of concern were postulated to occur at ages 4 and 14, and a slow but constant increase from adolescence to old age was noted.

In the 1930's Paul Schilder was the central figure in a series of studies involving attitudes toward death. The methods used were the questionnaire and the depth interview. In three separate papers Bromberg and Schilder reported the attitudes of psychoneurotics,[9] murderers,[41] and a group of normals composed largely of college and professional school students.[8] The results of these studies were interpreted in terms of psychoanalytic doctrine. Conscious reports concerning death were tied to libidinal and ego needs. What is of interest here is that in the normal group it was reported that these people rarely thought of death spontaneously. Most of the subjects reported that it was difficult to think of their own death, and roughly three-fourths of the sample felt their own death to be an improbable event. When asked whether they were constantly aware of death in the dim reaches of consciousness, the dominant response was negative. From these results Schilder found little evidence to support an existentialist position.

Middleton[33] in 1936 reported the results of a questionnaire study on attitudes toward death in a population of 825 college students. He found that 93 percent of his subjects reported that they think about death, but only very rarely or occasionally. Dreams about death or dying were denied by 63 percent of the group, and of the remaining 37 percent only 2 percent had such dreams more than rarely or occasionally. Only 12 percent of this population indicated fear or horror of death, 25 percent said they were unafraid, while 62 percent reported indifference.

Later studies by Stacey and his associates,[44, 45] using a modified form of the Schilder and Middleton questionnaires, have demonstrated that various sub-groups in the population (e.g. normal and subnormal adolescent girls, students in different fields of specialization, forestry, law and engineering, and penitentiary inmates) respond differently as groups to a great many of the questions asked. These studies, however, offer no explanation of the results. They give only the questions on which the groups differ. Feifel[16] added similar information on the aged.

The material from empirical sources reveals that on a conscious, verbal level people in our culture do not seem to be seriously concerned with thoughts of death. Is it a reflection of a basic indifference? Or, perhaps, are these results a function of the kind of measurement that was made? Or is it a matter of conforming to a cultural expectation of fearlessness and fortitude? It was to the broad question, whether death is a matter of indifference, that we first turned our attention.[1]

EXPERIMENT A

We sought a method that would eliminate the major difficulties encountered in the verbal-questionnaire type technique. Our search was for a technique that was quantitative, reliable, easy to employ, and also one that had the advantage of keeping from the subject that which we were most interested in measuring. We found the word-association task to be readily adaptable for our purposes. With appropriate modifications we utilized the experimental approach of Jung and his students, introduced some fifty years ago.[27] Response time and psychogalvanic responses were recorded to a list of 27 carefully selected stimulus words.

Word list: The list contained three sets of words: basals, a priori affectives (sex and school words), and death words. The basals are general samples from the language, of varying affective meaning for different subjects, used as the base line against which to measure change in affect. The reasoning is as follows. Words related to sex and also to school are assumed to be capable of inducing increased affective response in a college population. The comparison between basal and the combined sex-school category is the first that is made, and to the extent to which our premise is true we have a sensitive measuring instrument. The critical measurement is then made between responses to basal words and responses to death words.

All words were chosen from the Thorndike and Lorge Teacher's Word Book of 30,000 Words.[50] The sub-groups were closely matched for word-frequency counts, length of word, and number of syllables. A random procedure was used to determine the position of a word on the list. The only restriction imposed was that critical words (non-basals) were not allowed to follow each other. A selection from the word list follows. Sex: romance, maiden, lover. School: college, lecture, scholar. Death: funeral, death, burial. Basal: sunset, insect, criminal.

Subjects: The subjects, 31 male Princeton undergraduate students, were volunteers. They were all known to one or another of the experimenters, and upon superficial analysis seemed to represent typical members of the undergraduate population. None were known to have had psychiatric histories and all were naive with respect to the purpose of the experiment.

Procedure: After being comfortably seated, the subject was told that the purpose of the experiment was to determine the efficiency of a particular recording device in measuring skin responses. His head was placed in a fixed position and he was instructed to respond into an adjacent telephone receiver with the first word that came to mine upon presentation of a stimulus word. The experimenter manually initiated an electric timer to coincide with the onset of the stimulus. The timer was interrupted by the subject's response into the telephone receiver which acted as a voice key. Measurements of the difference in voltage generated between the palm and the dorsal surface of the hand were made and recorded on a Sanborn 2 channel recorder. A wet electrode, rubdown technique described by Bitterman et al.[5] was used to bring the basal resistance of each subject to comparable levels. The time interval between word presentations fluctuated between 45 seconds to one minute, depending on how soon the subject returned to a resting level. A preliminary, practice word group leading right into the experimental list was given to accustom the subject to the task and to the apparatus.

Results: The results clearly indicated that death words call forth an increased affective response in our subject population. Latency of response time and PGR distributions, originally skewed, were normalized by logarithmic transformation. Means were determined for each subject on each of three sets of words, and the differences among means was assessed by the analysis of variance technique. Table 1 contains a summary of these results.

TABLE 1—*Analysis of variance of PGR and response time scores*

Source	PGR				Response time			
	Sum of squares	df	Mean square	F	Sum of squares	df	Mean square	F
Total	12.30	92			4.25	92		
Between word groups	.2	2	.1	8.55†	.07	2	.035	4.86†
Between individuals	11.4	30	.38	32.48‡	3.75	30	.125	17.36‡
Discrepance	.70	60	.0117		.43	60	.0072	

†$p < .05$
‡$p < .01$

What is portrayed here from an examination of the F ratios is that the several word groupings are responded to differently by the subjects as a group and that the individual subjects differ significantly from each other in their responses to these three sets of words.

The analysis among word groupings was made by a t-test of difference distributions and is presented in Table 2. Responses to the selected affective words differ significantly from basal

TABLE 2—t *Values for word group comparisons on both response measures*

Comparison	PGR	Response time
Basal vs. affective	4.60†	2.73†
Basal vs. death	3.85†	2.66†
Affective vs. death	.09	.61

†p<.01

words on both measures and thus provide some expression of validity for the technique. Responses to death words are also significantly different from basal word responses on both response measures. Response time is increased as is the magnitude of the PGR. Comparison between death words and affective words reveals chance differences.

Discussion: What we learned from these observations is that despite expressions of indifference and minimum concern reported by earlier investigators,[8, 33] death words have the ability to bring forth increased affective responses from a group of normal, male, college students. It is as though our culture teaches us to be little involved, and this is the way we behave verbally. Yet, on a more primitive physiological level we act as though we are more intensely involved. A clear illustration of this process was provided by a test subject who was used in a preliminary phase of the experiment. This person gave unusually long latencies and large PGR deflections to the death words. When questioned at length informally, he expressed no preoccupation with thoughts or feelings about death. It was only by chance that he indicated that he was a diabetic whose life depends on the administration of a drug each day. While it is an inference that extreme test responses and disturbed medical states are causally related, it is certainly an hypothesis that is open to empirical check.

THE CHILD AND DEATH

Encouraged by the possibilities of the method we turned our attention to another aspect of the problem about which some evidence has been gathered, namely the child and the concept of death.

The earliest references to the child and death are to be found in the writings of psychologists who recorded various aspects of the development of individual children, usually their own.[30, 38, 39, 47] These observations, common to the experience of most parents, indicated that almost all children at some time within the first six years of life become intensely interested in death and especially in its meaning for them personally.

In later studies dealing with children two basic approaches were taken. One traces the development of the death concept in light of the more general development of logical thought, as in the work of Piaget.[38] The other is more concerned with the antecedent causal conditions of emotional attitudes towards death, as in the work stemming from psychoanalytic theory. In either case controlled, quantitative data are almost nonexistent.

Anthony[4] studied parents' written accounts of children's spontaneous interest in death, the results of a story-completion test, and responses to the items on an intelligence test in which material relevant to death appeared. She found that death thoughts appear frequently in children's fantasies. Roughly half of the subjects introduced death into their story endings although this concept was not suggested in the story stems. As a result of her investigations, Anthony distinguished five stages in children's thoughts about death, ranging from ignorance of the meaning of the word to clear definition in logical or biologically essential terms. At age 3 no meaning is attached to the concept, by age 10 almost all children use a causal-logical explanation.

Nagy[35] studied written compositions, drawings, and recorded discussions of 3 to 10-year old children. Three stages of response were differentiated to the question "What is death?" In the youngest group, under 5 years, death is at first reversible, then later gradual and temporary. Between 5 and 9, death is most often personified. It is perceived as an aggressive act contingent upon the behavior of others.

Cousinet[13] noted that at first there is a refusal on the part of the child to accept the idea of death. This stage is followed by an attempt to substitute severe but curable illness for death. At a later age, death simply disappears as a troublesome concept. Cousinet holds that this last stage may precede an understanding of death in naturalistic terms.

While there seems to be reasonable agreement about the succession of stages in children's thinking about death, there is controversy when discussing their feeling states and the conditions from which these feelings derive.

Schilder and Wechsler[42] reported that normal children rarely show fear of death. They deal with the idea in a realistic manner. When fear occurs it is likely to be related to aggression and deprivation, states to which they unconsciously connect death.

Other writers have been concerned not so much with the frequency of death fears in a children's population as with its origin. Anthony[4] relates it to a fear of retaliation for one's own aggressive impulses. Harnik[23] offers the fear of suffocation resulting from early difficulties in breathing as a possible source. Chadwick[12] questions the orthodox psychoanalytic belief that castration anxiety is a root of the death fear. She believes that the converse relationship may be true and relates fear of death to such conditions as excessive physical restraint, masturbation guilt, fear of darkness, and especially to infantile separation anxiety. Others[10, 31, 34, 37] have invoked fear of pain, fear of the unknown, unpleasant experiences associated with death and burial, guilt and disappointment over unfulfilled potential, and influence of adults with morbid superstitions about death as explanatory concepts.

EXPERIMENT B

Our study was designed to provide information on the affective response to death in children and young adolescents.

We were concerned with the relationship of the development of the affective response to the information available on the development of logical thought. We were also concerned, as in our first experiment (A), with the apparent discrepancy in reports about affective involvement in children. On the one hand there are the statements of an indifferent attitude shown by children: matter-of-factness, reality orientation, and lack of fear.[42] At the same time there are reports of defensive denials, morbid concern, and undue stress in fantasy production.[4]

Word list: The method, except for a few essential modifications to suit the particular population studied, is the one that was used in the previous study. The word list was selected from a manual for the teaching of spelling published by New York City's Board of Education.[48] The word levels in the manual were based on word frequency counts of written English for elementary and high school children.

The 27-word experimental list contained three sets: affectives (words related to sex and family), basals, and death words. The sub-groups were equated for such relevant variables as length, frequency, etc. A sampling from each group follows. Basal: dress, brave, happy, star, deep, animal. Affective: mama, papa, child, love, married, kiss. Death: buried, kill, dead.

Rationale: The experimental rationale followed that of the earlier work. The comparison between basal and affective words was a check on the measuring technique. The critical comparison was between basal and death words. It is to be remembered that basal words were by no means chosen to be innocuous or words low in affect. They are samples from the language having the possibility of calling forth affect from individual subjects. Our concern was whether death words call forth an increased affective response.

Subjects and procedure: The subjects, 108 males, ages 5 to 16, were all summer campers in a Settlement House Camp. Almost all of the subjects were from low-income families; Negroes and whites were represented. None of the children were known to have psychiatric histories, nor was there any reason to believe that intelligence was distributed atypically in any age grouping. All subjects were volunteers selected in the following manner. A group of children living together in a group would be scheduled for testing during an activity period in a special room not used by the children for any other purpose. An introductory period was used to introduce the purpose of the experiment. The children were told that they were helping to determine whether a new recording machine was sensitive enough to record activities in the cells of the body. Comparisons with various measuring instruments, e.g. stethoscope, EKG, etc., were made in accord with the experience level of the group. Following this interval, a group demonstration of the procedure was provided with the counselor serving as subject. This opportunity generated great enthusiasm among the subjects as is evidenced by a 95 percent volunteer rate.

Each child was tested individually in essentially the same manner described in Experiment A. This time, however, change in basal resistance was measured as was time to respond. For more technical details of this particular procedure the reader is referred to a separate publication.[2]

Results: For the analysis we divided our subjects into three age groupings: 5 through 8 (N=29), 9 through 12 (N=48), and 13 through 16 (N=31). Our rationale was based on the natural divisions that seem to be evident in the development of logical thinking,[38] the results of the previously mentioned work of Anthony[4] and Nagy,[35] and the developmental stages as described in the theory of Harry Stack Sullivan.[46]

As a check on the validity of the technique for measuring affect in children the first comparison was made between basal and affective words. T tests for correlated measures were computed for both response indices and were found to be significant (P_{pgr} .01, P_{time} .05). The affective word category was then eliminated from further comparisons.

The analysis of variance technique was used to assess the contributions of the various component factors to our total result. A summary of the findings is presented in Table 3. Let us first discuss the PGR variable. It can be seen that the group as a whole responded differently to the two sets of words, basal and death. The F ratio for treatment is 4.1 which is significant beyond the .01 level of confidence. Age in itself is not a critical factor in the PGR to word stimuli, ($F_{\text{age groups}}=.54$). However the different age groups responded differently to the two sets of words. This aspect of the analysis we shall expand presently.

TABLE 3—*Analysis of variance of PGR and response time scores*[*]

Source	PGR N=88				Response time N=108			
	Sum of squares	df	Mean square	F	Sum of squares	df	Mean square	F
Treatments	.41	1	.41	4.1[†]	1.62	1	1.62	14.73[†]
Age groups	2.69	2	1.35	.54	20.48	2	10.24	15.28[†]
Treatments x age groups	1.74	2	.87	8.7[†]	.21	2	.11	1.00
Subjects	213.35	85	2.51		69.93	105	.67	
Treatments x subjects	8.85	85	.10		12.01	105	.11	

[†]p<.01

[*]The treatments x subject variance is used as the error term for treatments x age groups. The subjects variance is used as the error term for age groups. See Wilk and Kempthorne.[52]

The N's differ for the PGR and response time measures. In twenty cases PGR records were either not obtainable or not scorable. No one sub-group contained a preponderance of such subjects.

With regard to response time, the entire group responded differently to basal and death words. Age brought about a decrease in response time, and the different age groups responded in a relative fashion in much the same way despite the general decrease in response time. This last relationship may be seen more clearly from an examination of Table 4.

Table 4 presents the basal-death word comparisons for the three age groupings. What is indicated here is that there is a decrease in skin resistance to death words in the youngest (5-8) and oldest (13-16) groups. The middle group (9-12) responds similarly to both basal and death words. Response time, however,

TABLE 4—*t Values for word group comparisons by age groups
on both response measures**

Age group	PGR	Response time
5-8	1.65*	4.74†
9-12	.10	3.17†
13-16	3.47†	2.80†

*p<.05
†p<.01

*Personal communication from Josey of hitherto unpublished material.

remains significantly longer for death words for all three age groups.

DISCUSSION

In our early considerations we selected response time and the sweat gland activity of the palm as response indicators without any real attention to what particular aspects of the individual's functioning they may represent. Our only criterion was that they had been found to be reasonable indicators of affect even though the relationship of these measures to one another was not known to be strong. The results of this study led us to postulate that perhaps these measures tap different levels of functioning. Response times to death words remain consistently longer; perhaps this reflects the general cultural prejudice against dealing with the subject of death, no matter what one's own feelings may be. The PGR, on the other hand, is more likely to reflect the emotional response of the individual, the involvement of the autonomic nervous system. Were we to assume this hypothesis, our PGR results would fit very nicely with descriptive notions on the serenity and storm of the various stages of personal development. The early school years and the early adolescent years are both times of great change. New patterns have to be learned, new demands are made on the individual, and the picture of the self is more likely to be subjected to severe test. It is in these periods that death is responded to with increased affect as though one's response was a function of *ego stability*. The pre-adolescent years, on the other hand, have been portrayed as a time of relative calm, a settling down period when new skills are acquired, when friendship patterns are rather stable and satisfying, where little of the jockeying for position that is common to the immediately earlier and later stages takes place. At such a time the ego is relatively stable. It is immersed in the new-found joys of increasing ability to handle the problems of everyday living. It is this kind of situation, where the ego is in firm control, which seems to be necessary to keep affect about death to a minimum level.

Summary and new hypotheses: The considerations involved in these first two experiments have led to a series of speculations which shall provide the basis for further empirical work. Let us review these and introduce some further thoughts.

In the first instance we shall suppose that death becomes a realistic problem for children, at least in western culture, between the fourth and sixth year of life. This problem has tied to it a state of negative affect which motivates the child to seek a set of relieving conditions. These conditions can vary from a more intense identification with protective adult figures, both real and fictional, to denial, or repression, or masking of the death possibility. The resolution of any particular child will be in part a function of the degree of ego strength that is built up as a result of the kinds and qualities of early relationships. The more ego strength during these formative years, when death first becomes a conscious problem, the greater the probability that the individual will be able to keep out negative affect about death except in extreme circumstances.

In general then we shall suppose that death and its attendant negative affect will become more conscious the more difficulty the ego has in coping with the problems of life. We shall further suppose that this condition will hold for both the individual in times of internal or external stress, and for mankind in general.

Thus we could expect increased death anxiety in the so-called critical periods of life: puberty, entrance into adult economic culture, the climacteric, old age, as well as in the imposed conditions of war, famine and pestilence.

RESOLUTIONS OF DEATH ANXIETY

Two considerations led us into our third study. One was a recognition of the limited information that could be extracted from our method. Thus, in addition to the word association task we sought to apply other quantitative techniques to the problems. A second consideration was the wide individual differences observed in people's responses to death. Some subjects showed a great increase in affective response, others little or none. Perhaps these differences were due to the fact that we had only a single somatic representation of affect while people are known to have different somatic patterns for affective display, e.g. increased blood pressure, heart rate, etc.[32] Another possibility was that the apparently unmoved subjects had found successful ways of handling the concept of death, at least to the extent that they were not disturbed by having to respond with an immediate association to death words. This latter possibility provided the focus for our next investigation.

Religion and death anxiety: It has been an axiom of some psychological systems that man operates on a principle of order; that he is compelled to give meaning to the various aspects of the universe with which he comes in contact. Inability to order or give meaning to events especially critical to the well-being of the individual is likely to create an affective condition known as anxiety. The operation of this process has been clearly spelled out by Goldstein.[20] A simple way for man to handle recurrent anxiety-provoking problems is to seek a ready-made set of beliefs that reflect on the nature of his problems and provide in their logic a solution. One such category of beliefs especially concerned with man's mortal nature is religion. The promise of eternal life in a heavenly paradise as a reward for belief is a prominent feature of many of the world's religions. Death is not pictured as the end but rather as the beginning of a far more glorious existence.

With regard to religion and its relation to anxiety about death much has been written. Durant[14] writes of Schopenhauer who called fear of death both the beginning of philosophy and the cause of religion. G. Stanley Hall[22] declared that a salient feature of Christianity was that it served as a psychotherapy to alleviate the fear of death, converting this fear into a friendly hope. Gordon Allport[3] indicated that religious supplication results in answer to the demands brought about by the insecurity fostered by death. These are but a few of the many in philosophy and religion who have noted the role of religious belief in reducing death anxiety.

It was our intention to provide information on the effectiveness of a religious solution for this purpose. The attempt was made not with the idea of resolving so vast a question but rather to give a first approximation of an answer in limited and controlled circumstances and to point out some possible methods for gathering further evidence on this question.

EXPERIMENT C

This study was based on the assumption that one could select two populations, similar in all relevant respects save their contact with, belief in, and devotion to religion.

We sought, in the religious group, people with strong positive religious sentiments that resulted from a way of life established and maintained early in the home and family. In the non-religious group we wanted people whose contacts with religion were minimal as a result of both family patterns and present choice. Our concern was with people who were little influenced by formal religious training, not with those who had rejected some particular church doctrine.

Subject selection: The parent population was a group of 315 undergraduate males at Princeton University from which were culled 25 who met the "religious" criterion and another 25 who met the "non-religious" standards.

Initially all students were given the Josey Scale[26] of "religiosity," which consists of 59 items relating to positive religious attitudes, beliefs, and experiences. The subject rates the importance of each item to him on a five-point scale (0-4). The total score is a simple summation of the individual item scores. Reliability and validity data for the scale are reported and indicate that the scale is sensitive to such things as church attendance, church membership, and preparation for a professional career in the ministry. In addition, the subjects were asked to complete a prepared questionnaire which dealt with background material including the religious attitudes and practices of the subject and members of his family.

The scores on the Josey Scale were used as the first criterion for inclusion in the study. Subjects in the upper and lower quartiles of the distribution were selected as possibilities and processed further. The second stage of selection involved the examination of the background questionnaire material. To eliminate two possible sources of variation, not immediate to our central problem, the experimental sample was confined to Protestants and also to subjects who had not suffered the loss of a member of the immediate family. Further selection was based on church membership, church attendance, religious education, and family practices. When doubt arose as to the inclusion of any subject in either group, a personal interview was held at which time only matters pertaining to the subject's religious history were discussed. Eighty-one members of the original population met the selection criteria, and were put through the experimental battery. Final selection rested on an evaluation of religious attitudes and sentiments expressed in the free interview portion of the battery. This material, which was recorded, was assessed by three independent judges including a member of the clergy. Only those subjects on whom the judges unanimously agreed were included in the final groupings. In all, there remained 25 subjects in each of the two groups.

These final groups were then compared on a number of nonreligious background variables to assess their relative composition. Age, class in school, scholastic achievement, size of family, position in family, and family income level were all investigated.

In general the groups were quite similar except for income levels. The majority of the non-religious group indicated family incomes above $10,000, whereas the religious group fell mainly in the $5000-$10,000 bracket. This may represent real class differences or may be somewhat artificial since several of the fathers of the religious subjects were ministers, a high-prestige, low-paying occupation. Two further checks on the composition of the groups were made. The Rotter Incomplete Sentences Blank,[40] a neuroticism scale, showed a similar distribution of scores for the two groups. In addition, the Tucker Goals of Life Inventory,[51] which includes a "religious" dimension, served as an independent check on the adequacy of the entire selection procedure. The results of this test clearly differentiated our two groups on the religious dimension.

Procedure: For the experimental session each subject was scheduled separately. The general plan was to assess responses to death on several levels of awareness and to measure manifest anxiety as a function of serious discussion about death. The basic question under consideration was the efficacy of the religious solution in reducing death anxiety.

The procedure was as follows. The subject, after being told that the purpose of the experiment would be explained to him at the end of the session, was given a word-association task similar to the one described in the earlier experiments. Following this, Part 1 of the Cattell Manifest Anxiety Scale [11] was administered. The scale is reported to be sensitive to situational changes in manifest anxiety level.* Scores on this part of the scale were used as a base against which to measure the impact of the remainder of the experimental procedure.

Upon completion of the first half of the anxiety scale, the subject was introduced to the semantic differential technique devised by Osgood.[36] This technique purports to measure the connotative meaning of words. Here the word-association list items were rated on a large number of seven-point bi-polar adjective scales whose factorial characteristics are described by

---

* Various scales of the Cattell battery sensitive to manifest anxiety were selected after personal communication with Cattell and Scheier.

the terms "evaluative," "activity," and "potency." Thus each of the adjective scales has a loading for one of the three factors. By plotting the results of the subjects' judgments it is possible to get a picture of the "meaning" of the judged word in this factorial space.

Next, the subject was asked to complete a prepared question-naire on death similar to the one used by Schilder[8] and Middle-ton.[33] This was followed by an open-ended interview divided into three sections. The first dealt with the subject's notions about heaven and hell, the purpose of life, and the effects of his at-titude towards religion on his feelings about death. The second section dealt with early thoughts about death, the death of rela-tives and its effects on the family members, and the general attitudes taken by the parents toward death. The third section called out the subject's feelings about his own death, the death of loved ones, and some speculation about the time and circum-stances of his own death.

The final measure was the second part of the manifest anxiety scale. Although a variety of procedures was employed, the individual sessions were between one and one-half and two hours in length.

Hypotheses: Relative to the basic consideration of the role of religion in reducing death anxiety a number of hypotheses were generated.

1) Religious subjects when compared with non-religious sub-jects should show less disturbance in responding to death words on a word-association task.

2) Religious subjects should put death words in a semantic space of "good," "potent," and "active," and the values attached to these factors should be more extreme than for non-religious subjects.

3) Manifest anxiety as a function of discussion of one's own feelings and attitudes toward death should increase more for non-religious than for religious subjects.

Results: The results in general do not support the hypotheses, and in this limited test situation cast doubt upon the idea that a religious belief is more effective in reducing death anxiety than any other "solution." Let us take up our findings in turn.

Word association: On the word-association task given prior to the time that the subject was aware of the nature of the investigation, we find that each group shows an increased psychogalvanic response to death words, but that the groups do not differ from one another. Both religious and non-religious subjects respond alike in all respects on this task—on their responses to neutral words, as well as to death words. As in our earlier work, there is every indication that death is not an affect-free concept for normal, intelligent, moderately successful young people, and this appears to be true no matter what the strength of their religious convictions seems to be.

Semantic differential: With regard to the "meaning" of death words as seen in Osgood's semantic space, our hypothesis turned out to be an extremely complex one for which the evidence cannot clearly decide. Religious subjects order these words in a space that can be described as "bad," "potent," and "active." The discrepancy from our set of expectations lay in the finding that death words were placed on the negative side of the evaluative factor rather on the positive side as we had predicted. This may have been due to the particular words that we chose to represent the death concept, a possibility which shall be discussed in a later section.

The non-religious subjects place the death words in a space that is "bad," "potent," and "passive." Immediately a qualitative difference is seen with respect to the activity factor. Religious subjects see death as essentially "active," a finding in line with an after-life concept. Non-religious subjects reflect their belief in death as the end of things by placing death on the passive side of the activity factor.

To make more accurate comparisons of the one group with the other, it may be necessary to use the semantic differential space for neutral words for each group as the base line. We find that both groups put words in general on the "good" side of the evaluative factor, but the non-religious group see neutral words as less "good." Both groups also place words slightly above the mid-point on the potency factor toward the most potent end, but the non-religious group does this to a lesser extent.

On the activity factor both groups place neutral words above the mid-point toward the most active end of the scale, but again the non-religious subjects see words as less active than do the religious subjects.

All of the above differences between the two groups on the neutral words are reliable as assessed by a sign test. If we use the responses to neutral words as the base line, it appears that death is judged more toward the "bad" end of the evaluative factor by the religious than the non-religious group. In addition, the concept is even more "potent" for the non-religious than for the religious group, and the differences between the two groups on the activity factor are somewhat reduced, although the religious group continues to remain on the active side and the non-religious group on the passive side of the factor's mid-point.

To summarize these findings, in a three-dimensional semantic space the religious group describes death as bad, potent, and slightly active. The non-religious group sees it as bad (but less bad), potent (but more potent), and slightly passive. The magnitudes of these differences are not large although the trends are obvious. For a small sample such as ours these differences are not reliable. The only inference that one can draw from these responses is that the groups do not differ. Both religious and non-religious subjects perceive death in roughly the same semantic space.

Manifest anxiety: The evidence on our third hypothesis, regarding the change in manifest anxiety as a function of discussing death, runs counter to our prediction. In our sample, manifest anxiety increases reliably more for the religious than for the non-religious subjects after the prepared questionnaire and open-ended interview concerning death. Thus, it seems that our religious subjects are more disturbed by the concept of death than are their non-religious counterparts. An interesting finding, and one taken into consideration in the above analysis, is that the non-religious group showed greater manifest anxiety to begin with, that is, in the portion of the scale that was administered immediately following the word-association task. What this suggests is that death anxiety is much closer to consciousness in the non-religious subjects and may even be stimulated by an innocuous task containing death words, whereas one must go to more direct techniques to bring out these feelings in the religious group. An alternative hypothesis that this non-religious sample had in general more manifest anxiety is rejected on the basis of the similarity of the two groups in the word-association task using both response times and the PGR as criteria. In addition, some expression of a difference between the groups in manifest anxiety might have been expected to appear on the Rotter Incomplete Sentences Blank if an initial difference had existed. This, however, was not the case. The two groups were almost identical in both mean and median scores on the Rotter test.

Discussion: The most general conclusion called for by this set of findings is that death anxiety, as we measured it in this particular sample, is by no means dissipated by a religious approach to life. However, an examination of the words we used to represent the death concept in the word-association and semantic differential tasks may illuminate why our initial hypotheses were not substantiated and what role an after-life concept might play in attitudes and feelings towards death.

The critical stimulus words (coffin, funeral, corpse, death) all relate to the immediate conditions surrounding the cessation of life. These are words that are more likely to tap feelings about dying rather than what happens afterward. In such a case we find that there is an increase in affective response in both populations and the two groups see the actual departure from life as relatively bad and potent.

What then is the psychological role of a belief in an after-life? Basically it seems to be a defense in which the undesirable aspect (death as pain or departure) is allowed to remain in awareness but never made the focus of conscious thought. For our religious subjects, death is more likely to be a topic of conversation and indeed earlier memories about death may be more easily recalled. This material came to light in the free interview situation. However, the emphasis is always on the positive aspects of the concept: revelation, reward, peace, and contentment. It is as though, in the Lewinian sense, one has a positive-negative conflict where one must go through the negative zone in order to achieve the positive goal. One possible solution is a reorganization of the field where the negative becomes embedded in the positive, and this seems to characterize the religious group's attitude.

In the non-religious group the most likely defense is repression. One speaks less and thinks less about death. One cannot remember very early memories related to this topic. The forces of repression may be very easily overcome by any kind of reference to death, whereas one must speak directly of the act of dying and its consequences to involve the general affect of the religious group. However, when one's own death is the topic for discussion, more anxiety results in the religious than in the non-religious subjects.

It becomes more and more apparent from the increased volume of clinical reports that death is a problem that man does not find easy to handle. In some instances [24] the fear of death is a primary symptom of pathology, in others it is a concomitant of a more general inability to handle life's problems.[49] That it seems to be so prevalent in pathological conditions makes it quite likely that death anxiety is latent in all humans and simply manifests itself in a wide variety of ways. For some it can be the underlying, guiding theme of the life effort, as in the followers of an Epicurean philosophy, or in the explorer's search for the fountain of youth, or in the scientist's inquiry into the origin of life. For others, deeply repressed, it is only to be dealt with in times of crisis.

SUMMARY

In reporting this series of investigations a serious effort has been made to present death as a meaningful psychological problem. Standard psychological techniques have been indicated as feasible for use. In general, what we have found is that death is a concept to which normal subjects, varying from nursery school through college age, respond to with increased affect. Only in the so-called latency period, from 9 through 12 years, is this finding not upheld. Additionally we have tested, in a limited setting, the effectiveness of a religious way of life in reducing anxiety connected with death. There is no evidence in our data to suggest that the concept of death induces less affect in religious than in non-religious subjects. It is postulated that both groups have comparable negative feelings about the act or process of dying. Only the defense against these negative feelings differs. Religious subjects tend to escape to the satisfying concept of an after-life. Non-religious subjects are more likely to banish the topic from consciousness.

References

1. Alexander, I. E., Colley, R. S., and Adlerstein, A. M. Is death a matter of indifference? *J. Psychol.*, 1957, 43, 277-283.

2. Alexander, I. E. and Adlerstein, A. M. Affective responses to the concept of death in a population of children and early adolescents. *J. genet. Psychol.*, in press.

3. Allport, G. *The individual and his religion, a psychological interpretation.* New York: Macmillan, 1950.

4. Anthony, S. *The child's discovery of death.* New York: Harcourt, 1940.

5. Bitterman, M. E., Krauskopf, J., and Holtzman, W. H. The galvanic skin response following artificial reduction of the basal resistance. *J. comp. physiol. Psychol.*, 1954, 47, 230-234.

6. Blackham, H. J. *Six existentialist thinkers.* London: Routledge and Kegan Paul, 1952.

7. Bottome, P. *Alfred Adler, a biography.* New York: Putnam, 1939.

8. Bromberg, W. and Schilder, P. Death and dying. *Psychoanal. Rev.*, 1933, 20, 133-185.

9. Bromberg, W. and Schilder, P. The attitudes of psychoneurotics toward death. *Psychoanal. Rev.*, 1936, 23, 1-25.

10. Caprio, F. S. A study of some psychological reactions during pre-pubescence to the idea of death. *Psychiat. Quart.*, 1950, 24, 495-505.

11. Cattell, R. B. and Scheier, I. Personal communication.

12. Chadwick, M. Notes upon the fear of death. *Int. J. Psychoanal.*, 1929, 10, 321-334.

13. Cousinet, R. L'idee de la mort chez les enfants. *Psychol. Abstr.*, 1940, 14, 499.

14. Durant, W. *The story of philosophy*. New York: Pocket Library, 1954.

15. Eissler, K. R. *The psychiatrist and the dying patient*. New York: International Univ. Press, 1956.

16. Feifel, H. Some aspects of the meaning of suicide. In Shneidman, E. S. and Farberow, N. L. (Eds.), *Clues to suicide*. New York: McGraw-Hill, 1957.

17. Freud, S. Thoughts for the times on war and death. In *The complete psychological works of Sigmund Freud*. Vol. XIV. London: Hogarth Press, 1957.

18. Freud, S. *Beyond the pleasure principle*. London: Hogarth Press, 1950.

19. Fromm, E. *Man for himself*. New York: Rinehart, 1947.

20. Goldstein, K. *The organism*. New York: American Book Co., 1939.

21. Hall, G. S. A study of fears. *Amer. J. Psychol.*, 1896, 8, 147-249.

22. Hall, G. S. Thanatophobia and immortality. *Amer. J. Psychol.*, 1915, 26, 550-613.

23. Harnik, J. One component of the fear of death in early infancy. *Int. J. Psychoanal.*, 1930, 11, 485-491.

24. Hoffman, F. H. and Brody, M. W. The symptom, fear of death. *Psychoanal. Rev.*,1957, 44, 433-438.

25. Jones, E. *The life and work of Sigmund Freud*. New York: Basic Books, 1953-57.

26. Josey, C. C. A scale of religious development. *Amer. Psychol.*, 1950, 5, 281. (Abstract)

27. Jung, C. G. *Studies in word association*. London: Heinemann, 1918.

28. Jung, C. G. *The integration of the personality*. New York: Farrar and Rhinehart, 1939.

29. Jung, C. G. *Two essays on analytical psychology*. New York: Pantheon Books, 1953.

30. Katz, D. *Gespräche mit Kindern*. Berlin: Springer, 1928.

31. Kotsovsky, D. Die Psychologie der Todesfurcht. *Psychol. Abstr.*, 1939, 13, 134.

32. Lacey, J. I. The evaluation of autonomic responses: toward a general solution. *Ann. N. Y. Acad. Sci.*, 1956, 67, 123-164.

33. Middleton, W. C. Some reactions towards death among college students. *J. abnorm. soc. Psychol.*, 1936, 31, 165-173.

34. Moellenhoff, F. Ideas of children about death. *Bull. Menninger Clinic*, 1939, 3, 148-156.

35. Nagy, M. The child's theories concerning death. *J. genet. Psychol.*, 1948, 73, 3-27.

36. Osgood, C. E., Suci, G. J., and Tannenbaum, P. H. *The measurement of meaning.* Urbana: Univ. of Illinois Press, 1957.

37. Osipov, N. W. Strach ze smrti. *Psychol. Abstr.*, 1935, 9, 534.

38. Piaget, J. *The language and thought of the child.* London: Routledge, 1952.

39. Rasmussen, V. *Child psychology.* Vol. II. New York: Knopf, 1922.

40. Rotter, J. B. and Willerman, B. The incomplete sentences test as method of studying personality. *J. consult. Psychol.*, 1947, 11, 43-48.

41. Schilder, P. The attitudes of murderers towards death. *J. abnorm. soc. Psychol.*, 1936, 31, 348-363.

42. Schilder, P. and Wechsler, D. The attitudes of children towards death. *J. genet. Psychol.*, 1934, 45, 406-451.

43. Scott, C. A. Old age and death. *Amer. J. Psychol.*, 1896, 8, 67-122.

44. Stacey, C. L. and Marken, K. The attitudes of college students and penitentiary inmates toward death and a future life. *Psychiat. Quart.* (suppl.), 1952, 26, 27-32.

45. Stacey, C. L. and Reichen, M. L. Attitudes toward death and future life among normal and subnormal adolescent girls. *Except. Child.*, 1954, 20, 259-262.

46. Sullivan, H. S. *The interpersonal theory of psychiatry.* New York: Norton, 1953.

47. Sully, J. *Studies of childhood.* New York: Appleton, 1914.

48. *Teaching Spelling: Course of study and manual.* Board of Education for the City of New York, Curriculum Bull., 1953-54 series, No. 6.

49. Teicher, J. D. "Combat fatigue" or death anxiety neurosis. *J. nerv. ment. Dis.*, 1953, 117, 234-243.

50. Thorndike, E. C. and Lorge, I. *Teacher's word book of 30,000 words.* New York: Teacher's Coll., Columbia Univ., 1944.

51. Tucker, L. R. Factor analysis of double centered score matrices. *Educational Testing Service Research Memorandum*, R.M. 56-3, 1956.

52. Wilk, M. B. and Kempthorne, O. Fixed, mixed, and random models. *J. Amer. Statist. Ass.*, 1955, 50, 1144-1166.

53. Wittels, F. *Sigmund Freud: His personality, his teaching and his school.* New York: Dodd, Mead, 1924.

54. Zilboorg, G. Fear of death. *Psychoanal. Quart.*, 1943, 12, 465-475.

Noël Mailloux

and

Leonardo Ancona

IV

A Clinical Study of Religious Attitudes and a New Approach to Psychopathology

INTRODUCTION

ON THE BASIS of broad clinical observations, a general reformulation of present-day theory of neuroses might well be considered. Of course, this does not mean that the now widely accepted· dynamic interpretation is not valid. Beyond the merely descriptive classification of symptoms, it represents an extremely penetrating attempt at rendering the best defined syndromes more intelligible, articulate, and explanatory. A meaningful interpretation was gradually substituted for a purely factual nomenclature. One cannot help noticing, however, that we are still confronted only with generic frames of reference.

We have long been accustomed to think that it is almost immaterial whether the content of a phobic or obsessive system appears to be of a sexual, social, or religious nature. What is regarded as most essential is the particular manifestation of the neurotic disturbance with which we are dealing, not the specific conflict provoking its appearance. On the other hand, it may be more justified to assume that if a given conflict, e.g. of a sexual nature, is liable to produce either a phobic, obsessive, or delusional condition, this might well be due to the influence of some more or less casual factors, developmental, dynamic, or economic, which determined the adoption of this particular pattern of expression.

Such an assumption implies that the conflict itself constitutes the real core of a neurotic disturbance, and that its specific content should be carefully studied independently of, but in connection with, the pathological manifestations through which it is expressed. This kind of approach was suggested by our repeated observation and study of specifically religious problems. First then, on the basis of a broader concept of the object love relationship, we shall attempt to redefine the hypothetical areas of neurotic conflicts. Second, we will present a still sketchy clinical picture of what we consider the most basic moral and/or religious conflicts. This is intended to illustrate the need for a more careful investigation of the particular content and structure of inner conflicts, as well as to stress the implications and importance of such content and structure for the general theory of neurosis.

A BROADER CONCEPT OF THE OBJECT LOVE RELATIONSHIP

The theologian has always set himself the complicated task of defining explicitly the basic norms which are supposed to regulate human conduct. In the process of trying to accomplish this task effectively, he came to examine the sources whence human conduct derives its main dynamic orientations. Although having to rely merely on his own psychological acumen, he was nevertheless able to attain insights the comprehensiveness, preciseness, and depth of which deserve the admiration of the modern clinician. Only the theologian ventured, in the one gaze, to extend his horizon wide enough to embrace all four of those spontaneous inclinations whose specific and composite impact on an adequate interpretation of human behavior is just beginning to be suspected by empirical science, namely: existentiality,* sexuality, sociability, and religiosity. Whenever he at-

---

* The authors are purposely choosing this term in preference to the much more familiar one of *self-preservation*. The latter, indeed, has some rather static, negative, or defensive connotations, which tend to obscure the more basic propensity toward self-realization or progressive expression of one's vital potentialities, even through the other above-mentioned inclinations.

tempted to describe the structure, the development, the functioning, and the dynamic interplay of what might be called the *moral apparatus,* the theologian considered all of the fundamental object relations as they emerge from these natural inclinations and are regulated by a whole array of connected virtues.

Thus far, the psychologist has unfortunately shown persistent reluctance to envisage the complete realm of object relations. Voluntarily restricted clinical observation has enabled him to clarify how, from autoerotism, there slowly arises, via narcissism (and thus in relation to the self), the capacity to establish individual object relations.[3] Then, another decisive step was taken when the fact was borne out by clinical evidence and clearly stated[11] that sexual object love does not reach the stage of normal maturity as long as it is not primarily imbued with the desire for parenthood. Here, let us try to dispel a rather common and harmful confusion of notions. The organization of human sexuality is not completed when the primary of genitality is established, i.e. when the infantile sensual impulses more or less subside and become subordinate to genitality. There is still far to go before biological maturation has taken place and genitality can be *effectively* exercised. As the *basic* spontaneous capacity for establishing object love relationships becomes more differentiated, it concomitantly leads to the integration of genitality into an increasingly conscious sexual love relationship, which is normally characterized by the primacy of the parental attitude. For obvious reasons, not extraneous to wide spread biased conceptions of marriage, such an evolutive process was constantly disregarded, in spite of cumulative findings deriving from psycho-pathological research.[2, 9, 10] Too many scientists, as well as moral thinkers who should have known better, continued to assert that mature sexuality coincides with the ability to perform satisfactory intercourse with a person of the other sex and that, both from theoretical and practical viewpoints, the desire for parenthood should be considered merely as one of its incidental or arbitrary components.

Still, the fact that one has stepped beyond the bounds of narcissistic identification and is able to manifest genuine object love, or even display a mature parental attitude, does not imply that he has become *socialized* in the full meaning of this term. An irreducible distance separates the relatively simple process of altruistic love from a nascent social attitude through which one begins to perceive himself as a responsible member of a structured group and to think in terms of its common good. While dedicating himself to his family, man soon realizes that he is expressing an inclination which, although it derives from the original desire to perpetuate his own existence, has much broader implications. Similarly, the more diversified aspirations which develop in the enlarging circle of the family inevitably lead to the pursuit of ideals and goals, utilitarian or cultural, which are realizable only within the context of a larger, more highly organized society. Thus, to secure for himself, as well as for the ones he has begotten, the totality of the human good, appears to be a sufficiently strong motivation to make a man look beyond the immediate horizons of the home, and develop a specifically new interest in the community as a whole. Psychopathology now tries to elucidate the most crucial conflicts encountered in this late phase of human development, just as it has elucidated the conflicts comprising a failure of the reality principle, which interferes with the assertion of existentiality, and the conflicts which involve an inability to maintain an adequate object love relationship, which leads to sexual deviations. Following in its steps, social psychology has recently engaged in a fresh and rather energetic attempt to cope with this tremendously complicated problem. After much rambling, it has supplied, at least on an operational level, some articulated frames of reference which appear to be increasingly useful for a phenomenological description of group dynamics. Much information has been gained about the developmental aspects of mature group functioning, as well as about the various conditions which favor, or interfere with, the appearance of genuine reciprocity, of autonomous solidarity, and of harmonious productiveness among its members.

However, in spite of the results accruing from these recent investigations, modern psychology is still unable to point out what makes an individual capable of integrating himself into society and of playing therein a responsible and creative role. Similarly, no satisfactory dynamic interpretation can be offered of typical social deviations, even as serious as repetitive delinquency, when they are not embodied in one of the gross so-called neurotic or psychotic syndromes. No wonder, then, that the empirical scientist, when confronted with the highest expressions as well as with the superstitious or pathological distortions of religiosity, often becomes either entangled to the point of utter confusion or else ends in naïve simplifications. To make things worse, in the first systematic observations derived from psychopathology where religious phenomena—often closely knit with neurotic formations—assume such queer patterns, Freud [5] himself recognized that many individuals affected by mental illness tended to develop a private religion of their own. But, instead of concluding, on such a narrow clinical basis (as he unfortunately did), that universal religion is just another illusory manifestation of these same symptomatic distortions, many contemporary psychologists have begun to tackle the problem from the opposite angle. To them clinical data merely supply an illustration of the fact that, as a spontaneous human inclination, religiosity is subject to conflictual tensions, regressions, and deviations, just like sociability, sexuality, and existentiality.

With his shrewd insight Freud was not slow in realizing the intensity of man's quest for happiness. But, having misconstrued the real nature of the latter, whose definition falls beyond the realm of empirical science, he was unable to see in it the highest and most comprehensive expression of human love, the search of God, as an infinite good, which ultimately regulates and transcends our self-love as well as our increasingly expansive object love. After having encompassed our quest for happiness in the narrow formulation of the *pleasure principle*, he was soon compelled to recognize in it a constant threat to existentiality and was led with painfully faltering awareness to assert the primacy of the death instinct, of *Thanatos* over *Eros*.[4, 6]

Admittedly, in cases where magical thinking continues to prevail over rational thinking, the infantile feeling of omnipotence often gives rise to an illusory desire to play God. But it is surprising that such a feeling was not understood earlier as an undifferentiated assertion of the human will's capacity for autonomous determination. Similarly, it is quite true that the traumatic discovery of one's extreme dependence and helplessness may crystallize in the ego-dissolving experience, nowadays described as an "oceanic" feeling and characterized by inhibition of will power or by passivity. Under normal circumstances, however, the increasing awareness of one's limitations only leads to the recognition of his contingent condition as a creature. Involving a new all-embracing object love relationship, dependence on God is not perceived as impotence. Lived as a universal dynamic attraction, it channelizes towards its transcendent object all the above-described inclinations. Also, it gives to human free will its initial impulse, which, according to Boutonier,[1] will permit it to surmount the anxiety arising from its original indeterminacy as well as the rigidity imposed by the ego's mechanisms of defense, and to display in its mature functioning all the initiative and decisiveness deriving from serene hope.

HYPOTHETICAL AREAS OF NEUROTIC CONFLICTS

In the light of this more comprehensive dynamic construct, emerging from evidence gathered in the borderline territory of psychopathology, the methodological reductionism implied in the pansexual interpretation, or for that matter, in any other unilateral interpretation, will have to be discarded. Neurotic conflicts are prone to occur within the scope of any of the typical realms of object relations outlined above. In the realm of sociability and religiosity, especially, a whole array of peculiar reactions will have to be closely examined, which are ordinarily disregarded because they fall outside the categories of the familiar pathological syndromes. As is well known, the objective study of sexual disturbances met with considerable resistance. Similarly, many feel strongly reluctant to question the normality of the often upsetting behavior displayed by certain social leaders or of the pseudoreligious, antireligious, and/or irreligious attitudes and practices adopted by some fanatic individuals. An initial attempt in that direction was made by one of us,[7] who, after a systematic analysis of interview material supplied by a group of twelve cases, arrived at the conclusion that moral scrupulosity should be considered as a symptom *sui generis*, i.e. as a manifestation of the malfunctioning of religious conscience as such.

From this study it appears that the various phenomena, which, according to the theologians, constitute the broad spectrum of moral scrupulosity, cannot be considered as mere manifestations of an obsessional condition. The interpretation suggesting that we are simply dealing with obsessive systems having a moral or religious content is inadequate. In a certain number of cases an obsessive-compulsive functioning is apparent; in an equal proportion of others there is a clearly phobic, depressive, or paranoid picture. To offer a satisfactory explanation of this concrete fact, three working hypotheses might well be proposed and tested. First, it is possible that at least some moral and religious disturbances merely reflect the pattern of severe primary neurotic and even psychotic disorders, rooted in some other sphere. Second, it may well happen that such neurotic or psychotic conditions are occasional concomitants of moral and religious deviations and rapidly become closely interwoven with them, although we continue to be dealing with two basically distinct syndromes. Third, it is also plausible that neurotic conflicts, in whatever sphere of psychic life they happen to occur, always express themselves through a limited number of pathological reactions which tend to present the same typical patterns, some already familiar and others still to be defined.

The fact that a review of the material supplied by the twelve cases mentioned above has led to the formulation of these hypotheses indicates that we were confronted with intricate pathological constellations, which could not be restricted to the narrow scope of the usual interpretations. In severely disturbed cases, such as those ordinarily coming under clinical observation, the typical abnormalities resulting from basically moral and religious conflicts are almost inevitably blurred by gross neurotic structures deriving from more familiar sources. We could soon discern a variety of trends, similar to what has been observed in recent studies of delinquency. At one time, if one could see any relationship between criminal behavior and some diagnosed neurotic condition, one felt that it was sufficient to carry out some adequate treatment of the latter to ameliorate social attitudes and prevent further offenses. Although this may be true in the case of a limited number of individuals, nowadays our conceptions of this relationship have changed considerably, and we know that the type of abnormality which is at the source of antisocial behavior may appear or persist independently of the classical neuroses and requires a different kind of treatment.

A CLINICAL STUDY OF MORAL AND RELIGIOUS CONFLICTS

An initial attempt has been made to determine whether some parallel picture could be found in the field of morality and religion. Eight other cases were carefully selected on the basis that their complaints referred exclusively to moral or religious difficulties which could not be overcome through ordinary means and seemed to be rooted in some unconscious conflict. These individuals, four males and four females, were young adults from 23 to 40 years of age. Besides coming from excellent Catholic families and having received adequate religious training, most of them had pursued their general education up to the professional level, had been markedly efficient, and were highly regarded in their immediate environment. Four were married and already had two or more children, two were contemplating marriage in the not too remote future, and two had performed religious vows. Without exception they had been practicing their religion conscientiously and were striving constantly to live up to their high moral standards.

The following complaints were verbalized: "In spite of all my good will, I cannot bring myself to pray as I used to." "Sometimes, I wonder whether my faith is waning, because I feel dreadfully indifferent." "Whenever I attempt to listen to a sermon, to enter the confessional, or to go to the altar rail, I am overwhelmed by a sudden fear and I feel like running away." "I know that I should dedicate myself completely to some ideals and goals that I have deliberately chosen, but I feel desperately hampered from doing so by insuperable inhibitions." Since many would be readily inclined to see in all this nothing more than the expected manifestations of the vicissitudes inevitably encountered in one's spiritual development, it is necessary to recall that such an expert master as Saint John of the Cross[8] long ago recognized that such disturbing reactions may be symptomatic of a morbid subjective condition, like "melancholia." Insofar as the cases here studied are concerned, there were obvious signs of latent pathological conflicts, although the neurotic patterns emerging therefrom, usually involving unsuspected variables and unexplainable reactions, never appeared as clear-cut as the ones with which we have become familiar.

THEORETICAL FORMULATIONS

At this stage any attempt to grasp the precise nature and content of religious conflicts or to circumscribe the typical symptomatic constellations emanating from them would evidently be premature. However, from the wealth of data which have already been collected, it seems possible to propose a tentative formulation of the characteristic attitudes which precipitate the emergence of moral and religious conflicts.

In the first place, an acute anxiety is apparent which blurs the ultimate meaning of human existence and of all activities, often even of those chosen and engaged in with unquestionable poise and eagerness in the past. All the subjects express the disquieting feeling of having lost their general orientation in the world of spiritual values. They can no longer see why they should maintain any particular interest or why they should try to achieve anything at all. For them ideals and goals, which formerly seemed to inspire their decisions and mold their personality, are now completely devoid of their once powerful attractiveness. A paralyzing uncertainty obscurely pervades their conscience, threatening to undermine their secure faith and their admired virtues. They do not change their philosophy or way of life, because of the painful feeling of being incapable of taking any decision. In such inertia, a decisive factor is a latent or conscious fear of death, the mere idea of death being loaded with the whole morbid uncertainty with which they face the problem of human destiny.

Under the impact of such deep-seated anxiety, mature theological thinking is soon abandoned. As in any other type of neurosis, the path of regression is readily followed, leading to prelogical, concrete, symbolic, and magic thinking. In the field of religiosity, this predominance of phantasy obviously means that superstitious ideas will begin to play a determining role in the genesis and evolution of emerging conflicts. Concomitantly, an emotional regression also takes place, explaining the revival of the same narcissistic motives which dominate the specific picture of the various pathological conflicts, namely: fear, shame, guilt, and disgust. As an initial step in this investigation, which aims at formulating an adequate dynamic interpretation of religious conflicts, we will be satisfied with a brief description of ensuing neurotic attitudes, more amenable to clinical observation.

It is clear enough that, in certain individuals, religiosity is totally pervaded by an overwhelming *fear*, which finally crystallizes into full-blown phobic conditions. Such individuals look at religion as at some mysterious world, inspiring the inhibiting awe of the unknown. To them venturing into this spiritual world involves the same risks as venturing into some unexplored territory, and they prefer to remain in or withdraw to the familiar world of matter where they can rely on experience or, perhaps, on science to achieve predictable control, satisfaction, security, and even omnipotence. They feel a strong reluctance to enter a church, to attend a religious service, to receive the sacraments, to listen to religious instructions, or to talk to a priest. Whenever they are exposed to these situations, they feel just as much fear as does an agoraphobic who finds himself in the middle of the street or in the midst of a crowd.

For the obsessive compulsive perfectionist, on the other hand, religion consists mainly in a set of formalistic practices and rituals which have to be performed with punctilious precision. He soon discovers in it a powerful means to satisfy his narcissistic cravings for admiration and praise. Perhaps, while kneeling in the first pew, he will phantasy himself as a model of sanctity in the eyes of the crowd. Unfortunately, imagining oneself as perfect is of little help towards actually becoming perfect. When such individuals come to realize that, through casual distractions, they may indulge in ridiculous performances, or that, under the spell of temptation, they are unable to control their impulses, they are irremediably submerged by *shame* to the point of feeling doomed to annihilation. Henceforth, they will tend to abandon the generalized practices, through which normal mature believers express their religious devotion towards God, and to fall back on puerile, more or less superstitious, private rituals. For a time, they will find some compensatory narcissistic gratification in trying to fulfill them with exacting punctiliousness. But, as this proves also impossible, they will find themselves under the necessity of restricting their religious life to the performance of some few trivial and void gestures, if not of dropping it entirely.

Although much has been said concerning the depressed self-accuser who proclaims his irremissible *guilt,* his case would need a thorough reconsideration from our viewpoint. While he is displaying his despair, he is obstinately denying the reversibility of human free will and expressing the feeling that there are no alternate ways of fulfilling one's religious and moral duty in the service of God. He insists that he has missed his unique spiritual vocation and has engaged himself in an impasse which permits of no substitutions. All his other crimes are the inevitable consequence of this initial sin and are considered as its justified punishment. Strangely enough, while such individuals deny the possibility of changing their mind and of making a fresh decision about the present course of their spiritual life, they would like to straighten out some unique events of their life cycle which obviously cannot be repeated. They claim that they should be married or ordained anew, or that their whole spiritual life has been ruined from the time of their first communion or first confession. Some will go as far as saying that the only way of being saved would consist of being born anew and starting their life all over again, which, they desperately admit, is impossible.

For the theologian, who recalls the universal orientation implied in the first moral decision of a human conscience and the tremendous influence it may have on future more particular decisions, this striking lack of integration will appear as especially significant.

Finally, there is a category of mildly paranoid individuals, the study of whom may contribute much to our understanding of the early phase of religious development. The subjects who happened to come under observation were of extremely high intellectual ability and, in spite of their very serious religious disturbance, their Rorschach protocols appeared remarkably good. It took a long time to recognize that they were cautiously hiding a deep and tenacious mistrust, even towards those for whom they displayed great respect and admiration, behind a show of *disgust*. Either with humor or with open violence, they expressed their chronic contemptuous displeasure with everything religious: the church, the priest, the sermons, the religious attitudes and practices of others, etc., only to end up by admitting that they were mainly disgusted with themselves. After years of almost angelic impeccability, they had the impression of lapsing into a state of alarmingly cold indifference or of being filled with rebellious ideas and impulses. Going to confession, attending Mass and receiving Holy Communion, to say nothing of prayer in general, appeared increasingly difficult to them, if not indeed altogether impossible. At some early period of their development, all of them had strongly identified with some intensely hated person whom they felt somehow compelled to regard as a model of sanctity. They also kept the vivid impression that this could be achieved at the terrific cost of sacrificing all manifestations of an innocent, although vigorous, vitality. As time went on, they slowly discovered that the idealized person was far from being disinterested or was even trying to get away with violations of standards strictly imposed on others, and then they could not help feeling terribly deceived and cheated. Since, through the process of identification, this person has been incorporated in their ego and superego, these individuals often remain faithful to their ideals, although they do so with a felt lack of conviction. Little wonder then that they feel as disgusted with themselves as with the one who has ruined their whole spiritual life, and that they meet with almost insurmountable difficulties whenever they try to establish a loving and confident relationship with God. To them God appears to be nothing but an unreliable, arbitrary, and cruel tyrant, or as one put it in the following bitter sentence, "I don't dare to pray to Him, because, each time I do so, I am sure that something terrible is going to happen to me."

SUMMARY

On reaching the end of this chapter, the reader will be aware of its limitations. It carries one step further the study of moral scrupulosity, which constituted the subject matter of an earlier report,[7] in that it suggests the possibility of reconsidering the problem of religious pathology in the light of some fresh hypotheses. The theoretical considerations that have been formulated, supplemented, and made explicit by the clinical data that we have been able to assemble, may provide a useful basis for a dynamic interpretation of religious conflicts and a genetic explanation of religious attitudes.

References

1. Boutonier, Juliette. *L'angoisse*. Paris: Presses Univ., 1945.

2. Deutsch, Helene. *The psychology of women; a psychoanalytic interpretation*. Vol. II: Motherhood. New York: Grune & Stratton, 1945.

3. Fenichel, O. *Collected papers*. New York: Norton, 1953.

4. Freud, S. *Civilization and its discontents*. London: Hogarth, 1946.

5. Freud, S. Obsessive acts and religious practices. In *Collected papers*. Vol. II. London: Hogarth, 1948.

6. Freud, S. Beyond the pleasure principle. *Complete psychological works*. Vol. XVIII. London: Hogarth, 1955.

7. Mailloux, N. The problem of scrupulosity in pastoral work. In *Proceedings* of the Institute for the Clergy on Problems in Pastoral Psychology. New York: Fordham Univ., 1955.

8. Saint Jean de la Croix. *Oeuvres sprituelles*. Paris: Seuil, 1947.

9. Zilboorg, G. The dynamics of schizophrenic reactions related to pregnancy and childbirth. *Amer. J. Psychiat.*, 1929, 8, 733-766.

10. Zilboorg, G. Depressive reactions related to parenthood. *Amer. J. Psychiat.*, 1931, 10, 927-962.

11. Zilboorg, G. *Mind, medicine and man.* New York: Harcourt, 1943.

Gerald S. Blum

V

Psychoanalytic
Behavior Theory:
A Conceptual
Framework for Research*

INTRODUCTION

"BEHAVIOR THEORY," a currently popular phrase in psychological parlance, is almost as loose in connotation as it is elusive in realization. Approaches grouped under this heading vary greatly in scope and focus. They differ in the nature and number of behavioral domains pursued, in level and comprehensiveness of explanation sought, and in methods of investigation. Emphasis may be given to learning, motivation, perception, cognition, or action. Individual differences and personality variables are central to some; in others they receive little or no attention. Even the range of potential experimental subjects, traditionally including man and lower animals, has been extended in general systems theory all the way from viruses to galaxies.

It is appropriate therefore to preface any formulation by pointing out its broad guidelines. Stated in the most general terms, our approach seeks to integrate within a systematic framework certain aspects of academic psychology and psychoanalysis.

* This manuscript is a product chiefly of the joint efforts of a research team composed, in addition to the writer, of Justin Weiss, Research Associate; and Robert Goldstein, Abram Minkowich, and Sidney Perloe, Research Assistants. Other members of the project staff who have contributed materially are Esther Helfman, Mary Lee Pierce, Helen Sherman, and Ann Vroom. Financial support has been provided by grants from the National Institute of Mental Health (USPHS M-1286) and the Ford Foundation Mental Health Program.

We have set our sights on the understanding and prediction of human behavior, studied at the individual psychological level, with special concentration on dimensions of personality as they relate to behavior in a variety of domains. For a particular domain we aim to specify in detail the conditions bearing on the complex processes which occur between original stimulus and final response. Put in the jargon of electronic computers, our hope is to "write the program" by which human beings process information from input to output.

The major stages in a stimulus-response sequence, with corresponding requirements deemed essential by us for eventual success in predicting behavior, are presented in Table 1. In the First Stage it is important to know the sensory qualities

TABLE 1—*Stages in the behavioral sequence and accompanying requirements for prediction*

Stages	Requirements
1. Input (stimulus)	Properties of stimulus must be known
2. Activation of memory traces	Stimulus-relevant memory traces must be mapped as fully as possible
3. Processing of ideas	Processing principles must be developed and spelled out in detail
4. Output (behavioral response)	Behavior for which prediction is desired must be clearly specifiable and relatable to the stimulus input

(e.g. intensity) of a stimulus and also those properties (e.g. message content) which are involved in its comparison with previous stimuli. The requirement accompanying Stage 2 is more stringent than what other theories usually require. We feel that it is not sufficient to state in a general way that past experiences relevant to a particular stimulus are likely to be mobilized, or that a "strong hypothesis" must have been present, and let the matter drop at that point. We can be much farther ahead if we attempt in advance to assess, with the maximum inferential precision possible, the cognitive, affective, and motoric characteristics of all those registered experiences in memory which can be expected to share some kind of similarity with the new input. Underlying Stage 3 is the conviction that success can be achieved only if efforts are directed toward the explicit formulation of principles governing the unobservable processing of ideas within the psychic system. The fourth requirement stresses the seemingly obvious but often neglected caution that the behavior for which prediction is sought must have been instigated by the stimulus input. If one is unable to pin down the conditions which initiate a particular sequence culminating in the behavioral output under study, it is not likely that the intermediate links will be discovered.

Program research in behavior theory typically follows certain strategies. At times these strategies may be carefully planned prior to any collection of data. More often they exist in vague, implicit form and do not take shape until a later phase, and in some cases may continue in effect without attention ever being focused on them. Our own program, which for the past ten years has dealt with the operation of psychosexual conflicts and defense preferences in various behavioral settings, has now reached the point where we feel ready to formalize a long-range perspective to guide future lines of research.

The steps in our strategy for developing a behavior theory can be outlined as follows:

I. A comprehensive working model is constructed from general background material drawn from academic psychology, psychoanalysis, and to some extent physiology.
   A. Such a framework, although tentative, points systematically to problem areas where research is needed.
   B. The working model later provides a structure within which to incorporate principles suggested by research findings.

II. A miniature behavioral system with known inputs and outputs is analyzed.
   A. Selection is made of a diversified sample of domains of behavior (e.g. memory, perception, reasoning) where the behavioral output can be clearly related to the stimulus input.

    B. Operational measures are developed to tap each domain.

    C. With precise knowledge of inputs and outputs (Stages 1 and 4, respectively, in Table 1), it is then possible to attack Stages 2 and 3.

        1. Stage 2, the mapping of stimulus-relevant memory traces, involves the best estimation of memory traces existing prior to experimental stimulus inputs plus recording of new traces formed after presentation of experimental stimulus inputs.

        2. Stage 3, the derivation of principles according to which activated memory traces are processed, constitutes the crux of the problem. These principles are to be inferred by filling in the gaps which follow Stages 1 and 2 and precede Stage 4, all of which are now known.

    D. The working model is next revised to fit the principles inferred in Stage 3.

III. The revised model is applied to the prediction of Stage 4 within the miniature behavioral system.

    A. Knowledge of Stages 1, 2, and 3 is utilized to predict output.

    B. These predictions are then checked against the actual recorded output.

    C. Further revision and refinement of the model is made as necessary.

IV. The model is finally tested for its ability to predict a wide range of behaviors outside the miniature system.

    A. Extensions are made to a variety of stimuli other than those already employed.

    B. Extensions are made to domains other than those already sampled.

A WORKING MODEL

We have said that the first step in our strategy requires the formulation of a comprehensive working model capable of encompassing concepts of academic psychology and psychoanalysis. The fact that no such framework is readily available can be attributed at least in part to the minimal past interaction of the two disciplines. Freud himself never did put together a complete theory, a failure which he felt very keenly according to Jones.[6] At various phases of his career he tried to develop theoretical models, beginning with a neurophysiological one, discarding it in favor of a reflex arc interpretation of the mental apparatus involving the structural systems of Ucs, Pcs, and Cs, and finally switching to the so-called "hydraulic" model based on division of the personality into Id, Ego, and Superego.* Within academic psychology, an effort to link the two disciplines was made by Dollard and Miller[4] who sought to translate some Freudian concepts into Hull's system, but by and large psychologists have tended to ignore or reject psychoanalysis in their own theorizing.

The influences of the *Zeitgeist* on a particular endeavor are generally mysterious and difficult to unravel. The precipitating circumstances surrounding the origin of the present model, though, can be clearly traced to late December, 1955, at which time the writer asked his brother-in-law† if a section of Freud's paper "A Note Upon the 'Mystic-Writing Pad' "[5] was not reminiscent of electronic principles. The ease with which the latter subsequently diagrammed the description of perceptual and memory processes led the two of us to embark on the task of developing a complete behavior theory analogue, consisting of block diagrams as used for electronic devices. After many hours of collaborative effort, this first formulation was exposed to the light of day—more precisely to the critical appraisal of other psychologists. The light proved to be strong enough to fade much of the dittoed sketch in which it appeared and over a two-year period a series of major revisions has taken place.

A few introductory comments about the current version are probably in order. First, it must be recognized that it is not a formal model which attempts to analogize from an intricate set of electronic principles to behavior. We have no interest in details of electronic construction nor do we dream of someday

---

* See Colby[3] for an excellent discussion of the evolution of Freud's theoretical models. Colby's own scheme, which came to the writer's attention shortly after completion of the first version of the one to be presented in this chapter, is described as a "cyclic-circular" structural model and is represented by three-dimensional diagrams. Earlier, a scholarly attempt to construct a theoretical framework for psychoanalysis was undertaken by Rapaport,[8] who specified primary and secondary models of cognition, conation, and affect.

† Irving W. Wolf, Electronics Division, General Electric Company.

building a machine to simulate behavior. Instead it is a tentative framework, still serving primarily heuristic functions, and borrowing from electronics only a few conceptual operations like scanning, mixing, and amplification. In fact, the trend through the various revisions has been away from the use of complicated electronic structures and toward a relatively simple scheme based upon specification of psychological conditions underlying behavior.

Second, our attitudes concerning physiology should be spelled out. Although we feel that the ultimate model for behavior theory must be a neurophysiological one, enough is not yet known about the operation of the human brain to launch at that level the type of full-scale research attack on the prediction of behavior which we consider essential. We seek to avoid incompatibility with the existing facts of physiology but do not wish to be limited in our theorizing by the many gaps in that knowledge. The exciting recent advances in neurophysiology are of general interest to us insofar as they point to possible neural mechanisms for several of the operations in our system. These potential congruences will be alluded to briefly after the model has been described.

Third, we are not trying to preserve any conceptual ties with psychoanalytic theory or to translate its formulations into a new framework. We deal with personality dimensions (based on aspects of psychosexual development) which psychoanalysis has shown to be significant and we intend eventually to account for those clinical phenomena to which it has directed attention. The principles which hold promise of testable validity are of course borrowed where pertinent, others which do not pertain or offer no possibility of test are omitted from consideration.

But enough disclaiming of electronics, physiology, and psychoanalysis. It is time to state what we are interested in, i.e. the complex processes occurring in what we shall call, for lack of a better term, the psychic system. The diagram in Figure 1 shows the psychic system, enclosed by a broken line, and four outside systems which connect to it. In the following section we shall first supplement the diagram with a condensed overview of the whole framework and then proceed to discuss detailed, concrete illustrations in the context of ongoing research inspired by the model.

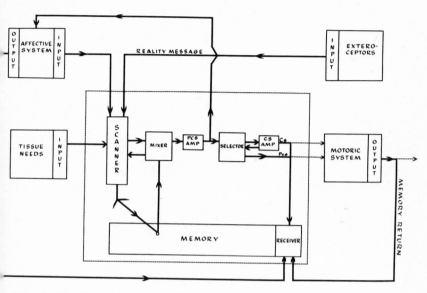

Fig. 1. Psychoanalytic behavior theory: a conceptual framework for research.

1. *Systems in communication with the psychic system.* The connecting systems are the exteroceptors (upper right), affective system (upper left), tissue needs (middle left), and motoric system (middle right). Each of these "black boxes" is a complete and complex organization in its own right, with many varied functions, but our only concern is with those inputs and outputs bearing on the psychic system. The exteroceptors pick up stimuli originating in the outside world through the media of seeing, hearing, touching, smelling, and tasting. These stimuli are converted to a form appropriate for transmission to the psychic system as reality message inputs. Tissue needs are an internal source of input sending converted messages relevant to hunger, thirst, elimination, sex, etc. A third input is from the affective system, which is seen autonomously transmitting messages stemming from currently active emotional states, like fear, anger,

grief, or joy, built up from previous experience. In addition to this input function, we know that emotional discharges, e.g. crying, laughing, sweating, are triggered by signals reaching the affective system and these output discharges are themselves registered in memory (see line from affective system designated as memory return). Finally, the motoric system, which receives signals from the psychic system and translates them into action, also has its motoric discharges registered via a memory return.

2. *Scanning and memory.* The three input messages just described activate the scanner to search memory for traces matching the input in some way. Once a similar trace is located the scanner accomplishes the release of a *signal* emitted by that *trace* and the signal goes to the mixer. The released signal may also be fed back from mixer to scanner and itself can serve as a fourth input to initiate subsequent scanning. The mixer, which now has received a signal from memory in addition to the original input message relayed by the scanner, is the major locus of processing operations, but before we attempt to delve into its mysteries we must specify the contents of memory in more detail.

Memory is a storage place for the countless past experiences of an individual. These experiences include acts, conscious ideas which never culminated in action, and preconscious thoughts which were readily available but for some reason did not enter consciousness (e.g. attention not directed to them) or the motoric system. Each separate experience exists in the form of a trace, a unit with several component parts. Every trace contains a *cognitive* component, which is the content or informational aspect, and can also have *affective* and *motoric* potentials. The latter two components, typically but not necessarily present in a trace, have the capacity for triggering discharges in the affective and motoric systems, respectively, once the trace has been activated and its released signal processed through the psychic system.

Cognitive components vary along an intensity dimension which we label *vividness*. Their complex patterns can share varying degrees of overlap or *similarity* with other traces. Affective components, not as numerous in kind as the cognitive, also vary along an intensity dimension, referred to as amount of *loading*. These potentials for emotional discharge range from positive to negative, but we shall pay particular attention to anxiety, a type of negative affect of special import for the processing of signals. The motoric or *motility* potential represents the likelihood of a signal reaching the motoric system and eventuating in some form of action. Figure 2 schematizes two hypothetical memory traces according to their component parts.

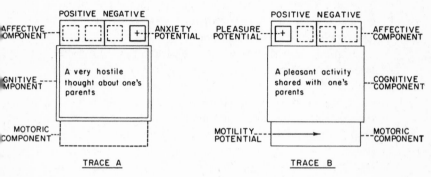

Fig. 2. Schematic representation of component parts of a memory trace.

Trace A has a very vivid cognitive component (double lines) along with a loaded potential for an anxiety reaction, in contrast to trace B whose cognitive component is less vivid and is accompanied by an affective potential for the experience of pleasure. In A the motility potential is absent (broken lines), due to the fact that the signal of this trace has not previously been given motoric expression in either word or deed, whereas in B the potential is present as a result of earlier acts and possibly verbalizations. The broken line boxes in the affective components indicate that other kinds of affective potentials, sometimes found in traces, are not present in the illustrations.

A trace, once registered, remains available in memory unless its original intensity was so low that possible dissipation over time renders it too weak to be detected by the scanner. Upon activation by the latter, the trace itself does not leave memory; only its released signal is picked up by the mixer. A trace can be scanned for either cognitive, or affective, or perhaps even motoric patterns depending on the input message. Three of the four input channels—exteroceptors, tissue needs, and feedback from mixer to scanner of a just activated memory trace—ordinarily lead to scanning cognitive components for possible similarities to the message. But the autonomous input from the affective system impels a search of affective components for similarities. Scanning on such a basis would result in a seemingly bizarre sequence of thoughts, since the signal of a trace is *always released in its entirety no matter which component part was responsible for its selection.*

Implicit in the foregoing discussion is the notion that no inter-trace organization exists in memory. Instead there is a built-in capacity for category formation as a consequence of shared similarities or overlap among traces. It is in the mixer that the matching and combination of signals for processing is accomplished. Thus memory is merely an aggregate of registered experiences or traces, conceptualized as having cognitive, affective, and motoric components. Next we must consider the operations performed upon signals of activated traces and follow the course of new combinations through to their own ultimate recording in memory.

3. *Unconscious processing.* Signals of similar traces released during the scanning of memory join the input message in the mixer where all are assembled or fitted together into a resultant combination of signals. Those parts of signal patterns which coincide are superimposed and thereby boosted in intensity—a crucial factor in subsequent transmission through the system. A particular mixing operation ceases with the rapid dissipation of available signals or with the introduction of a new reality message which initiates another sequence.

Once mixing has taken place the combined signals are "broadcast" to the preconscious amplifier. The various parts of the combination differ in intensity (both as a function of original vividness, loading, or motility of the memory trace as well as similarity matching to the input message), so there is not an equal likelihood for all parts to be picked up by the amplifier. The strong are received first, the medium next, and the weak probably dissipate en route. The first stage of amplification therefore is dependent upon signal intensity.

Strong parts of combined signals in the mixer are also likely to be picked up by the scanner in addition to the Pcs amplifier. This fourth input channel, mentioned earlier, leads to a process of *successive scanning* in which traces similar to the immediately prior ones are activated. If another strong signal is brought up, it in turn can initiate a new sequence and so continue the chain reaction. Successive signals, then, are *derivatives* of ones which instigate scanning in this way.

So far we have considered the transmission of mixed signals only in terms of their intensity. A second regulating principle, central to the operation of the psychic system, involves the special processing of signals containing loaded anxiety potentials. The organism strives to minimize the triggering of painful discharges in the affective system and accordingly must avail itself of a mechanism to prevent potentially disruptive signals from being amplified. If *inhibition* is not invoked, the loaded signal proceeds automatically from the Pcs amplifier to trigger an emotional response (see diagram for line originating between Pcs Amp and Selector and going up to Affective System). Inhibition consists of a momentary shutting off of the first-stage amplifier. During this shut-off period it is possible for a moderately loaded signal to dissipate completely in the mixer before amplification is resumed. A highly loaded one, however, takes longer to dissipate and may still remain sufficiently strong, after the temporally-fixed inhibition phase ends, to be picked up by the Pcs amplifier and thence relayed to the affective system. It should be added that the inhibitory mechanism does not interfere with feedback of the loaded signal to the scanner.

Inhibition is a function of the amount of loading of a signal's anxiety potential. If the latter exceeds the organism's tolerance limit for anxiety discharge, amplification is shut off. If the signal is within the limit, it is processed the same as all other signals, the only difference being that a minor affective discharge is triggered after first-stage amplification. This tolerance limit of an individual, set in terms of past emotional experiences and possibly constitutional factors, is geared to the sensitivity of the affective system, which in turn can be altered by the overall state of arousal of the organism. A highly sensitive affective system requires a more stringent limit in order to minimize disruptions. All these conditions have implications for failures of inhibition and consequent breakthroughs of loaded signals, but inasmuch as speculation about psychopathology cannot be included within the scope of this presentation, we must return to the sequence of system operations.

4. *Preconscious and conscious processing.* A mixed signal which has been amplified is sent next to the selector (see diagram) in addition to being picked up by the affective system as described above. In the selector, operations which determine its ultimate destinations are carried out. Alternative outcomes are to remain in the preconscious stage or to attain conscious awareness after second-stage amplification. Either channel can result in action if the signal reaches the motoric system and triggers a response. Also, both routes automatically lead to storage of the mixed signal in memory.

The selection of signals to be fed into the Cs amplifier depends upon their intensities and similarity relationships. Since signals emerge only one at a time into conscious thought, even a rapid succession of changes in attention cannot prevent some piling up in the selector. In the absence of similarity relationships, the strongest signal is most likely to enter consciousness first (i.e. picked up by the Cs amplifier). The next one in succession is chosen on the basis of similarity to its immediate conscious predecessor, whose signal is already fed back to the selector for matching purposes, and so on. It is also possible that a very strong signal, unrelated to the conscious predecessor, may interrupt the chain of thoughts by achieving second-stage amplification.

Thus consciousness, according to our view, is merely an end-state with respect to the processing of a current signal, but plays a vital role in determining the order of signals to be selected subsequently. It also has special relevance for later mixing operations by virtue of the fact that conscious signals are amplified more than preconscious ones and therefore exist in memory as traces of greater intensity.

Registration in memory is mediated by the receiver (see diagram), which picks up memory returns from output discharges in affective and motoric systems in addition to direct signals transmitted through Cs and Pcs channels. In fact, simultaneous receipt of return and direct signals is another basis (along with mixing) for new trace assemblies and hence learning. These temporal pairings are routinely stored as traces in the same manner as signals processed directly through the psychic system.

We have stated earlier that some dissipation over time probably occurs in memory traces. Of course such deterioration is relatively slow and cannot be compared at all to the rate of disappearance of fleeting signals active in the system. Recently stored traces, not exposed as long to decay, tend therefore to be stronger on the average than traces antedating them. As a consequence their signals, if released by the scanner, are more prominent in mixing and transmission.

We recognize that a highly condensed description of an ambitiously comprehensive framework like the one just outlined can do little more than raise numerous questions in the reader's mind. For us such questions, which have continually forced themselves upon our attention while constructing the still tentative working model, have proven valuable assets in pointing systematically to research directions. Next we shall list some of the major issues confronting us and then devote the rest of this chapter to actual research approaches illustrating our current efforts to clarify a few of these problems.

5. *Suggested problem areas for research.* The problems which have occurred to us fall into a number of categories. First, there is the usual host of methodological considerations. How are we to assess strength of anxiety potentials, determinants of vividness, factors influencing similarity? Second, there are basic questions concerning the interdependence of component parts of a memory trace. For example, what is the relationship between loaded anxiety potential and overall signal intensity? Third, the operations within the system raise another series of issues. What conditions underlie cognitive vs. affective scanning of memory? Is there also motoric scanning? What rules govern

the interaction of similarity and intensity in mixer and selector? Are there specifiable constants in the system, such as an unvarying amount of amplification or a fixed time-period of inhibition?

Then there are other problems relating to affective aspects. We speculate that the organism is exceptionally responsive to internal affective inputs under certain special circumstances like sleep or sensory deprivation where reality messages are kept to a minimum, and consequently dreams or thoughts emerge in the alogical manner Freud described as "primary process." Is there good evidence for or against postulating these relatively autonomous (we do not have reference here to the controversy over whether some non-specific sensory stimulation is always necessary for cerebral activity) inputs from affective system to scanner? If the answer is affirmative, we find ourselves incorporating features both of the James-Lange and Cannon-Bard theories of emotion. We can also add to this list the study of the influence of various states of organism arousal on anxiety tolerance limits and inhibition, for which hypnosis and drugs offer promise as research techniques; the relationship between amount of anxiety loading and strength of consequent emotional discharge; effects of activated anxiety potentials on performance; and transmission priorities of signals with pleasure potential compared to those without affective loading.

Finally, we have allowed several general areas only cursory and incidental consideration thus far. Our preoccupation currently is with the development of processing principles which apply to the relatively normal, structurally mature organism. Later, attention must be paid to developmental features of the system, to all the problems involved in human learning, and to conditions resulting in psychopathological breakdown. Ultimately, as has been mentioned before, we must also take into account neurophysiological counterparts.

Some potential congruences are already on the horizon. For example, the exciting recent advances involving the reticular formation of the brain point to both amplifying and inhibitory functions. "Gating" mechanisms seem pertinent to the shutting off of Pcs amplification and the operations in Cs selection. Especially relevant are some comments by Penfield.[7] Describing a permanent record of past experiences preserved in amazing detail within the brain, he speculates that "at the time of the original experience, electrical potentials passed through the nerve cells and nerve connections of a recording mechanism in a specific patterned sequence, and that some form of permanent facilitation preserves that sequence so that the record can be played at a later time." The "interpretive cortex" of the temporal lobes makes possible "the scanning process by which past experiences, however scattered they may have been in time, are selected and made available to the present for the purpose of comparative (automatic) interpretation." Following along these lines, we might append the thought that a well worked-out psychological model can perhaps point to new areas for neurophysiological investigation.

ONGOING RESEARCH

Our long-range plan for developing a behavior theory calls first for a comprehensive working model, followed by empirical analysis of a miniature behavioral system with known inputs and outputs. We are currently in the midst of the latter phase, which has occupied our research attention for the past year. This step (II on p. 109) demands a reciprocal interplay of model and data: the conceptual framework points to basic problems for research and to crucial variables for which operational measurement is required; subsequent findings in turn suggest modifications and refinements in the model.

An initial decision concerned the sample of behavioral domains to be selected for investigation and the type of stimulus inputs to be used. Fortunately a sufficient number of techniques, devised during our earlier studies of conflict and defense, is available to encompass a broad and diverse group of domains, including memory, reasoning, fantasy production, association of ideas, self-percept, visual perception, humor, and preference behavior. The underlying dimensions on which the techniques are based grow out of psychoanalytic theory. These dimensions are tapped by the Blacky pictures,[1] which portray in semi-structured fashion certain aspects of psychosexual development and relationships to significant familial figures.

By having a wide variety of behavioral tasks revolve about the use of Blacky pictures as stimuli (e.g. asking experimental subjects to identify the pictures flashed tachistoscopically; to recall them from memory; or to rank defense preferences on each picture), the construction of a miniature system becomes feasible. Known stimulus inputs, along with their specifiable behavioral outputs, readily merge into a connected system when they can be related across domains. Such a system is "miniature" only in the sense that behavioral tasks involving primarily the Blacky pictures are tied together, for it is obviously large in the number and scope of domains covered. Presumably the processing principles which mediate the stimulus-response sequence should not change with the particular content (an assumption to be checked later in step IV), and the prospect of discovering them seems, in our view, infinitely brighter if they can be pursued in a well-defined setting.

The above tactics began to take concrete form with the collection of data from 28 male and 34 female college students, each seen for a total of approximately ten hours over a series of several individual sessions and one small-group meeting. Recruitment was accomplished by posting notices and advertising "a psychology experiment" in the university newspaper, with participants paid at the rate of one dollar an hour. When individuals telephoned to volunteer, they were told that they would be exposed to "a number of personality tests and a physiological measure." At that point no one was wise enough (or perhaps rich enough) to be dissuaded by the warning. On our part we rejected only students who had taken psychology beyond the introductory course or who were not free at any of the scheduled times. Almost all those agreeing to come did appear at the first session.

At the present writing, the data bearing on just a few of the projects have been fully analyzed. For illustrative purposes we shall select two to describe in more detail—one a methodological contribution essential for operationalizing the system, the other an example of the reciprocal interplay of model and findings in the prediction of behavior—and then, in the space remaining, simply mention some of those whose analysis is still in progress.

1. *Assessment of anxiety potential.* According to the model, a major determinant of signal transmission is the anxiety potential of an activated memory trace. Signals emitted by traces whose affective components are highly loaded with anxiety potential automatically invoke the mechanism of inhibition (shutting off of Pcs amplification) because they exceed the organism's anxiety tolerance limit. Signals which are transmitted and still contain some anxiety potential trigger discharges in the affective system after amplification. So the first research objective was to devise a set of procedures to assess, for every individual, the strength of anxiety potentials inherent in traces relevant to each of the eleven Blacky pictures. The other attributes of memory traces—cognitive vividness, motility, and shared similarities—were felt to pose less formidable measurement problems.

Previous work with the Blacky pictures, as with most other instruments, typically made use of disturbance scores based on *inter-individual* comparisons for a given dimension. For example, an individual might be assigned to the lower part of the disturbance distribution on masturbation guilt (picture V) and to the upper part of another distribution on sibling rivalry (picture VIII). It was not possible to establish *relative* degrees of disturbance along the dimensions *within* an individual, since a low score on V might reflect more actual disturbance than a high score on VIII if overall the two distributions differed on an absolute scale. In the current series of studies we wished to concentrate instead on the more powerful level of *differential predictions within the individual* as a function of relative strengths of his various anxiety potentials.

Toward this end, each subject was individually administered several procedures as part of the first experimental session, which lasted about three hours. Initially he was asked to tell spontaneous stories (SS) about Blacky's actions and feelings in all the pictures, given in the conventional order. Next he was shown the pictures again, in a different order, and told to describe "what human experiences correspond to Blacky's, and wherever

possible illustrate with a first-hand experience of your own"
(HE). Sometime later in the session he was interrupted while
working on other tasks and required to give his self-insights on
each picture, presented in still another order. The instruction
was to answer "what problem area you think the picture is
supposed to represent; how much of a problem it is for you;
and why you think it is or is not a problem for you" (INS). All
these procedures were tape-recorded and afterward transcribed
verbatim, including exact timing of pauses and notation of
laughs, sighs, throat-clearing, stuttering, and mumbling. In addition, the subject's non-preferred hand and forearm were connected by electrodes to a galvanic skin resistance apparatus
(GSR), whose activity was continuously recorded on chart
paper.* Near the conclusion of the session he was asked to
point quickly to the "three pictures disliked the most."

From the responses to these Blacky tasks a sizable number
of commonly employed clinical and experimental indicators of
anxiety were set up. In addition to the expressive ones mentioned above and several GSR measures, a series of blocking
indices was developed. Criteria for scoring all the variables,
worked out mostly on a pretest sample of a dozen subjects, were
based on intra-individual rankings of the eleven pictures and
generally consisted of assigning checks to the top one or two
pictures in an individual's rank order on each variable. For
example, on the variable SS reaction time (timed delay between
presentation of picture and beginning of subject's story about
Blacky) the eleven picture-delays for a given individual were
ranked and the longest one checked. Using this intra-individual,
within-task approach to scoring, the GSR variables—initial drops
upon presentation of pictures and number of drops during period
of talking—were largely free of the methodological complications
besetting that field of measurement (i.e. individual differences
in baseline and reactivity; changes in baseline over time and

---

* Equipment was the standard Fels Dermohmmeter and accompanying
Esterline-Angus recorder. Synchronization between GSR and tape-recording
was accomplished by simultaneously feeding a signal into both every ten
seconds, and also by manual operation of an event marker on the Esterline-
Angus at prescribed points in the procedure.

with temperature and humidity deviation; difficulty in ascertaining which stimulus causes the drop).

After all subjects had been scored individually on the anxiety indices, the latter were intercorrelated across subjects and factor-analyzed (quartimax method) separately for the male and female experimental samples. This was done in order to derive a relatively pure set of measures for inclusion in the ultimate battery. The first factors in male and female analyses were sufficiently alike (statistically significant in similarity according to Burt's formula[2]) to permit their combination in assigning weights to the variables loading on them. Table 2 shows the final variables, the weights reflecting magnitude of their loadings on the factor, and a brief summary of rules for scoring them.

Using these factorially derived weights, it was then possible to compute anxiety potential scores for each individual on all eleven pictures, precisely the type of information we were seeking. In this connection it is interesting to note that our original reluctance to apply inter-individually based scores to intra-individual analyses is supported by the fact that certain pictures are more likely than others to produce anxiety responses, despite wide individual variation. Leading the list is masturbation guilt (V), followed by oral eroticism (I) and anal sadism (III). Those least likely to be accompanied by high scores are identification (VII), ego ideal (X), sibling rivalry (VIII), and guilt feelings (IX). In the middle range are castration anxiety (VI), oral sadism (II), love object (XI), and oedipal intensity (IV).

The composition of the obtained factor itself is important in interpreting the meaning of the computed scores. Those variables loading most heavily, namely, absent or minimal verbal output, are reflections of an inhibitory process—the very mechanism which the model predicts should be invoked when strong anxiety potentials are activated. The minor contributions of the remaining variables may represent some transmission of signals still containing sufficient anxiety potential to trigger affective discharges (GSR drops during periods of no verbal output) and to result in subjective awareness of unpleasant discharges (disliked pictures). Thus the scores, based as they are on variables reflecting primarily inhibition and some affective breakthrough,

TABLE 2—*Derived measures of anxiety potential*

Variable	Wt.	Rules for scoring
SS-Pause	2	Picture in spontaneous stories with largest absolute sum of pauses, provided sum is greater than 10 sec and ratio of pauses/talking time is 0.8 or more; picture with largest ratio, provided it is at least 0.8
SS-Talk time	2	Picture in spontaneous stories with shortest amount of actual talking time (pauses not included), provided the amount is less than 25 sec and at least 2 sec less than the next shortest picture
HE-Talk time	2	Same as SS-Talk time, except applied to pictures in human experiences procedure
HE-Pause	1	Same as SS-Pause, except applied to HE procedure
SS-Reaction time	1	Picture in SS with longest time between presentation and beginning of talking (must be at least 2 sec longer than second longest picture, or else of 10 sec duration or more)
SS-Initial GSR drop	1	Two pictures with largest drops between presentation and beginning of talking
INS-Initial GSR drop	1	Two pictures in insight procedure with largest drops immediately following instruction to begin telling self-insights
Disliked pictures	1	Three pictures chosen as most disliked

appear to provide *estimates of differential probability of release of signals with high anxiety potential* when the various pictures are shown to an individual.

With this enigmatic attribute of the memory trace now under

operational control, we can proceed to study how it, along with the accompanying attributes, influences other behavioral outputs. The next section describes the findings of an investigation which illustrates such an approach.

2. *Predicting the recall of Blacky pictures.* One of the behavioral domains in which we desire to make successful predictions is memory. At three points during the initial experimental session our subjects were asked to "name the Blacky pictures as fast as you can, in any order—just a short phrase so we know which picture you mean." A stopwatch was held on the table and each recall was halted after thirty consecutive seconds without a new picture being brought up. Total time spent on a recall task typically ranged between one and two minutes. Thus far the data for the first recall, which followed immediately after the SS and HE procedures, have been analyzed.

The first and second columns of ranks in Table 3 presents the eleven pictures according to 1) the frequency with which the group of 62 subjects as a whole recalled them; and 2) their mean position in the recall sequence when they were remembered. These two sets of ranks are criterion behavioral outputs in response to the stimulus input "name the Blacky pictures." Following the dictates of our strategy, we were led to explore the processing principles which mediate the S-R chain, in the hope of arriving at a theoretical formulation capable of fitting the obtained data.

A logical beginning seemed to be to examine the attributes of memory traces in which the various pictures were imbedded. Those attributes figured on *a priori* grounds to have most relevance for performance on this task were cognitive vividness, strength of anxiety potential, and shared similarity among picture traces. The motoric potential, possibly involved in the choice of label by which pictures are verbalized, was not pursued (rightly or wrongly) because the subjects were under no constraint to use labels felt to be offensive.

Pictures designated beforehand as likely to be especially vivid were I, III, and IV. Oral eroticism (I), first picture exposed in SS, was referred to by the examiner as "picture

TABLE 3—*Blacky pictures ranked according to recall frequency,
recall position, similarity index, and anxiety potential*

Picture	Recall frequency (1=recalled most often)	Recall position (1=earliest mean position)	Similarity index (1=highest similarity)	Anxiety potential (1=highest mean anxiety score)
I Oral eroticism*	4	3	5	2
II Oral sadism	8	6	9	5
III Anal sadism**	1.5	1	6	3
IV Oedipal intensity***	1.5	2	4	7
V Masturbation guilt	9	7	11	1
VI Castration anxiety	7	4	10	4
VII Identification	10	9	7	10
VIII Sibling rivalry	3	10	3	11
IX Guilt feelings	11	11	8	9
X Ego ideal	5	5	1.5	8
XI Love object	6	8	1.5	6

*vivid due to primacy
**vivid due to surprise
***vivid due to recency

	with Recall frequency	with Recall position
Similarity Rhos	.58	.04
Anxiety Rhos	.11	.61

number one" and portrays Blacky at the very start of his
ignominious career. Anal sadism (III), third in the SS order,
is typically greeted with surprise, if not dismay. Subjects do not

expect to view a drawing of a defecation scene (the picture is introduced with the comment "here Blacky is relieving himself") and almost always experience difficulty in verbalizing a story. Oedipal intensity (IV) was the last picture given in the HE series, just prior to the recall instructions. Table 3 indicates the striking effect of cognitive vividness in promoting both recall frequency (the three pictures occur in the top four ranks) and early position in the sequence (the first three ranks).

Next the similarity attribute was investigated. On the assumption that consistently paired pictures should be similar in some way, an index was calculated by inspecting the three recall lists of each individual and noting those pictures which were named adjacently on all three occasions. The number of systematic "contiguities" for every picture was added across subjects and then corrected for total number of times remembered, since an instance of forgetting precludes the possibility of three adjacent mentions. Table 3 reveals that similarity correlates with recall frequency (rho=.58), i.e. pictures with high similarity to other pictures are more likely to be remembered, but does not correlate with position in sequence (rho=.04). A comparable Blacky study relating similarity to recall, done on a male sample several years ago, yielded essentially the same result (rho=.64) and roughly parallel picture-ranks.

Thus both vividness and similarity contribute to recall in ways predictable from common sense as well as from the many experiments dating from Ebbinghaus. However, neither source provides us with a clear expectation regarding the effects of relative loadings of anxiety potential on frequency and position. At the gross level of recall ranks, Table 3 demonstrates that pictures with high mean anxiety scores, computed according to the methods described in the preceding section, are likely to be named early and ones with low mean scores to be named late (rho=.61). The correlation between anxiety potential and frequency of recall is negligible (rho=.11). Breaking down the anxiety (A) scores into finer categories, though, does divulge a systematic relationship to frequency and elaborates the position finding.

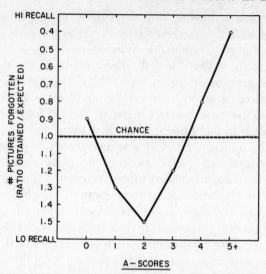

Fig. 3. Recall frequency vs. anxiety potential scores broken down by categories.

Figure 3, derived from the same raw data as the ranks in column 1 of Table 3, reveals a curve along which A-scores of 0 appear to have no bearing on number of pictures forgotten; moderate scores of 1, 2, and 3 are accompanied by more forgetting; and high scores of 4, 5, and over go with greater remembering. The ordinate scale consists of ratios of obtained number of forgotten pictures within an A-score category divided by a weighted expected number for that category. In the denominator, differential forgetting among the various pictures is taken into account. The corresponding chi-square table is significant at less than the .05 level of confidence, pointing to special effects of strength of anxiety potential on recall *frequency* with all other influences controlled.

Further analysis of the *position* data broken down according to A-score categories corroborates the earlier result that loaded anxiety potential is tied to accelerated mention in the sequence —but only up to a point. A-scores of 5 and over are accompanied by *delay* rather than acceleration. Since there are fewer extremely high than middle scores, the overall relationship is the one reflected in the rho of .61. In summary, then, we are confronted by what appear on the surface to be paradoxical trends: in the case of very high A-scores, greater remembering but delay in sequence position; with moderate A-scores, greater forgetting but acceleration in position when remembered. Obviously an intriguing set of findings for model-building!

Before pursuing theoretical implications, it is worth mentioning that assignment of numerical weights to the variables of vividness, similarity, and anxiety potential, according to their obtained effects, provides almost perfect prediction to the criterion variables of recall frequency and position ranks of the pictures. Of course such an approach (akin to a multiple regression equation) requires cross-validation in order to be substantiated, but the goodness of fit is nevertheless encouraging.

With these data available as checks, we can now "plug in" the model (see Fig. 1 again) and, at the conceptual level, consider what might be taking place in the psychic system in response to the stimulus input "name Blacky pictures."

First this reality message, emerging from the exteroceptors, reaches the scanner and causes the activation of those memory traces in which the pictures have recently been imbedded during the SS and HE tasks. Signals of the activated traces are then released to the mixer, where they are all combined and broadcast. Signals arrive in the mixer with varying overall intensities, and further differentiation in strength results from the combination process. Overlapping parts of originally separate signals are boosted in intensity, accounting for the dominance in general of picture-parts of signals over other cognitive, non-picture-parts as a natural consequence of the greater frequency of the former in the traces activated. Within the class of combined signals of given pictures there is apt to be wide variation in strength.

During the broadcasting phase, signals of the strongest pictures are picked up earliest by the Pcs amplifier, followed by those of medium overall intensity. The weak have a low probability of ever being picked up. In the absence of inhibition the sequence is maintained in the course of transmission of amplified signals to the selector. From that point the strongest signals reach the Cs amplifier first, proceed to the motoric system, and come out as verbal responses identifying certain pictures. The early signals are also fed back from Cs amplifier to selector to be matched with other signals currently arriving. If a similarity match can be made to one of these, its signal is amplified next into consciousness. If no similar signal exists, the order of subsequent transmission depends upon relative strengths of the signals still present in the selector.

In the interim another process has been set in motion by the mixer's broadcasting of signals, namely feedback to the scanner. The latter also picks up the strongest picture signals and immediately starts a new search of memory, now for traces specifically matching this new input. Released signals, automatically boosted in the mixer by combination with the instigating signal, then proceed directly through the system and typically achieve verbal expression some time after the first series described in the previous paragraph.

Once the supply of signals has been exhausted, the original reality message is repeated (often the examiner has to prod the subject to continue if the thirty-second blank period has not expired; other times subtle cues induce further efforts at recall) and a second round is initiated. Now the recently named pictures, just stored in memory, are brought up along with other signals and reach the selector readily because of their previously amplified state. However, they are usually not sent again to the motoric system (repetitions do occur occasionally) because that would run counter to the reality-based expectation that pictures are to be named only once. As a consequence of this inability to verbalize new responses at the output end, successive scanning instigated by strong signals continues to activate new traces in memory. Failing to locate additional similar pictures, the scanner automatically searches for traces similar to the picture signal just released and begins a chain of signal associations which is no longer linked primarily to picture-parts of traces. Derivatives brought up in the course of such scanning may sometimes lead indirectly to the discovery of new pictures, which are then processed and eventually verbalized. These would naturally appear very late in the sequence.

So far we have discussed only the transmission of signals containing anxiety potential loadings which do not exceed the organism's tolerance limit. What happens when the loading is high enough to invoke the inhibitory mechanism of shutting off Pcs amplification? We have already said that some dissipation of signals occurs in the mixer during the fixed time period of the inhibition phase. Picture signals of moderate overall intensity are likely to dissipate completely and never achieve amplification. Very strong ones, although reduced by dissipation, may still retain sufficient strength after the cessation of inhibition to be picked up by the Pcs amplifier. Thus they proceed through the system but are delayed in the sequence.

In light of the above theoretical expectations, let us turn to the observed fate of specific pictures in terms of their recall position and frequency. The special vividness of I, III, and IV, doubtless important determinants of overall intensity, fits with the fact that they tend to be processed first. For the next batch of pictures (VI, X, II, and XI, trailed closely by VII) we have no *a priori* hunches about cognitive vividness, but if the A-scores can be assumed to relate to overall signal intensity it follows that they should be found in the middle ranges. The one seeming exception is V, which has the highest mean A-score and occurs seventh in the sequence. However, V also has by far the largest number of very high A-scores, so inhibition is presumed to be invoked more often in its case with a resulting delay in position. The invariant adjacency of X and XI whenever both are mentioned can be traced to operations in the selector. The striking physical similarity of the two, their juxtaposition as the last two pictures in SS, and their fairly close mean A-scores all suggest that if one reaches the Cs amplifier, the other is readily available in the selector to be transmitted next as a consequence of feedback from Cs amplifier to selector.

The last two pictures in the recall order are VIII and IX. Both, judging by the A-scores, appear to be weak in overall signal strength. However, the former is rarely forgotten (only 4 out of 62 times) whereas the latter is often forgotten (33 out of 62 times). The explanation clearly lies with similarity. Picture VIII has a very high similarity index (ranks third after X and XI) and its predominant pairing is with IV (both depict family scenes with Blacky left out). Here we see the operation of feedback to the scanner described above. When IV, one of the most vivid pictures, is in the mixer its signal is picked up by the scanner, which now almost always selects VIII from memory and starts its late transmission through to verbal response. Picture IX, on the other hand, is low in similarity as well as intensity and its chances for being brought up depend largely upon a derivative with mediating similarity being hit upon during the course of successive scanning. Picture VII suffers from the same liabilities, though probably to a lesser extent.

The assumption which enables the foregoing to make sense is that a positive correlation exists between A-scores and overall signal intensity, so the higher the A-score, the stronger the signal. One of the basic questions for research raised earlier concerns precisely this relationship of anxiety potential to signal strength. The A-scores themselves are presumed to represent estimates, for the various pictures, of differential probability of release of signals with high anxiety potential. It is theoretically possible for released signals causing inhibition all to be of comparable strength, a condition which would make for absence of correlation. By drawing hypothetical curves which fit the A-scores to the obtained recall data, we can gain some insight into the true nature of the correlation.

Figure 4 has for its abscissa a theoretical continuum of overall signal intensity. The stronger the signal, the more probable is its subsequent amplification. The ordinate is a theoretical continuum of anxiety potential, with a tolerance limit fixed at some point beyond the medium range. All signals above this limit are inhibited, all those below are transmitted if strong enough to be picked up by the Pcs amplifier. The three curves, portraying separate categories of A-scores across pictures, are drawn to fit the data: (1) A-scores of 0 show no marked relationship to frequency or position, for they are composed mostly of moderately strong signals, which may or may not be picked up, plus counteracting amounts of weak and fairly strong; (2) pictures with A-scores of 1-4 have the greatest likelihood of complete dissipation by inhibition, yet, when the

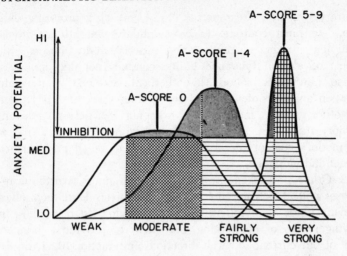

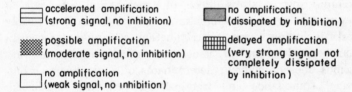

Fig. 4. Hypothetical curves fitting anxiety scores to obtained recall data.

tolerance limit is not exceeded, their signals are apt to achieve early amplification because of their strength; (3) pictures with A-scores of 5-9, fewer in number than the other two distributions, have relatively more chance of invoking inhibition, but sufficient strength usually remains for them to be recalled eventually.

Thus Figure 4 suggests, in answer to the basic question, that A-scores are positively correlated with overall signal intensity, though the three distributions probably overlap considerably. Also, the seemingly paradoxical findings are no longer so strange when the model is called into play. We do not wish, however, to convey the impression that the problem of predicting recall behavior is solved to our satisfaction. Quite the contrary, we view the reported study only as a promising first step. We must continue to cross-validate weighting systems, manipulate orders of presentation experimentally, observe the effects of altered tolerance limits, conduct detailed inquiries, devise new tests of our hypothetically-deduced relationship between anxiety potential and signal intensity, etc. Until these and other projects, including the mapping of a person's relevant memory traces, are accomplished, we cannot hope to arrive at the model's goal of successful prediction of recall performance in each individual case.

3. *Other projects in progress.* The ten hours' worth of responses collected from each of the 62 subjects lend themselves to many kinds of investigation. The following list of studies, in varying stages of completion, may help to provide a broader view of our current research directions: interaction of vividness, similarity, and anxiety potential in a perceptual task requiring identification of Blacky pictures flashed tachistoscopically at very rapid speeds; stress effects of experimental activation of traces containing anxiety potential on performance in a variety of tasks including sensory discrimination, sensory-motor coordination, reasoning, rate of associative verbal output, and preconscious decision-making; determinants of, and affects accompanying, compliance and transgression responses in Blacky stories and inquiry items; construction of measures to reflect extent of ambivalence toward parents and siblings existing in memory traces; determinants of rankings of defense preferences relevant to the Blacky dimensions; prediction of pictures ranked as problem areas in self and others; analysis of chained word-associations to the pictures; factors influencing enjoyment and recall of humorous cartoons whose contents parallel Blacky dimensions; psychological concomitants of GSR responses to Blacky stimuli.

SUMMARY

This chapter has described a research program aimed at the eventual formulation of a theory of human behavior growing out of the fields of academic psychology and psychoanalysis. We began by stating our opinion that successful prediction of behavior requires detailed spelling out of the complex processes which intervene between original stimulus and final response. As strategic steps in this direction we proposed the construction of a comprehensive working model, to be checked and revised in light of analyses of a miniature behavioral system of known inputs and outputs, and finally to be applied to the broad range of human experiences. The rest of the chapter was then devoted to a condensed exposition of a working model and some illustrative research approaches related to it.

In retrospect it may seem that we have moved too far afield from psychoanalysis to feature the word in our title. To some extent this is true, inasmuch as we have made no systematic attempt to translate Freudian notions into the framework. Certain key concepts are handled differently; repression, for example, is subsumed under a general mechanism of inhibition, and other classic defenses are included in the category of derivatives of inhibited signals. Our experimental methods clearly deviate from the psychoanalytic tradition. However, the dimensions tapped by our stimulus situations, the series of tasks built around the Blacky pictures, are specifically oriented toward the theory of psychosexual development. Also, we have incorporated Freud's primary emphasis on unconscious mental functioning and the central role assigned to anxiety.

On the other side of the fence, we work in the time-honored domains of academic psychology—memory, reasoning, perception, et al.—and employ its brand of research techniques. Yet the substantive content is quite alien. We study recall performance and, to be sure, note the effects of primacy and recency, but at the same time we also devote major attention to the interaction of such factors with anxiety potential attached to affectively-loaded psychosexual stimuli.

Weaving one's way through such a middle course can increase exposure to the mines and booby traps belonging to both sides, but so far we are optimistic enough to believe that we are not destined to remain in no man's land.

References

1. Blum, G. *The Blacky pictures.* New York: Psychological Corp., 1950.

2. Burt, C. The factorial study of temperamental traits. *Brit. J. Psychol.*, 1948, 1, 78-203.

3. Colby, K. *Energy and structure in psychoanalysis.* New York: Ronald, 1955.

4. Dollard, J. and Miller, N. *Personality and psychotherapy.* New York: McGraw-Hill, 1950.

5. Freud, S. A note upon the "mystic writing pad." In *Collected papers.* Vol. V. New York: Basic Books, 1959.

6. Jones, E. *The life and work of Sigmund Freud.* Vol. I. New York: Basic Books, 1953.

7. Laurence, W. Science in review. *N. Y. Times,* 1957, Nov. 24.

8. Rapaport, D. *Organization and pathology of thought.* New York: Columbia Univ. Press. 1951.

A. R. Luria

VI

Experimental Analysis
of the Development of
Voluntary Action in Children

INTRODUCTION

THE PROBLEM OF VOLUNTARY ACTION, its formation in the course
of development and the objective analysis of its laws, has always
been one of the most important topics of Soviet psychology. The
concept that voluntary action is a primary attribute of mental
life, to which scientific analysis cannot be applied, has always
been alien to Soviet psychology. Relying on the traditions established by Sechenov,[14] the famous 19th century Russian physiolo-
gist, Soviet psychology regards the analysis of the formation of
voluntary action in the course of development as its fundamental
task.

Almost a quarter of a century ago, the outstanding Soviet
psychologist Vygotski[15] outlined the principal ways of investigating the formation of the most complex voluntary forms of
behavior unique to man. He formulated the concept that voluntary action arises in the process of the child's relationship with
the adult, and passes through a number of successive stages in
its development. Originally taking the form of the fulfillment
by the child of the adult's verbal instruction, it is gradually
—with the development of the child's own speech—transformed
into a system of self-regulating acts in which the decisive role
is played first by external and subsequently by internal speech,
the chief mechanism of voluntary action.

The purpose of this chapter is to report and discuss one in
our series of studies examining the principal stages of the

development of voluntary action and illustrating the main phases of the regulatory role of speech.

VOLUNTARY ACTION AND EXTERNAL SIGNALS

Study of the formation of voluntary action in children should begin by analyzing the way in which a child accomplishes the adult's verbal directions. The child's capacity to subordinate its movements to instructions given by others eventually turns into a capacity to regulate its movements to orders formulated in internal speech. With the development of the regulatory role of speech, there arises a form of organization of action that we call voluntary movement.

Observations indicate that the regulatory role of speech is not formed all at once. At early stages of development, at age 1½ to 2 years, the adult's verbal instruction may easily call forth an adequate movement in the child. Everyone knows, for example, that the child readily complies with the command "clap your hands!" However, as noted by Shchelovanov and his co-workers, an adult's verbal instruction can call forth proper action *only if it does not come into conflict with another dominating action of the child.* If this happens, the effect of the verbal instruction will be unspecific and will intensify the earlier performed action. For example, if a child of 1½ or 2 is busy removing rings from a bar and is then told to put one ring back on the bar, this will only intensify the action of removing rings, although under usual conditions a youngster will readily carry out the given instruction. Thus, at early stages of development the adult's verbal instruction can only start the action of the child; it can neither inhibit nor switch it to some other activity.

It is also impossible at this stage to form in the system of the child's speech a preliminary conditioned connection which would lead to future action at the appearance of a conditioned signal. For example, you give a rubber ball to a child of 2 or 2½ with the instruction to squeeze it at the flash of a red electric bulb. On hearing the words "when the light appears," the child immediately begins to look for this light; with the words "you will squeeze the ball," it begins to squeeze the ball at once without waiting for the signal. Even when, after a training period (of which we shall not speak here), the child succeeds in squeezing the ball only at the appearance of the signal, action is not limited to a single squeeze. The continuing stimulation of the ball in the child's hand cannot be inhibited by verbal instruction. It produces numerous involuntary, unceasing motor reactions; there is no quiet waiting for the signal to be given. It is of interest that all attempts to inhibit these superfluous movements with such verbal instructions as "Enough!", "No more!" do not produce the desired effect. They either act unspecifically, that is, intensifying the diffused involuntary squeezing, or completely inhibit the child's movements.

It may be asked whether it is possible to overcome these involuntary movements and obtain a *model of well-regulated voluntary action* even in those instances in which direct speech has no inhibiting influence. Practice shows that this is quite possible, but the conditions of the experiment must be changed.

In our usual experiments the optical signal only started the movement; the muscular sensations originating in the child's own movement, and reinforced by the influence of the verbal instruction ("no more!"), served as an inhibitory signal for discontinuing the movement. But, the neurodynamics of the child's motor reactions were too diffuse, the muscular sense too underdeveloped, and the influence of the speech system too weak to crown our experiment with success. To ensure a desirable result, we had to rearrange our experiment so that the child's motor reaction could evoke a distinct exteroceptive stimulation which would serve as a signal of adequate action and *inhibit any further movements in accordance with the feedback principle.*

Such an experiment proved to be quite feasible. The child was told to squeeze the ball and thereby ring a bell, or turn off the light at the appearance of the optic signal; in this way we ensured experimental conditions under which the child's motor reaction itself produced an exteroceptive signal. Yakovleva's[16] observations of 2 and 2½ year old children have shown that it is possible to obtain distinct movements coordinated with the signal and to prevent superfluous involuntary impulses (Figure 1).

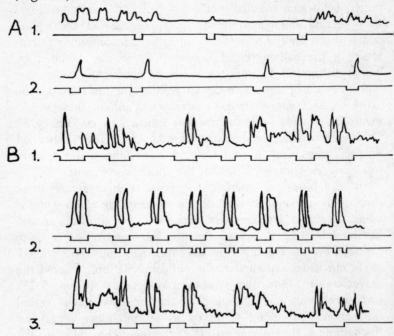

Fig. 1. Control of superfluous involuntary action through an exteroceptive signal with feed-back effect. A. (1) Simple motor reaction: when a light—squeeze, (2) plus feedback: pressure switches light off. B. (1) Simple motor reaction: when a light—squeeze twice, (2) plus feedback: every pressure gives a sound signal, (3) without feedback.

The exteroceptive signal called forth by the child's own movement acted according to the feedback principle, serving as a signal to discontinue the action and inhibit all further motor excitation. Thus was obtained *the simplest model of voluntary action,* producing an effect that could not be achieved by direct verbal instruction.

VOLUNTARY ACTION AND INTERNAL SIGNALS

We have described the simplest process of developing voluntary action. Is it not now possible to pass to the next stage and obtain a considerably more perfect process? Can we go from external signals to a system of internal signalization, which is always at the child's disposal and can help it attain *self-regulation*?

Let us try to replace the system of additional external signals, originating from the movement of the child, with the child's own *speech signals* which can reinforce the necessary movement and, according to the feedback principle, inhibit all superfluous impulses.

We shall tell the child (who must respond with motor reactions to the conditioned optical signal) to accompany each movement performed in response to the verbal instructions, with its own verbal command "Go!" If the dynamics of the nervous process, on which the system of speech is based, prove more perfect, more concentrated, and more mobile than the dynamics of the nervous processes which underlie the motor reactions, then the inclusion of additional speech signals, issuing from the child's own speech, will serve as a means of regulating its motor responses.

All attempts to produce such an effect in children at the age of 2 to 2½ (or in 3 year olds reared in conditions of insufficient speech practice) ended in failure: their speech system was too weak. Speech reactions became extinct too rapidly and were inductively inhibited by motor reactions. Attempts to introduce, at this age, the child's own regulatory speech into the experiment only led to a still greater derangement of motor reactions.

Quite different results were obtained in experiments with 3 to 4 year old children reared in kindergarten where their speech was systematically trained. As Peskovskaya and also Tikhomirov have shown, a child of this age was practically unable to respond with distinct motor reactions to the signals presented, producing numerous inter-signal reactions of which it was hardly conscious and which it could not inhibit at will. However, the neurodynamic processes, on which the child's speech reactions are based, proved at this age so perfect and mobile that the child could easily react to the corresponding signals with the words "Go!", "Go!", without giving any superfluous or persevering answers. When we then united the two reactions and told the child to say the word "Go!" while squeezing the ball at the appearance of each signal, the situation changed radically. The neurodynamically more perfect verbal reactions began to regulate the less concentrated and mobile motor reactions, the superfluous involuntary movements disappeared, and we obtained a *model voluntary movement*, this time *regulated by the child's own speech system*.

When we reverted to the experiment with silent motor reactions, all the defects appeared anew. Similar results were obtained in more complex experiments when the child had to react to each signal with two squeezes of the ball; again the verbal accompaniment of these reactions made their regulation quite easy.

THE REGULATORY INFLUENCE OF INTERNAL SIGNALS

What then is the mechanism of the regulatory influence of speech? Does it act by virtue of its elective connections, or is its action at this stage even more elementary and its regulatory influence determined by the fact that the child's verbal reactions create an additional system of innervation impulse? If we try to separate these two factors from each other in a special experiment we shall obtain a definite answer.

We found that a child reacting to an optical signal with the words "one, two!" is unable to perform the distinct double movement demanded by the verbal instruction. This regulatory influence originating from two separate verbal impulses cannot be retained, however, if we instruct the child to react to the optical signal with the words "I will squeeze twice!" In this case the regulatory influence will not come from the elective (significative) side of speech, but from its innervatory (impulse) side; when pronouncing these words, the child will accompany them by a single protracted motor reaction. For the same reason, attempts to obtain in a 3 or 3½ year old a regulative influence from the significative side of speech during more elaborate elective differentiated motor reactions are rarely successful. For example, if a youngster of this age, after being told

to squeeze the ball in response to a red signal and not to squeeze
at a green signal, shows a tendency to produce motor reactions
to both signals (Figure 2a and 2b), then, adding to these motor
reactions the verbal response "squeeze!" (at the red signal) and
"don't squeeze!" (at the green signal) still does not produce
any regulatory influence. The child accompanies the inhibitory
green signal with the words "don't squeeze!" and at the same
time squeezes the ball; the louder the child pronounces the
inhibitory command, the more intense the accompanying motor
reaction (Figure 2b).

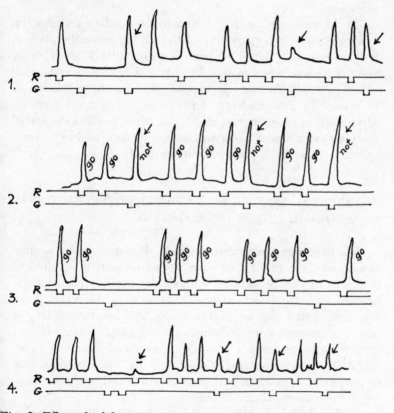

Fig. 2. Effect of inhibitory commands on impulsive reactions. Simple
system of reactions: (1) to red and green; (2) with speech reactions
of child; (3) with only positive speech reactions; (4) speechless. R=
red+; G=green−.

It can thus be observed that the regulatory influence comes not from the significative but from the impulse side of speech. Only if we eliminate the conflict, by telling the child to say "squeeze!" exclusively in response to the red signal and to silently inhibit movement at the green signal, will the regulatory role of speech become strongly apparent (Figure 2c). The predominant influence of the unspecific, impulsive side of speech will disappear at a later stage of development, at ages 5 to 6, when the child's motor reactions become regulated by the system of elective connections which by that time assume decisive significance.

At the same age the child begins to intermediate its responses to signals by *verbal rules,* formulated during the elaboration of motor reactions. The child now develops that kind of really voluntary movement which is directed and regulated by *internal speech.* As demonstrated in special experiments, regulation of movement by pronouncing a signal's meaning becomes unnecessary; it is often sufficient to train a child's adequate verbal reactions. Subsequent motor reactions, now regulated by internal speech, will begin to proceed quite normally.

EXTERNAL SIGNALS AS A COMPENSATING FACTOR IN ABNORMAL MOTOR DEVELOPMENT

We have some experiments which show that under normal conditions the regulation of voluntary movements in children of 5 to 6 years can be effected without the decisive participation of their external speech. However, as soon as these conditions are complicated the self-regulatory system becomes deranged and the compensatory influence of the child's own external speech again acquires a strongly pronounced character. This might be most convincingly illustrated by cases of abnormal development in children with weakened cortical processes leading to the cerebroasthenic syndrome.

If the child has suffered at a relatively early age from a trauma, infectious disease, or protracted dystrophy, the dynamics of the cortical processes may radically change. The force, stability, and power of concentration of the nervous processes are affected and the balance between the excitatory and inhibitory processess becomes upset. In such instance the child manifests heightened impulsiveness, which markedly complicates his normal education.

Without overstepping the limits of our experiment, we can see that such a child, while not revealing any appreciable intellectual defects but exhibiting a considerable instability of the nervous processes, possesses peculiar neurodynamic defects. The child preserves distinct differentiated systems of motor reactions to positive and inhibitory signals. If these signals are presented at an accelerated and shorter rate, i.e. if greater demands are made on the force and mobility of the nervous processes, the picture changes considerably; the child begins to produce inadequate impulse reactions to inhibitory signals, or does not manifest proper reactions to positive signals. In some children the number of wrong motor reactions may reach 40 or 50 percent. It is in these cases that the regulatory influence of the child's own speech may come to the fore.

As shown by the observations of Homskaya,[3] the neurodynamic processes, on which the speech activity of such children is based, often prove much more concentrated and mobile than the neurodynamics of their motor reactions. If the motor reactions to signals are replaced by verbal responses (for example, by "squeeze!" at the positive signal and "don't squeeze!" at the inhibitory signal), the child will give correct responses even when the conditions of the experiment are similar to those under which a considerable number of erroneous motor reactions are produced.

It is the greater stability of the neurodynamics of the speech system which can be used as a compensatory factor. Therefore, if we combine in such children their motor and verbal reactions (telling them to respond with the word "squeeze!" to positive signals and to simultaneously press the ball, and with the words "don't squeeze!" to inhibitory signals and to refrain from pressing the ball), the new functional system normalizes the course of these reactions. In some children it strengthens the inhibitory processes and in others it increases the tone of the excitatory processes; this leads to a considerable decrease in the number of erroneous reactions.

While regulating the course of motor reactions by means of external speech, an excitable child with weakened cortical processes retards its reactions and inhibits the superfluous impulse responses to negative signals. In similar conditions, a child that easily passes into a state of diffused inhibitions also strengthens its motor reactions with the help of the regulatory role of speech; the child accelerates and intensifies its reactions, and produces adequate positive responses. In both cases the child's external speech, by stabilizing connections and neurodynamics, normalizes the course of the nervous processes and becomes a powerful means of compensating neurodynamic defects.

SUMMARY

We have analyzed the complex process of the development of voluntary action in the child and cited several experiments showing the role of the second signalling system which, according to Pavlov,[12, 13] "introduces a new principle of nervous activity" and gradually becomes "the highest regulator of human behavior." Although these studies bear only a particular character, they bring us closer to the solution of important problems relative to the mechanism of the formation of voluntary movement in man and compensatory processes in abnormal motor development.

References

All references, except the works of Pavlov, are published in Russian.

1. Anokhin, P. K. The afferent apparatus of a conditional reflex. *Vop. Psikhol.*, 1955, No. 6.
2. Elkonin, D. B. Interaction of the first and second signalling systems in children of preschool age. *Trans. U.S.S.R. Acad. Pedag. Sci.*, 1954, 64.

3. Homskaya, E. D. Contribution to the question of the role of speech in the compensation of motor reaction. In Luria, A. R. (Ed.), *Problems of the higher nervous activity of normal and abnormal children.* Moscow, 1956.

4. Homskaya, E. D. The dynamics of the latent periods of motor reactions in children. *Proc. U.S.S.R. Acad. Pedag. Sci.,* 1957.

5. Lublinskaya, A. A. The role of speech in the mental development of the child. *Trans. Hertzen Pedag. Inst.,* Leningrad, 1955, 113.

6. Lubovsky, V. I. Some peculiarities of the higher nervous activity in oligophrenic children. In Luria, A. R. (Ed.), *Problems of the higher nervous activity of normal and abnormal children.* Moscow, 1956.

7. Luria, A. R. (Ed.) *Problems of the higher nervous activity of normal and abnormal children.* Moscow, 1956.

8. Luria, A. R. The role of speech in the formation of temporary connections in man. *Vop. Psikhol.,* 1955.

9. Meshcheryakov, A. I. The role of previous experience in the elaboration of new connections in man. *Vop. Psikhol.,* 1955.

10. Meshcheryakov, A. I. Participation of the second signalling system in the analysis and synthesis of the chain stimuli in normal and mentally retarded children. In Luria, A. R. (Ed.), *Problems of the higher nervous activity of normal and abnormal children.* Moscow, 1956.

11. Paramanova, N. P. Formation of interaction between two signalling systems in normal children. In Luria, A. R. (Ed.), *Problems of the higher nervous activity of normal and abnormal children.* Moscow, 1956.

12. Pavlov, I. P. *Twenty years of objective study of higher nervous activity of the animal.* Moscow: U.S.S.R. Acad. Sci. Publ. House, 1951.

13. Pavlov, I. P. *Selected works.* Moscow: Publ. House Foreign Languages, 1955.

14. Sechenov, J. M. *Selected papers.* Moscow: U.S.S.R. Acad. Pedag. Sci., 1952.

15. Vygotski, L. S. *Selected psychological papers.* Moscow: U.S.S.R. Acad. Pedag. Sci., 1956.

16. Yakovleva, S. V. The role of speech in the regulation of motor reaction in the preschool child. In Luria, A. R. (Ed.), *Problems of the higher nervous activity of normal and abnormal children.* Moscow, 1956.

17. Zaporozhets, A. V. The development of voluntary movements. *Vop. Psikhol.,* 1955.

18. Zaporozhets, A. V. The problem of voluntary movements in the light of the works of S. M. Sechenov. *Vop. Psikhol.,* 1956.

VII

Personality Research and Psychopathology: A Commentary

INTRODUCTION

FOUR OF THE FIVE CHAPTERS in this section are addressed to personality theory and research, and only one is concerned with psychopathology. That this distinction does not seem critical to the authors derives in large part from the influence of Freud. Four of the papers are directly concerned with issues raised by Freud, the colossus of personality theory and psychopathology who still exerts a profound influence. Only Luria's "Experimental Analysis of the Development of Voluntary Action in Children" could have been written whether or not there had been a Freud. This is also the chapter least concerned with pychopathology. It is in the best Russian tradition, which means an indebtedness to Pavlov and his co-workers. I will first discuss briefly each of the five chapters and then comment on the present state of psychopathology in general.

MILLER

The continuity of Miller's research with the past is obvious, but there is also real novelty here. He has, in an extensive program of research, explored in depth the interactions between social context and personality. It is only recently that we have begun to learn the full impact of the social context on psychopathology, and Miller is one of the pioneers responsible for this advance. Freud paid little more than lip service to sociocultural factors. Not only were the social sciences in their infancy at the end of the nineteenth century, but Freud was certainly more interested in the universals of the human situation than in the personality variations produced by sociocultural differences.

While Miller illuminates the significance of the social context he avoids a continuing pitfall in the psychological investigation of psychoanalytic concepts: to attain precision at the expense of content. Too many experimental investigations of psychoanalytic concepts have introduced experimental control and rigor by so restricting the field of inquiry that the question which is answered is not the one Freud raised.

Finally, Miller has reported unanticipated findings which are of interest. I refer to the fact that denial of both anger and failure varied significantly with verbal intelligence. Miller suggests, "If a boy is above a certain level of intelligence, he seems to rise above the handicaps of his background." This finding is certainly worth pursuing and particularly heartening in a democratic society.

ALEXANDER AND ADLERSTEIN

Alexander and Adlerstein have opened up for psychological theory and investigation a question of the same order of magnitude as of some of those raised by Freud. If this is so we may expect that the investigation of the prospect of one's own death will arouse as massive defensive maneuvers among psychologists as did the early investigations of sexuality and aggression.

The ubiquity and universality of the problem need no underlining. Its theoretical interest derives from the conjoint characteristics of remoteness (which varies in time) and ultimate unavoidability. It is as though one learned to cross the street with sufficient skill to avoid both death and the fear of death but with a dim awareness that no matter how much care one exercised he would ultimately be run over by the very automobiles he has no difficulty in keeping at a safe distance here and now. The techniques by which such a strain is met, its consequences for development and senility, its role in the etiology of mental disease, and the varieties of responses to death within the normal and abnormal population now assume significance.

Why did Freud not stress the significance of the fear of death? There is every reason to believe he was haunted by it and indeed he elevated it to the status of a regulatory principle—the death instinct. Was it because he could not face the *fear* of death with the equanimity he had when examining libidinal and aggressive wishes? I think not. It was because he could not free himself of the primary drive model—that he had first to demonstrate that the nightmares of the traumatic war neuroses were really *wish* (and therefore id, or drive) motivated, and ultimately that the wish behind aggression was self-destruction.

Although it was Freud who discovered the realm of affect, and particularly the role of anxiety, he was never able to assign a fundamental importance to affect because this was reserved for instinct or drive. Affect was only at the beginning equated with drive. It soon became the consequence of dammed-up drive transformed into anxiety, and in his later theory ended by being a *signal* that the ego uses to inform the person of "real" danger. To make aggression and the fear of death of more fundamental importance, he felt impelled to impute drive characteristics to each in turn. This is not the first time in the history of thought that an innovator has been partially trapped by the very categories he has generally revolutionized.

MAILLOUX AND ANCONA

Fear of death also assumes fresh significance in Mailloux and Ancona's clinical study of religious attitudes. They have discovered that crises of religious belief, marked by paralyzing uncertainty, are produced by a latent or conscious fear of death which is "loaded with the whole morbid uncertainty with which they face the problem of human destiny." On this point their study raises the same questions as Alexander and Adlerstein's— what is the relationship between coping with uncertainty in general and coping with death, which uniquely combines maximum ultimate certainty with maximum present uncertainty.

In a sense Mailloux and Ancona have also turned psycho-analytic theory against itself. If Freud exposed the infantile sources of religion, these researchers have exposed the infantile sources of *irreligion*. If God is the symbol of the father then it is a short step to show that fear, disenchantment, and hostility toward the father may determine an irreligiosity in no less neurotic a way than Freud demonstrated the positive transference. We are indebted to Mailloux and Ancona for this logical next step.

BLUM AND LURIA

Blum's chapter and that by Luria are not concerned with psychopathology proper. Luria reports on research with the development of voluntary action in children, and Blum deals with the "program" by which human beings process information from input to output. I have coupled them because both theorists employ the feedback principle.

Blum reflects, "It may seem that we have moved too far afield from psychoanalysis to feature the word in our title. To some extent this is true, inasmuch as we have made no systematic attempt to translate Freudian notions into the framework." He then goes on to show how much *is* Freudian in his theory. Luria makes no such disclaimer. He introduces the cybernetic model into the Pavlovian model with disarming directness. "To ensure a desirable result we had to rearrange our experiment so that the child's motor reaction could evoke a distinct exteroceptive stimulation which would serve as a signal of adequate action and inhibit any further movements in accordance with the feedback principle." Here then are a Pavlovian and a Freudian-electronic comrade, cybernetic bedfellows. This may be like having a large picture window in a Gothic cathedral. Can one engraft novelty upon an older corpus? It is, I think, the rule in ideology rather than the exception, that the large picture window *does* let in more light.

Even in the case of Freud it is clear: he carried a burden of 19th century conceptual baggage at the time he was forging some of the critical modern concepts. While discovering the extreme plasticity of the domains of affect and thinking he tied the transformable affects to the more fixed drive structures and the conceptual transformations to the same relatively stable, slow moving "primary" processes. Although he spoke in terms of information transformations, he could not rid himself of energy models, of "forces," hydraulic and somewhat inert in nature. His was a combined information and energy model. Blum has taken out some more of the energy characteristics and maximized the informational aspects.

Luria has modernized the Pavlovian model. Certainly that model lacked the flexibility of any cybernetic mechanisms—those made of wire and steel. It is time that the simpler "signal systems" have their loops extended beyond the skin, and also that they have a "return" channel, as in the feedback model.

Since we discovered that we can build intelligent mechanisms we appear to be more ready to accept "purpose" in man. It is paradoxical that American psychology was reluctant to admit the ingenious nature of man's own mechanism until he was able to externalize it in a "real" model. Now that we can externalize the inner circuitry, psychologists may be prepared to be bolder in conceiving the nature of their own design. Blum's model is one of a very great number of possible block diagrams. It is a carefully considered "circuit" and lends itself to empirical testing. We cannot ask more at this stage of communication network models. Any model which has sufficient precision to lead to testable consequences is a good one. We are here employing the feedback principle itself as a criterion of the scientific value of a theory.

PRESENT STATUS OF PSYCHOPATHOLOGY

The frontiers of psychopathology today extend in three main directions: the social context of psychopathology, the affective response mechanism, and the mechanisms of information processing. Paradoxically, Freud's "psychological" determinism has led to biochemistry and neurophysiology and engineering on the one hand, and to the social sciences on the other.

Social contexts: We are becoming increasingly aware that there are important differences in incidence of mental disease in different cultures as well as different subcultures, that a lower-class American schizophrenic is not exactly like a middle-class American schizophrenic, and that there are also sharp differences in readiness for different types of psychotherapy in lower and middle class Americans. Miller's chapter reflected the growing concern and knowledge in this area. It seems clear that important new insights await the social scientist who cultivates the domain of class, culture, and psychopathology. We may anticipate no serious resistance to the further exploration of this frontier.

Affective response mechanisms: Not so with the investigation of the affective response mechanism. Revolutionary discoveries in this area have caught us conceptually unprepared. We now know two vital facts. First, it is possible to stimulate specific subcortical centers which act as "joy" or "aversive" stimulation. An animal will work to continue stimulation to one center and to turn off stimulation to another center. Secondly, we know it is possible to so help a chronic, long-institutionalized schizophrenic with tranquilizing drugs, that he may become ambulatory and leave his mental hospital.

In such a case, we have not changed his "personality" in any fundamental way but we have helped him dramatically. The significance of the latter phenomenon has not been appreciated because we have believed, after Freud, that symptomatic relief is not "cure." Cure necessarily involves basic personality change (or so many of us believe) and tranquilizers are often regarded with some suspicion, if not hostility. Similarly, the discovery of the joy and aversive centers, while exciting to most psychologists, has nonetheless not been integrated into personality or learning theory.

Both of these embarrassments of riches stem from a single source: the century-old doctrine of the primary drives as the fundamental motivators. Only the biologists, Darwin, Cannon, Crile, and Selye, have addressed themselves directly to the problem of the emotions. In psychology proper they have constituted an isolated chapter in our elementary textbooks.

Only after Pavlov accidentally produced an experimental neurosis, and Freud began to influence American psychology, did there begin to be an enduring interest in one kind of affect-anxiety. It was studied for the most part, however, not as anxiety but as "avoidance behavior," i.e. what and how the animal would learn to reduce anxiety. This could be and was assimilated to the dominant American interest in learning theory. It did not increase our interest in the nature of the affect itself. The latter has been somewhat awkwardly labelled as "learned" drive or secondary drive.

I have argued that the apparent urgency of the primary drives is an artifact produced by the *concomitant* activation of the affective response mechanism which provides powerful amplification of the drive signal. The "excitement" of the sexual drive is in the chest, not the genitals, and when the affect is fear or satiation the sex drive does not appear to be so powerful, nor does it necessarily lead to sexual behavior. Further, excitement can and is "emitted" to a wide variety of stimuli and states other than sexual stimulation. Rather than suggesting that such interests represent "sublimation," I have argued that sexual excitement is a special case of the more general excitement. The same argument holds for the most compelling of drives—the need for oxygen. It is the accompanying panic which we have confused with the felt oxygen need. If the latter continues until euphoria is activated the individual may go to his ironic death with a smile on his lips.

The affective mechanism has generality of time and object. The drive mechanism does not. One can be hungry only periodically. If one were *always* hungry one would die, and so equally if one were *never* hungry. A human being may live his life always frightened or never frightened, always excited or never excited. It is because of this generality that affect can play such a monopolistic role in the economy of the individual.

If the affective system is a separate one from the drive system, and takes precedence over the latter, then the investigation of its nature opens very exciting possibilities for psychopathology. The reticular system and the drugs which can influence it now assume a primary significance for the understanding and control of mental disease. It is not unlikely that Freud's earlier views delivered in 1909 at Clark may have been more fundamental than the later metapsychology. He said then of the theory of hysteria, "We assign the first rank to the affective processes." Mental disease may well turn out to be a disorder primarily of the emotions in which thought disorders are the derivatives.

Information processing: The third frontier, we said, is the field of communication theory and information processing. Here the neurophysiologist, engineer, and mathematician are converging on possible brain models which may illuminate the circuitry within us. It is not altogether unlikely that the computers we build will bear some resemblance to our own information processing mechanisms. We cannot help but design these mechanisms in our own image even if we wished to do otherwise. They are inevitably "projections." It is clear, however, that this whole enterprise has alarmed many who feel man is being degraded by the analogy. Rather than admiring the externalization of man's intelligence these critics are fearful that either man will be subdued by his own creation or be humiliated by it. That this reflects a prejudice is clear from the contrary bases for rejection of the analogy: the machine that will degrade man by excelling him, as against the machine that degrades man by its inferiority.

From the neurophysiological investigation of the perceptual process has come the intriguing possibility that what Freud thought of as repression, i.e. the erecting of barriers to intolerable information, may in fact be a very general type of response in the handling of all information and particularly sensory information. Recent evidence here suggests that centrifugal inhibitory messages *prevent* sensory messages from reaching the cortex when the organism is busy attending to some other channel. It also appears possible that the ability to inhibit is directly related to intelligence.

The value of a more precise model of the information processing mechanism for psychopathology consists in the possibility of being able to plug in more effectively into the affective conceptual matrix than we can now. It was not until Mowrer illuminated the "neurotic paradox," the non-extinguishability of certain learned fears, that the problem of the *acquisition* of these responses appeared in a new light. Unless we can spell out in greater detail how an individual learns to be afraid, we have little hope of control and reversal of the processes. What is needed is a model which integrates the affective system with the information processing system.

SUMMARY

Almost all the chapters in this section reflect the continuing influence of Freud, although only one is directly concerned with psychopathology. Some of the major research trends in contemporary personality theory and psychopathology are illustrated. The three main frontiers today are the social context, the affective responses, and the mechanisms of processing information.

PART THREE

Person Perception

Franz From

VIII
Perception of Human Action

INTRODUCTION

IT'S ABOUT TIME, I think, we stop allowing behaviorism to scare us away from the study of behavior. If we want to learn something about human behavior, I believe the best idea is to start studying it in whatever way we can.

It's an excellent idea to study rats and their conditioned reflexes, if we want to increase our knowledge of rats. Studying displaced reactions of geese and gulls is laudable, too, if we are interested in precisely these topics. But, to study mice to know men is probably not one of "the best-laid schemes," in the words of Robert Burns, speaking o' mice an' men. In this chapter, then, I shall focus on human beings.

THE BEHAVIORISTIC FALLACY

To my mind other people and their behavior comprise one of the most important fields of modern psychology; this is in contrast to the earlier approach and its focus on the individual and his inner life. Somehow, research psychologists have not been very interested in the way we experience human actions. Behavior has been regarded as something independent of the observer, as if behavior were objective and the study of behavioral experience irrelevant.

A few psychologists have touched on the problem. Koffka[5] discussed how we experience our own behavior as "phenomenal or experienced." He termed our experience of other people's behavior "apparent behavior" but did not elaborate. Köhler,[4] in his volume on Gestalt Psychology, wrote about how we perceive other people's inner life from their behavior. Rubin[6] similarly considered the structure of our experiences of others. Noting that in daily life there is no sharp Cartesian distinction between body and mind, he suggested that when we perceive other people's behavior we experience almost undifferentiated entities which are not manifest as a mixture of something mental plus somthing material.

Suppose we take an everyday example. You see a man who has just stuck a cigarette between his lips put his hand into his pocket for his matches. You do not see—and it would in fact demand a special set (or *Einstellung*) to see—that he moves his hand downwards close to his thigh, then slightly upwards, lifting the edge of his jacket, and then downwards at an angle into his trouser pocket. You simply see him put his hand into his pocket to get his matches. (If you try to remember some of the things you have seen people do thousands of times, you realize how difficult it is to recall the precise movements involved; for example, when someone sits down on a chair or hangs up his jacket.)

We see the movements and purpose as one, and very rarely do we isolate in our experience of behavior the movements involved. The purpose is experienced as an integral aspect of the act, and we describe acts by naming the purpose, not by listing the movements concerned. This is true even when the movements are not human or are not even made by living organisms, but are movements of triangles and circles on a screen, as Heider and Simmel[3] have shown in their elegant experiments.

The fact that we so easily describe other people's behavior by naming the purpose we perceive in no way implies that the purpose is experienced as something separate, as something with an independent existence, "behind" the movements, so to speak, or in any other way divorced from the experienced movements. There is no dualism in our actual experience of the behavior, as Rubin pointed out, and in ordinary circumstances we do not experience people as composed of a mind and a body. We do not normally experience the behavior of others as consisting of something material (movements, body) and apart from that something mental (mind, e.g. purpose). The fact that no separation exists in our experience of behavior between body and mind, between material and mental, has caused considerable confusion among behaviorists. Watson,[9] for instance, thought that "the time seems to have come when psychology must discard all reference to consciousness; when it need no longer delude itself into thinking that it is making mental states the object of observation." Yet, when Watson tried to describe human behavior without mentioning consciousness, he employed terms that at the same time referred both to the material and the mental aspects of perceived behavior; the ghost of consciousness cannot be exorcized so simply. As Rubin[6] observed the behaviorists who base their descriptions on acts, rather than on a three-dimensional system of physical coordinates, escape the difficulties inherent in their theoretical approach, since by such descriptions they smuggle the mind back in again.

Because we simply see what people do, and because the experience of purpose is not the result of a conscious process of deduction from, or interpretation of, movements, but is something immediately apparent, it has been possible to make the peculiar mistake of regarding behavior with its inherent purpose as something belonging to the sphere of objective facts. And, in making this mistake, which might be called the behavioristic fallacy, the important task of elucidating *how* we *experience* behavior has, in my opinion, been grossly neglected.

THE EXPERIENCE OF PURPOSE

I'd like to discuss in more detail some of my experiments[2] on how we experience purpose and the role this plays in our experiences of actions. I used short films lasting about three minutes. Some showed the behavior of a single person; others were of groups.

One of the films, for example, presents a man sitting at a desk. He is working (writing). When the subjects experience that the man is doing some form of writing, this experienced purpose can function as a set, and influence the way in which the stimuli are processed. Or, I should rather say, corresponding to the experience of a purpose, an *Einstellung* has been aroused in the subject, which can determine the way the stimuli are processed. This can be seen when the man stops writing and does something else. In several cases the subject then experiences this behavior according to the *Einstellung* previously aroused. Even when the material aspect is altered (the man has stopped writing and has begun to do something else), the subject still experiences the same meaning: when the man gets up from his chair, several subjects report that he wants to get a needed book.

The purpose which the subjects experience the behavior to have does not necessarily change immediately because the material aspect of the behavior changes. The subjects may continue to experience the behavioral events according to the original set, which again corresponds to the purpose first perceived. A person may, in fact, continue to process events according to his original set in spite of very great changes in the material aspect, parallelling the constancy phenomena in the perception of size, shape, and color.

The experienced purpose, thus, functions as an *Einstellung* which may determine how we process the stimuli. When the subjects experience that the man in the film is drawing, a certain object is perceived as an eraser. Later, when he is lighting his pipe, the same object is perceived as a box of matches. A magician makes use of this phenomenon quite systematically. By letting us experience a purpose different from his "real" intentions, he makes us perceive events which do not actually occur.

The original purpose is, so to speak, retained as long as possible; but, naturally, the course of events may in the end force a change when it is no longer possible to harmonize the actions and the experienced purpose. Usually in such circumstances the subject sooner or later experiences that the man has a new purpose; the stimuli are then processed in agreement with a new set corresponding to the experienced new purpose.

There is one more detail related to the experience of purpose that I consider rather important. When the experience of a sequence of actions leads to the necessity of relinquishing a particular experienced purpose, because the later actions contradict it and prove that the subject was mistaken, we find, interestingly enough, that the original purpose does not always become completely inactive. It seems that it is kept ready, so that it will exert its influence again as soon as the course of events allows it to do so.

In some special experiments I used a film in which a man is seen sitting at a table, working. Very soon he gets up and puts on his jacket. Most subjects experience this as an intention on his part to leave the room, but he sits down again and continues working. Later on in the film, he leaves the table for a moment, but returns immediately with a book, which he opens. The subjects have thus twice had an opportunity to experience the purpose "he will leave the room," but in such a way that it later was contradicted.

It was especially interesting to note the way in which the subjects experienced the end of the film, where, in the final frame, the man is still sitting at the table. The distribution of the reports of the 44 subjects (Group A) taking part in these experiments is shown in Table 1. A third of the subjects experience that the man leaves the room at the end of the film, and if we include those who think he leaves but are not absolutely certain, we near the 50 percent mark. Only a quarter of the subjects experience that the man remains sitting at the table, which is what he does.

Next, I removed the two scenes in which the man gets up from his chair, so that the newly edited film shows someone who remains sitting at the table throughout. I showed this version to 28 subjects (Group B), and once again concentrated on how they experienced the end of the film. Their report distribution has also been recorded in Table 1. Now, no one experiences that the man leaves the room at the end of the film—and 82 percent

TABLE 1—*Film endings as experienced by two groups*

Response	Group A N=44	Group B N=28
He leaves the room	34%	0%
I think he leaves the room	14%	4%
He gets up, finishes what he is doing, replaces his books . . .	25%	11%
He remains sitting at the table	25%	71%
Cannot remember	2%	14%

of the subjects actually say that he is still working at the table. These results lend strong support to the assumption that the contradicted purpose played a role in the first film.

If we wish to discover how we experience behavior, therefore, it is not satisfactory merely to investigate the purpose we experience people to have at the moment. We must also study the previous, incorrect, purposes that have been experienced.

Another matter of importance for person perception is the peculiar tendency to "put the blame on others." One transfers his mistakes to other people in quite a naive manner because of what I have called the "behavioristic fallacy." We see what a person intends to do without any feeling of uncertainty, and when the person in question fails to act in accordance with this intention, then obviously the discrepancies must be due to his mistake; he has decided to do something else, or the like.

It is quite common for subjects to say that "he was about to leave, but then he remembered that he had forgotten something." Or, "he went to get the book, but it was not where he had expected it to be," or something similar.

EXPERIENCING ACTIONS OF OTHERS

There are important problems involved in the strangely "intolerant" attitude adopted by subjects when they cannot experience behavior as purposeful, and when the other person's behavior therefore appears to be meaningless. In my previously mentioned experiments the subjects did not experience that *they* lacked the necessary background for understanding the behavior if they experienced the man's behavior as meaningless; on the contrary, they experienced that there was something wrong with the man, that *he* was behaving aimlessly, was peculiar, or mad.

This tendency constitutes an important element in the intolerant attitude so often adopted toward people from groups with a different background whom we find difficult to understand. Such an attitude plays a role in the relationships between men and women, parents and children, employers and employees. It is quite usual to regard people from social classes different from one's own as peculiar. The same is true of nations and races. The greater the difference, the more meaningless we think the behavior is. The more primitive and undeveloped a person is, the less he understands the behavior of others, the more he will be liable to regard people as queer, and then tend toward intolerance.

Finding others peculiar often turns into finding them condemnable. It is not uncommon to regard all behavior not in agreement with *our* rules of conduct as more or less immoral.

As part of the more extensive investigation of how we perceive the behavior of others, I became interested in how we experience behavior breaking the usual rules of conduct. Offensive behavior seemed to be especially well-suited for this purpose.[2]

The following experiment was made: A student interrupted the speaker three times during a lecture, each time becoming more offensive and finally leaving the classroom in protest. After ten minutes the audience was informed that the incident had been planned. The 48 students attending were asked to write a report of the events and to describe how they had been affected. They were first-year psychology students.

There were several reasons why the students were told the episode had been prearranged: They could express themselves more freely; otherwise some might have been cautious so as not to hurt a fellow student. The very fact that the students were asked to write down what they had experienced might have provoked some suspicion that the whole thing had been pre-arranged. They might have imagined that it had been an experiment and this would have introduced an irrelevant factor; as it was, only two subjects reported a slight suspicion of play-acting. All but one wrote unsigned reports, but indicated their age and sex.

One of the subjects reported: "Right in the middle of an interesting lecture a student suddenly interrupts the lecturer, requiring him to repeat the last bit of his lecture '. . . as it wasn't clear to me.' At the time I felt extreme contempt for the interrupter. My first thought was something like 'the self-assert-ing fool—the silly idiot.' But it became even worse when a little later he persisted and stopped the lecturer in an even more offensive way. The majority of the audience now protested and assured the lecturer that they could easily understand him. The considerable tension created by the offender culminates when he very noisily collects his things, closes his briefcase with a smack, and leaves the room remarking that this is too much for him. I then vacillated between two theories: (a) there is a personal conflict between the lecturer and him, and he is unable to control his emotions; or (b) he is perhaps overstrained and mentally unbalanced. It never occurred to me that it might be play-acting."

Another student wrote: "Sometime during the first half of the lecture, there is an interruption by one of the students. He asked the lecturer to repeat his explanation of his drawings on the board; it had something to do with binocular vision. He then said that this was the first time he had attended lectures on this topic and therefore he had difficulties in following the lecturer. He asked for the repetition in a very impolite and arrogant tone. The lecturer explained what the student couldn't understand. A little later the same student interrupted again, this time in a much more insulting and offensive tone, saying that he did not understand anything at all. A certain uneasiness in the audience showed that it was against the interruptor. From all sides it was said that the explanation was clear enough. A moment later he got up, gathered his books with a lot of noise, and left the classroom saying something like 'I am sorry I have to leave; when you can't explain better, I might as well leave.' He was a boor and a beast."

All find his behavior queer and 80 percent consider it condemnable to a greater or lesser degree. Many condemn him immediately, finding his interruption irritating, impolite, foolish, and so on. Others make more allowances for him and find his first interruption forgivable, understandable or even justified. One applauds his first objection: "I was sitting right in front of the quarrelsome student and I turned around and said to him 'Very good' because I didn't understand the first explanation either. The next time he interrupted, he seemed very irritated and asked the lecturer in very sharp (it seemed to me impolite and improper) words to explain more clearly. This time I didn't understand his interruption; I found it embarrassing."

Another student sympathized with his unorthodox manner and "liked him for a while," but then dissociated himself from the student because his second interruption seemed aggressive: "His frankness was almost impudent."

In other cases a "Gestalt-factor" in experienced behavior appears to play a part. This is something which I have also found in other experiments. When behavior is experienced as having a certain meaning, this meaning will affect both the past and the future, and the entire sequence will be perceived as a whole with a homogeneous quality. In the present case the sequence is experienced as offensive, from the moment when he first opens his mouth to when he insultingly slams the door on his departure. His voice, gait, movements, looks, everything is part of the offensive whole; some even include his past, remembering that he was also argumentative before.

How, then, does this offensive person appear to his fellow students? To eighteen of them (37 percent) he is merely a type, "one of those who behaves in that way." As one subject says: "When he interrupted the first time, I thought that he was a self-asserting type, who does not underestimate himself in any way; an unsympathetic type." Often such classification serves as a pseudoexplanation, as for example when he is put down as "a very young person" (as the youngest subject wrote).

For twenty others (42 percent) he is an individual with his own character, while the remaining ten do not pay any attention to this problem. Those to whom he is a strong individual attempt an explanation of his behavior instead of merely taking offense.

The experience of inner life in others: As long as others in any given situation "do what is done," or their behavior in some other way follows directly from the situation, they are experienced without complications. Their inner life may appear in an indefinite and undifferentiated way—for example, when we experience our classmates during a lecture. As soon as a person does something which does not follow directly from the situation, his inner life may emerge in a more definite way, and we perceive, for instance, his wishes, desires, and intentions. However, in the experiment in which the student definitely breaks the rules of conduct, his inner life does not reveal itself sufficiently to make such behavior understandable.

In a number of social situations we are actively interested in understanding the behavior of others, and if this is not possible behavioristically, it is explained by our perception of the person's inner life. This can be seen in our experiment from the following examples: "He became furious when laughed at," "became embittered when his objections were not followed," etc.

Only a few subjects try this sort of explanation; a greater number, ten, directly experience his behavior as being due to his bearing a long-standing grudge against the lecturer. In other words, an action not understandable on the basis of the present situation becomes understandable when perceived as an actual manifestation of a more permanent emotional attitude, a "sentiment," as Shand uses the term.[7]

In the majority of cases, the experience is not so precisely differentiated. The person is simply seen as being in an *abnormal state*, this being the explanation of his *abnormal behavior*. He is nervous, ill, overstrained, mentally unbalanced, etc. As one has it: "My first thought was that he must be drunk or in some other abnormal state. I was very offended by his behavior which seemed impertinent and foolish."

The attitudes of the subjects in the situation: "Tout comprendre" is not always *"tout pardonner,"* which the experiment also shows very clearly: twenty-three students try to find some explanation for his behavior, but fifteen of these condemn his actions in spite of the explanation found. Often, explanations are used which are really condemnations in disguise, as when he is described as unintelligent, not quite right, abnormal, very juvenile, etc.

The reasons for condemning him vary. One student is irritated by the interruption in the middle of listening to the lecture. General irritation is expressed about his insolence, impudence, aggressiveness, etc. Many describe a more complex attitude. A girl writes, for example: "I squirmed and felt all queer inside— shame and dismay—deep sympathy with the lecturer—desire to remedy—look especially understanding. The comical element in the situation is, however, evident. I rejoiced a little because another dared—I had perhaps wanted to do so myself. But to leave in protest, that is too much—the whole audience is ready to side with the lecturer. He has now gone so far *outside* the group that one goes against him—this is the limit—one can not do a thing like that—poor lecturer!"

Several go so far as to want or expect the punishment of the offender, and while only one subject expresses understanding sympathy toward him, there is a general sympathetic feeling toward the offended lecturer. It almost looks as if the subjects were afraid of being suspected of siding with the offender, thus risking the anger of the offended authority and the displeasure of the majority. (Captain Castenskiold, M. A., carried out a somewhat similar experiment in a class of officers at the Military Academy. One of his subjects finished his report this way: "As far as I was concerned, the whole situation embarrassed me because I got the idea that the Captain might think that the officer who made the interruptions and the rest of the class had decided to try to provoke the Captain.") Without going further into the matter I would like to mention the theory of Westermarck[10] stating: "Again, as to acts which are supposed to arouse the

anger of invisible powers, the people are anxious to punish them
with the utmost severity so as to prevent the divine wrath from
turning against the community itself." We could also refer to
Durkheim's hypothesis [1] that the severity of punishment decreases as governments become less despotic.

During the expulsion of the offender, there are some who
describe how the others' reactions increased their own emotions:
"The others felt the same way as I did; this made me feel even
more offended." Each of us may have his own opinion about
the incident, but we feel supported when others think as we
do. As Adam Smith [8] said: "Our continual observations upon the
conduct of others insensibly lead us to form to ourselves certain
general rules concerning what is fit and proper either to be done
or to be avoided. Some of their actions shock all our natural
sentiments. We hear everybody about us express the like detes-
tation against them. This still further confirms and even exas-
perates our natural sense of their deformity. It satisfies us that
we view them in the proper light, when we see other people view
them in the same light."

This common feeling of embarrassment seems to link the
group members closer together. As one subject wrote in his report: "Afterwards a certain relief and fellow-feeling toward the
group and lecturer made itself felt. The tension ended in spontaneous laughter." Others find the laughter forced; as one subject says: "When the door closed behind him, we broke into
laughter, but I did not really think the episode funny, so the
reaction may have been somewhat artificial."

Many used the expression "painful episode." The situation
was dangerous in an indefinite way. One could suggest the
theory that the impending rupture of the group, more dangerous
because of the opposition to the lecturer's authority, creates an
intangible fear of finding oneself on the wrong side when the
group splits—it is impossible beforehand to be absolutely certain
whom the majority of the group will follow.

This may perhaps, in part, explain why so many feel "violent
anger, indignation, extreme ill-will, exceptional disgust, wrath,
dreadful irritation," and so on, or as one describes her reaction:
"I was stunned for a moment, then felt violent abhorrence for

the young man, and was extremely embarrassed on his behalf." Anger is aroused by his breaking the rules, desire is felt to show goodwill toward the offended party, one's own accord with the group is stressed. When the offender complained that the lecture was incomprehensible, many cried out that they understood it fully and one noted that "I was among the first who said aloud that I had quite easily understood the lecturer's exposition."

Here we recognize another attitude described by Adam Smith: [8] "We resolve never to be guilty of the like, nor ever, upon any account, to render ourselves in this manner the objects of universal disapprobation."

An emotion of the type here investigated offers a richly varied and complicated picture. I hope I have succeeded in sketching in some of the main lines. It appears to me that the *method employed* offers greater possibilities for the clarification of such problems than one gains from most of the usual experimental situations where the subject's attitude is supposed to be kept neutral.

With the present method the subject is personally and emotionally involved in the experimental situation. He plays an active part, and we can gain some insight into the complex way in which the ego is involved when we perceive the behavior of others. We see certain lines in the very complicated emotional pattern which develops in the individual, much like ice-ferns spreading over a window.

SUMMARY

Human behavior cannot be described purely in the language of physics; it is more than a series of physical events. So-called behavioristic descriptions, e.g. actions or trials, "smuggle" mind back in again, although behaviorists rarely realize that such entities always have a mental aspect.

I have tried to report on experiments showing how experienced purposes influence the way we experience behavior, and how rules of conduct may influence our perception of a series of human actions. The laws that govern perception have only begun to be investigated.

References

1. Durkheim, E. Deux lois de l'évolution pénale. *Ann. Sociol.*, 1899-1900, 4.

2. From, F. *Am Oplevelsen af Andres Adfaerd.* Copenhagen, 1953.

3. Heider, F. and Simmel, Marianne. An experimental study of apparent behavior. *Amer. J. Psychol.*, 1944, 57.

4. Köhler, W. *Psychologische Probleme.* Berlin: Springer, 1933.

5. Koffka, K. *Principles of Gestalt psychology.* New York: Harcourt, 1935.

6. Rubin, E. Bemerkungen über unser Wissen von anderen Menschen. *Exp. Psychol.* Copenhagen, 1949.

7. Shand, A. *The foundations of character.* London, 1914.

8. Smith, A. *The theory of moral sentiments.* London, 1804.

9. Watson, J. B. Psychology as the behaviorist views it. *Psychol. Rev.*, 1913, 20.

10. Westermarck, E. *The origin and development of moral ideas.* Vol. I. London, 1912.

Renato Tagiuri

IX

Movement as a
Cue in Person Perception*

INTRODUCTION

How PEOPLE PERCEIVE or know their human environment and
the way in which these processes are related to action is little
understood scientifically. The lack of comprehensive systematic
treatment of this problem is keenly felt in the analysis of interpersonal behavior, the very foundation of social psychology. Yet,
for all its importance, interpersonal perception is a relatively
new topic among the recognized areas in psychology.

This is not to say that students of behavior, from Plato on,
have not considered and written on this topic. It is, rather, that
it has never become a classical issue in psychology. Philosophers
have anticipated us here. A portion of the International Philosophical Congress of 1953, in Brussels, was devoted to the problem of the *connaissance d'autrui*, with major emphasis on the
nature of empathy, but in previous discussions of the problem
of how we know other minds, philosophers had not contributed
much to the *psychological* understanding of how we gain knowledge as to the *specific* content and nature of others' personalities.

* This work was done in the Laboratory of Social Relations and the
Graduate School of Business Administration, Harvard University, under
Office of Naval Research Contract No. N5ori-07670.

The author wishes to acknowledge the collaboration of Dean Peabody
and Edward Furash, both of whom contributed generously of ideas and
effort.

If we look at the psychological literature that has explicitly addressed itself to the problem of person perception, we find that, especially in the United States, the bulk of it is concerned with the problem of accuracy. Psychologists working in this area turned to quantification prematurely. In so doing they were caught in a veritable jungle of artifacts, the nature of which was, at first, unclear. However, students interested in process, such as Heider and Asch, threw doubt on the fruitfulness of such cognitive achievement-oriented research, and the mathematically sophisticated, Cronbach in particular, made a clear analysis of the factors involved.* These contributions have had their effect, for the emphasis on veridicality is decreasing and the tide is turning in the direction of analysis of the *processes* involved in knowing others.

In this chapter, we will attempt to contribute to this trend by speaking of the role of movement in the process of understanding other persons. By movement is meant the displacement through space of the *entire stimulus person,* and not what has sometimes been called expressive movement, such as gait, gesture, handwriting, and so on.

The strategy of inquiry in interpersonal perception is to find a point of attack that is neither hopelessly complex nor utterly trivial. The problem of what constitutes cues to inferences about other persons has, by and large, defied systematic treatment, for the relevant stimulus variables can seldom be described in terms of the classical dimensions of psychophysics. Movement, however, constitutes at least one important class of cues that can be studied under fairly rigid experimental conditions. Movement is, of course, an aspect intrinsic to several of the forms of stimulus used in research on interpersonal perception. What has not yet been done is an explicit analysis of the movement aspect of the complex configuration.

---

* It is very important to realize that the difficulties encountered in quantitative studies of *accuracy* cannot be eliminated by resorting to careful *qualitative* approaches. Such processes as real and assumed similarity, stereotype and differential accuracy, favorability sets and artifactual relationships, to mention but a few, apply to any kind of inquiry into person perception. The difficulties are inherent in any "dyadic analysis," in the sense of the phrase used by Cronbach in a recent paper.[3]

Except for Heider and Simmel,[6] students of interpersonal perception have not focussed on movement as a point of attack on the problem of person perception. However, investigators interested essentially in other problems have discussed the anthropomorphic meaning of movement. Michotte,[13] for example, describes the physical combinations of movement that correspond to various interpretations of human-like behavior, showing the extraordinary complexity and "depth" of meaning that can be conveyed by two rectangles moving variously in a straight line.

I think there are enough "obvious" reasons for considering movement an important source of cues. There are, however, others. Take, for example, the phylogenetic and ontogenetic evidence that perception of movement develops very early as a process distinct from perception of stationary forms. Or, the well-known fact that attention is extremely sensitive to movement in the peripheral field of vision—without necessarily involving the recognition of the *nature* of the moving object—and that this is followed by immediate turning and focussing of the eye upon the object. The potential injuriousness of *any* moving object makes discriminations in terms of movement prior in importance and, probably, in response readiness to, say, form or color discrimination.

METHODOLOGY

In our own work we have so far used two major methods of inquiry. In one—to which we shall refer as the "frozen path" method—we present a curved line as shown in Figure 1. The subject is asked to consider this line as a *path* described by a *person* moving in space from left to right; from point A, the *start*, to point B, the *end* or *goal* point. The instructions state that the movement was completely unencumbered by physical characteristics of the terrain and that it took place in daylight. The subject is to tell us what he can about the *personality* and *character* of an individual who would move in that particular way. In some conditions nothing about the goal is said in the instruc-

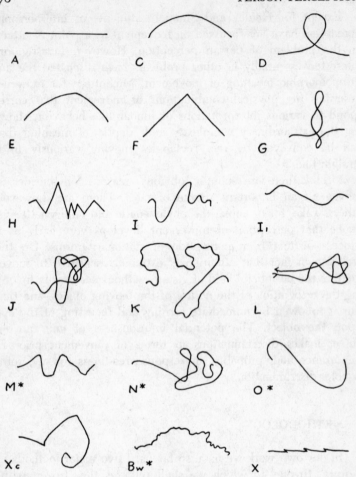

Fig. 1. Selected paths.

tions, in others the goal is described as desirable, or undesirable, or indifferent.

Similar instructions were used with a second method where the stimulus materials consisted of a film showing a dot moving from point A to point B. Essentially the same patterns were used for the films as in the "frozen paths." The speed of movement was held constant in this work, but it is obvious that change in speed is one of the most important sources of information about the person moving, and we plan to investigate it later.

A third method, used mostly for checking specific hunches, was to describe the person and the situation to the subjects and ask them to draw an appropriate path. This technique is particularly useful for discovering what *different* paths have *similar* meanings. All the methods described above were adapted for group administration.

Interviews were used in the earlier phases of the work to find out whether the techniques were practicable as well as to observe closely the behavior of the subjects. It was particularly important to ascertain whether the "frozen path" methods would be used at all, since we were leaning heavily on the cognitive contribution of the subjects to the stimulus situation. We can report that the subjects had no difficulty conceiving of the patterns as *paths of persons*. This is fortunate since the technique is very convenient in its simplicity. Nor was there much difficulty in relying on set, induced by means of the instructions, for obtaining variations in experimental conditions.

The *data* consist of free responses, mostly single terms descriptive of personality or character, often short phrases (e.g. "he is not sure of himself"). The subject was asked to indicate which of his responses he deemed most appropriate. We shall refer to the response so singled out as the "preferred" response. This report is based mostly on "preferred" response data.

The subjects were college students. Preliminary work with children suggests that the methods could be used with younger and less intelligent subjects.

THE NATURE OF THE DATA

To give, first, some impressions of the sort of data we obtain, let me list the *preferred* responses to two different patterns, where no information regarding the goal valence was given in the instructions.

The responses to the straight path (pattern A) are: *Well-reasoned, aggressive, persevering, determined, logical, purpose-*

ful, rational, knows where he is going, goal-oriented, practical, alert, unimaginative, resolute, ambitious, direct, economical, Good Christian, dull. Most subjects gave additional responses. These included many words or phrases that did not occur among the preferred responses, such as: *stubborn, cold, impatient, extrovert, conformist, honest, preoccupied, precise, witty, humorless, dogmatic, expedient, narrow-minded.*

If we now take the meandering pattern K, the preferred responses are: *immature, very emotional, stupid, irresponsible, vacillating, undependable, gay, careless, untrustworthy, confused, upset, sociable, unconcerned, wavering, wanderer, meticulous, prissy, disjointed, little sense of direction, happy-go-lucky, wandering mind, extremely indecisive to the point of confusion, extremely emotionally unbalanced, dependent on others to lead him, curiosity.* Again, among the additional responses we find many other items, such as *fear of accepting responsibility, unambitious, shy.*

There are a few general remarks I would like to make about these data, points that also apply to results obtained from other paths, and that will acquire relevance later on in the chapter.

There is, first, some question as to whether a line pattern conveys different information when interpreted as a path than it does when interpreted as a pattern-qua-pattern. Are the interpretations we obtain simple elaborations of the Ehrenfels qualities of the line? To investigate this we studied responses to the patterns when no reference to persons or "path" was made in the instructions. We find that the patterns are spontaneously viewed in one of several ways—simply as patterns to be described in terms of their physical characteristics, as symbolic representations of an idea, as symbolic representations of a person, and as the path of an object or person. In some cases it is possible to see that respondents structure the stimuli differently for these different sets. For example, the pattern shown below can be

viewed as an arch-like structure, suggesting *stability*. This is obviously quite different from conceiving of it as an *indirect* path, suggestive of *cautious approach*. Typical descriptions of pattern A, the straight line, are: *horizontal, level, straight, flat, even, smooth, direct, right, solid, sure*, and so on. Many responses, such as *straight* and *direct*, are clearly the type of response basic to more personalistic inferences obtained in reactions to paths. For pattern K, the responses, such as *rough, curvy, crooked, erratic, irregular, random, uncertain*, are often terms that can be applied to persons. In many cases the subjects spontaneously interpret the patterns as paths, irrespective of the instructions.

Our impression is that the meaning of a line pattern is often determined by the fact that it is spontaneously seen as a temporally organized event, and so interpreted. It may then be somewhat futile to attempt to distinguish *paths* from *patterns* for our purpose. The important fact for us is that subjects have no great difficulty responding to the patterns as paths, and that consequently this simple technique can be added to the repertoire of useful methods for approaching problems of interpersonal perception.

It is apparent that the interpretations of the patterns vary enormously in the extent to which they are removed from a literal description of the path. For the straight line, for instance, responses range all the way from the literal interpretation *direct* to such items as *logical, ambitious*, and *dogmatic*. Similarly, for pattern K, responses range from the literal description *wavering*, to *sociable, untrustworthy*, and *immature*.

This great range of inferential directness is interesting for at least two reasons. It shows, for one thing, how readily we infer from the simplest *physical* aspects of behavior to some of the most *inner* qualities. Whether in actual life these extraordinarily informative cues are taken seriously or not is an experimentally unanswered question. My belief is that they are. If I am correct, then my impression is that this source of information has not been given sufficient attention by students of person perception. This may be due partly to the fact that in actual life we have some access to the inner man. He or others tell us about him, or we make inferences from complex auxiliary evidence. Thus we fail to give explicit weight to the great many inferences we probably make from definitely external and relatively simple events of which movement is an important example. I am, in short, suggesting that we may not realize the extent to which our impressions of others are based on their movement, actual or symbolic.

The other interesting thing about the wide range of literalness in interpretations is that it seems possible to arrange the responses given by a number of subjects in a rough order of remoteness from the more literal interpretations. When this is done one has a composite reconstruction of what may be the steps implicit in the more indirect inferences of individual subjects. Thus for pattern K it can be seen that different series or groupings of inferences can be assembled from *indirect*, that is, from the most literal of the interpretations given.

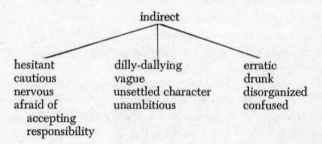

indirect

hesitant	dilly-dallying	erratic
cautious	vague	drunk
nervous	unsettled character	disorganized
afraid of	unambitious	confused
accepting		
responsibility		

These sequences or groupings of inferences can probably be "tested" for their plausibility by means of further experimental work. This type of analysis is of interest to the student of thinking as well as to the student of interpersonal perception, for here we have a chance to observe some of the processes of inference, processes largely inaccessible to conscious examination.

As a next general comment about the data, consider the heterogeneity of responses, that is the *disagreements* among the interpretations. The straight line, for example, is a path that, according to our subjects, could be traversed by an *alert* as well as by a *dull* person. The indirect path K can be attributed both to a *meticulous* as well as to an *irresponsible* person. What cannot be seen from the data in this report—consisting, as they do, of the preferred response of each subject—is that the alternatives

ath ce	A	E	K

Unspecified	Well-reasoned
	Aggressive
	Persevering
	Determined (2)
	Logical
	Purposeful (2)
	Rational
	Knows where going (3)
	Goal-oriented
	Practical
	Alert (2)
	Unimaginative
	Resolute
	Ambitious
	Direct (2)
	Economical
	Good Christian
	Dull
		Nonchalant
		Strong character
		Unstable
		Uncertain
		Conservative
		Relaxed
		Forceful
		Happy
		Drunk
		Fearful
		Unhurried (2)
		Unsure
		Undecided
		Not confident
		Casual
		Eventually gets work done
		  but takes time doing it
		Unhurried, casual
		Not quite sure of self
		  though perceptive
		Complacent
		Paranoid
		Direct
		Average
		Strong-willed
		Thoughtful
			Immature
			Very emotional
			Stupid
			Irresponsible
			Vacillating
			Undependable
			Gay
			Wanderer
			Meticulous
			Prissy
			Disjointed
			Careless
			Untrustworthy
			Little sense of direction
			Happy-go-lucky
			Wandering mind
			Extremely emotionally unbalanced
			Dependent on others to lead him
			Extremely indecisive to the point
			  of confusion
			Curiosity
			Confused
			Upset
			Sociable
			Unconcerned
			Wavering (2)

Desirable	Initiative
	Stuck up
	Strong
	Honesty
	Ambitious
	Purposeful
	Knows what doing
	Knows what after
	Determination
	Dull (horse w. blinders)
	Determined
	Self-confident
	To the point
	Direct
	Normal
	Straightforward
	Sighted his goal
	Perfect personality
		Leisurely
		Suspicious
		Sensible
		Optimistic
		Kind
		Varying personality
		Guided by thought rather
		  than emotion
		Aims beyond abilities
		Uses indirect methods
		Less stable (than path C)
		  but not too indecisive
		Sad person becoming happy
		  then disappointed and
		  again depressed
		Fairly well adjusted
		Not too confident but more
		  than others
		Indecisive
		Self-confident
		Lack of confidence
		Assured
		Fairly sure of self
			Disorganized
			Muddle-headed
			Erratic
			Mentally unbalanced
			Doesn't know what to do
			Likes to wander
			Aimless wandering
			Very nervous
			Unsettled character
			Knows what wants but no idea how
			  to get there
			Uncertain whether objective
			  desirable or not
			Lacks fortitude
			Unstable
			Drunk
			Unsure of goal

Undesirable	Determined
	Strong character
	Stubborn
	Knows what doing
	Straightforward (2)
	Courageous
	Even-tempered
	Strong character (goes
	  directly)
	Unafraid (though depends
	  on speed)
	Makes up mind quickly
	Determined but' fool-
	  hardy
	Uninformed or ignorant
	Hero complex
	Direct and frank
	Strong traits
	Steady
		Efficient
		Lofty ideals
		Half cautious
		Objective
		Cautious
		Lots of time
		Somewhat resolute but not
		  Spartan
		Makes mind up rapidly
		Resigned but not completely
		Happy-go-lucky
		Faces the inevitable
		Feels self-pity
		Hesitant about what to do
		A little indecisive
		Sensible
		Believes can rise above
		  unpleasant situations and
		  master of own fate
			Shy
			Nonchalant
			Aimless
			Has trouble deciding
			Daydreamer (2)
			Afraid
			Can't make up mind (2)
			Unable to decide
			Very young
			Realized had to go but lacked
			  courage to go directly
			Object very undesirable to him
			Weak though eventually faces
			  problem
			Afraid of object therefore
			  unreliable
			Avoids meeting object directly
			Fluctuating but not mixed up
			Completely lost and unaware of it

Fig. 2. Preferred responses given to Paths A, E, and K under three conditions of goal valence. (The numbers in parentheses refer to the number of subjects who gave a certain response. Data on other paths may be obtained from the author.)

given by the *same* subject are also often quite disparate. In short, we see that a path can convey many alternative things about the person moving. Clearly there are at least two problems. One is concerned with distinguishing paths in terms of their implications, and with the identification of the configurations related to the differences. The other problem is to distinguish the determinants of alternative interpretations made from the same path.

As to the first of these two problems there is no question about the fact that the inferences from the various paths differ, in spite of the heterogeneity within the responses to each path. As noted in Figure 2, paths can be distinguished in terms of the extent to which they yield inferences to such characteristics as *direct/devious, confident/unsure of self, purposeful/aimless, cautious/impulsive, rational/confused, strong/weak, rigid/pliable, afraid/unafraid, stable/unstable, calm/nervous, energetic/lackadaisical, orderly/disorderly*. These inferences can, in turn, be seen to relate to identifiable physical characteristics of the pattern, such as its straightness, oscillations in direction, angularity, uniformity, and so on, and above all, its directionality with respect to certain focal points. To this latter characteristic we turn next. Later on we shall give further consideration to the problem of the determinants of alternative inferences to the *same* path.

ANGLE OF MOVEMENT

Among the stimulus characteristics that appear to play a large, though not conscious, role in the inferences made about the person moving is the approach-avoidance relation a path bears to its start and end points. One can think of the direction of the path at any point X as forming an "angle of movement" with the line joining X directly to the *goal*. When the angle is zero, the movement is directly towards the goal (X_1 in figure shown below); for a 180-degree angle, it is directly away (X_2). A second basic angle of movement exists with respect to the *start* of the path. Movement directly away corresponds to a 180-

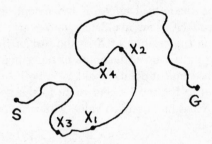

degree angle (X_3) while direct return to the start corresponds to a zero angle (X_4).

We have the impression that the meaning of movement *at any point on the path* is judged on the basis of these two angles, and that the approach-avoidance characteristics of the path as a whole are dependent on some kind of unconscious integration of the meaning of the successive points constituting the path. These two angles, however, play roles of different importance, depending on the definition of the situation in terms of movement "towards" or "away." Judgments are made with particular reference to the start or to the goal, depending upon whether the movement is understood as *ab*ient or *ad*ient, respectively. In our work we have defined the situation mostly as *ad*ient movement, the path being *towards* a goal.

In goal-determined, or adient, movement the perpendicular at point X to the line joining X to the goal constitutes a perceptual benchmark. Psychologically, this is the axis on one side of which movement proceeding from point X involves a *decrease* in distance from the goal, while on the other side it involves an *increase* in distance from the goal. It is our impression that the psychological geometry corresponds, in this case, to actual geometry, and that this line represents the critical locus about which psychological *approach* and *avoidance* are perceived, with the correlative family of less and less obvious inferences of *desire, purposefulness, persistence, eagerness* on one side and *dislike, fear*, etc., on the other.

It seems, however, that, while the perpendicular to the line joining point X to the goal may be a crucial basis of perceptual orientation, the theoretical angle of movement separating psychological approach from avoidance may vary, within limits, depending upon the relation of X to the rest of the path. Thus, for the circling path shown, the angle of movement with respect to the goal is the same at points X and Y. In both cases movement is at 90 degrees to the most direct route to the goal. Yet movement at point X has an approach value while movement at Y has an avoidance value.

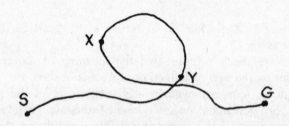

It is possible that the difference in meaning at X and Y can be accounted for in terms of the *curvature* of the path at points X and Y, as implying a *plan of moving toward* and *away* from G respectively. It is also conceivable that there may be some effect, though probably small, due to movement *toward* (at X) and *away* (at Y) from a hypothetical line joining the start and the goal.

Finer empirical distinctions can be made as to the meaning of angle of movement. Thus the range in which the angle of movement signifies approach can be differentiated, for instance, into *direct, purposeful* approach, and approach with *caution*. Similarly, the avoidance angles can be differentiated into *direct* avoidance or *escape* and *cautious withdrawal*. These rather literal interpretations of the angle of movement can be translated into less and less direct inferences (e.g. indirect approach →caution→suspicion). Thus, reversing the process, most inferences made from movement can, in principle, be translated into more direct ones and, in turn, into angle of movement.

Here than we have a possibility for some quantification of seemingly ephemeral aspects of behavior.

This schema helps somewhat with the meaning of movement at any one point, but there is a problem of understanding how the meaning of the entire path develops. Here we venture the highly speculative suggestion that the meaning of the whole path depends on the distribution of the values of its angle of movement. For example, if a path consists of half approach, half avoidance it suggests vacillating progress and hence a hesitant, insecure person. A spiral around the goal, on the other hand, would fall entirely into the "approach with caution" angle, signifying a steady but careful progress, thus persistence, and so on. It is possible that patterns of quite different appearance may have the same meaning when their distribution of movement angles are the same.

These comments are based on the overall impressions gained from the complex of observations made by means of various devices, and of course on the inevitable interaction of these with our personal experience. As such they are offered as tentative hypotheses to explain the data. But these speculations have one healthy property: they are amenable to careful testing by means of simple laboratory procedures.

SIGNAL FEATURES OF PATHS

In the course of working with stimulus materials, with responses and comments to the various paths, one gains the impression that certain features are singled out and very quickly identified as having a signal, or specific, function in the interpretation. By and large, these features seem to consist of common, easily perceptible sequences whose meaning is understandable in terms of the above discussion of the angle of movement. In these cases one is dealing with commonly experienced *sequences of values* of such angles for which a ready response is available. Such, for example, is the case with any change in sign of the curvature in the path. This always means *change,* more or less drastic. It may be an intensity change within approach or avoidance or it may be a change in polarity. Any crossing of the path, such as in forming a loop, is another signal feature. A crossing implies, of necessity, a full change in orientation with respect to the goal or the starting point.

There are, however, characteristics of the path that have intrinsic meaning somewhat apart, but perhaps not fundamentally, from the relation of the path to its start or goal. Let me give some examples. Take a path or a portion of a path where the person is moving in one direction, then makes a very sharp change in direction. The impression is one of *abruptness* since, as our subjects point out, people usually do not turn this way when the course of their movement is free. The sharp corner stands out, and is, so to speak, kept in mind as something important in forming the overall impression. The specific inferences obtained may vary a great deal, and in some cases it may not be immediately clear how they came about. The man may be described as *scatterbrained, impulsive, fickle, rude, sharp, inconsiderate, distracted, devious.* Inquiry discloses the specific, common basis of these inferences. *Impulsive,* for instance, is inferred from the fact that the two directions of movement are taken to be related to different plans of action. The change in plan takes place without the expected transition—gradual or wavy, depending upon whether there is conflict during the change. *Distracted* has an entirely different meaning but the same configurational basis. The person was doing something (i.e. moving in one direction) when *suddenly* he remembered that he should have been doing something else. He pulls up short and goes to it. This man had forgotten; hence he is *distracted.*

These are some of the path characteristics that seem definitely to strike a chord in the subject; if he is carefully interviewed he will eventually indicate that one (or more) of these particular features of the path was at the basis of his inference. Once explained, it all becomes *obvious.* Yet in many cases both the investigator and the subject have a feeling that is expressed well by the phrase, "isn't this interesting, I had never thought of that before." These signal features of the path are, if you wish, abstracted from the total thing and given special meaning. They may represent some of the basic perceptual components of a path. Components, that is, relative to a certain level of integration at which frequent combinations of still more basic components are assembled.

DEPENDENCE OF MEANING UPON FIELD CONDITIONS

A path may be thought of as having a meaning dependent exclusively upon its shape. Thus a path may be *direct, indirect, wavering, smooth, rough.* If the inferences about the person moving were made directly from the intrinsic qualities of the path then our task of understanding the inferential process would—at least operationally—be relatively simple. The data, however, make clear that this is not so and any explanation based on such a direct analogic principle is bound to fall short in accounting for particular inferences. This is not at all to say that a *straight* path ceases, under certain conditions, to have the meaning of *straightness,* but, rather, that *straightness* differs in implications depending on conditions. Thus, it may suggest *alertness* in one case, *obtuseness* in another.

The fact is that the inferences made from a specific path *include* considerations of the surrounding conditions. A direct path from A to B implies information not only regarding the person moving but also the nature of the object toward which the person is moving, and similar things. The inferences that can be made from a path about 1) the moving person and 2) features of the field, such as the valence of the goal object, are not independent of each other. In his studies of the meaning of movement, Michotte[12] has shown that an understanding of the perceptual or interpretive process necessitates the consideration of the *relationship* between the moving parts. Shor[17] has demonstrated that, with a given pattern of movement in the interaction of two symbolic persons, the attributes assigned to one person depend upon those assigned to the other. So, too, in our case, the meaning of variations in the characteristics of the path must be considered in connection with field characteristics.

Indeed, a path has a variety of possible meanings, and we have suggested above that these stem from common, more literal descriptions. The choice of appropriate meaning in a specific instance, however, depends upon such factors as whether the movement is seen as a movement *away* from a point (*ab*ient) or a movement *toward* a point (*ad*ient), upon the characteristics of the moving person, and upon the nature and valence of the object of interaction.

VALENCE OF GOAL OBJECT

I shall now consider in some detail the last mentioned determinant, the valence of the goal object, and the effect of specifying it as desirable or undesirable in the instructions.

Figure 2 shows the effect of changing the valence of the goal object for a number of different paths. Take the straight line, path A. Some of the inferences, such as *determined* and *direct*, which are close to the inherent physical qualities of the path, are compatible with both positive and negative goals. Applicable to desirable goals only are such traits as *purposeful* and *confident*. When the goal is undesirable, on the other hand, such inferences as *unafraid* and *courageous* are made. We see how the meaning changes with the sign of the valence from *determined, direct, purposeful, confident*, to *determined, direct, unafraid, courageous*.

These data become somewhat understandable in terms of the following assumptions about the path-goal interdependence mentioned above. A direct path towards a point implies with high probability a desirable object, and a desirable object implies with high probability a direct path. An *un*desirable object, on the other hand, implies a path *away* from the goal, and vice versa. Or, if the path *has* to end at the undesirable point, a tortuous, indirect path is expected, reflecting hesitancy, postponement, discomfort. A path is judged as "more direct or less direct than expected" under the given circumstances. In many situations, however, this normally expected articulation, or unit, between path and object is violated to different degrees. It becomes necessary then for the subject to introduce *explanations* for the unusual state of affairs. These explanations take the form of attributing to the moving person qualities that would account for the "deviation" or of spontaneous and largely unconscious imaginary elaborations of the field conditions.

The case of the *straight* path *towards* an object with negative valence illustrates such a violation of expectancy. Avoidance *or* a very indirect route is the expected type of path. But the given path is straight. *Unafraid, courageous* "explain" the anomaly. Another favorite explanation—somewhat implied in *courageous* —is that the person is *forced* to go to the goal by outside forces.

Pattern E illustrates an instance that fits the normal expectancy when the valence is negative. This case is particularly interesting when the goal is described as desirable. The inference *suspicious* can only be understood as an explanation of the failure to move more expeditiously towards a desirable goal.

It is as if the components involved in the inference process were as shown in the following scheme: (a) consideration of the goal valence; (b) a comparison of the path expected—given the valence of the goal—with the path observed, resulting in a judgment of more direct or less direct than expected; and (c) utilization of the cognitive contingency between goal valence and directness.

(a)	(b)	(c)
+	as direct as expected →	normal approach to positive goal (purposeful, active)
	less direct than expected →	abnormal failure to approach positive goal (purposeless, inactive)
—	less indirect than expected →	abnormal approach to negative goal (fearlessness)
	as indirect as expected →	normal avoidance of negative goal (fear)

For the experienced organism, these are extremely well practiced contingencies, readily accessible for use in "package" form. The movement itself and the field conditions are seen as a whole and the interpretation is based on the idiosyncratic interaction. Perhaps the highly informative quality of movement derives exactly from the fact that the same movement can have so many meanings, depending on context.

Most paths have somewhat different meanings with positive and negative goals. However, in several cases variations due to goal differences are minor. In these instances the patterns may be of particular interest if the absence of variation indicates that the essential meaning is "carried" by the path. Should this be true, confidence in judgments based on such movement patterns might be particularly high, dependence on field information low.

Directness is only one aspect of the path. Other variables, such as *smoothness*, enter in the expected articulation between path and goal object, but these will not be considered here.

CONCLUSIONS AND SUMMARY

Out of personal interest, as well as on the basis of the fact that movement is biopsychologically an important form of stimulation, and in reaction to the relative neglect of this problem, I have tried to show that it might be rewarding to pay more attention to movement as a source of information about other persons.

There may be objections as to the relevance, for the study of interpersonal perception, of such simplified and dehumanized situations as we used. My reaction to such doubts is that the real issue is not one of relevance but of what the investigator does with the information he obtains. If he uses it as a source of insights which he tests as best he can on actual persons, or if he uses the simple situations to test hypotheses developed from observing real people, then, I think, the approach is both fruitful and sound.

Furthermore, the study of the meaning of movement in very

simple symbolic situations appears to be a useful way of bringing to light certain processes of inference that are too rapid and unconscious in the complex medium of real life or facsimiles of real life. It is one way of slowing down the process so that we can take a look at it. When faced with simple movement the subject may be able to say that the "person" is afraid "because" he circles the object instead of going directly to it. In a comparable real life situation he might be unable to abstract the movement component of his judgment, yet he may have used it. The analogic and metaphorical tendencies in human thinking provide the bridge between the inferences drawn in our simple laboratory situations and inferences drawn in actual complex situations. Persons are always moving—in literal or symbolic ways. The usefulness of studying inferences from movement in simple symbolic situations may consist, in part, in making explicit and accessible for analysis modes and bases of judgments largely buried under the extraordinary cognitive achievements of ordinary men.

The meaning of movement depends upon a great number of factors besides the essential characteristics of the movement itself. The nature of the movement is but one of the factors involved. The same pattern of movement may convey different meanings, or *different* patterns may have the *same* meaning depending upon field conditions. In addition, there is considerable substitutibility or equivalence in meaning among different stimulus configurations. The problem of the meaning of movement in person perception, then, is in the analysis of the interpretations of the interplay between movement and field characteristics. Since high consensus appears to occur when conditions are specified, some well-established perceptual and cognitive principles must underlie the process.

The impressions or inferences we draw from a person's movement depend on what Michotte[11] called the "functional connections" existing in the overall perceptual structure. Michotte showed this to be true in the case of perception of causality and intentionality in movement patterns. Our observations certainly support this view as far as inferences from paths to personal characteristics are concerned. This is not to say that kinetic structures do not have an intrinsic meaning of their own. We are saying, rather, that where the problem is one of making inferences about a person, it is one of the *particular* meanings of the intrinsic meaning that is important. The particular meaning takes the field into consideration.

The importance of free movement as a cue derives, then, from the fact that it represents the essence of the unique functional relationship between the person and his field. Since, in ordinary life, the observer is usually fairly well informed about the field conditions, as well as about some of the characteristics of the person, the path of the movement affords an excellent source of information about the "inner state" of the person moving.

References

1. Allport, G. W. and Vernon, P. E. *Studies in expressive movement.* New York: Macmillan, 1933.

2. Bruner, J. S. and Tagiuri, R. The perception of people. In Lindzey, G. (Ed.), *Handbook of social psychology.* Cambridge, Mass.: Addison-Wesley, 1954.

3. Cronbach, L. J. Proposals leading to analytic treatment of social-perception. In Tagiuri, R. and Petrullo, L. (Eds.), *Person perception.* Stanford: Stanford Univ. Press, 1959.

4. Furash, E. *The meaning of path: a study in perception.* Unpubl. Undergrad. Honors Thesis. Harvard Univ., 1956.

5. Gemelli, A. La percezione visiva del movimento. *Riv. Psicol.,* 1957.

6. Heider, F. and Simmel, Marianne. An experimental study of apparent behavior. *Amer. J. Psychol.,* 1944, 57, 243-259.

7. Koffka, K. *Principles of Gestalt psychology.* New York: Harcourt, 1935.

8. Köhler, K. *Gestalt psychology.* New York: Liveright, 1929.

9. Leeper, R. W. *Lewin's topological and vector psychology.* Eugene: Univ. of Oregon, 1943.

10. Lewin, K. *Dynamic theory of personality.* New York: McGraw-Hill, 1935.

11. Michotte, A. The emotions regarded as functional connections. In Reymert, M. L. (Ed.), *Feelings and emotions.* New York: McGraw-Hill, 1950.

12. Michotte, A. *La perception de la causalité.* Louvain, 1946.

13. Michotte, A. A propos de la permanence phénoménale: Faits et théories. *Acta psychol.,* 1950, 7, 298-322.

14. Muybridge, E. *The human figure in motion.* London: Chapman, 1901.

15. Ruesch, J. and Kees, W. *Non-verbal communication.* Berkeley: Univ. of California Press, 1956.

16. Scheerer, M. and Lyons, J. Line drawings and matching responses to words. *J. Personal.,* 1957, 25, 251-273.

17. Shor, R. E. Effect of preinformation upon human characteristics attributed to animated geometric figures. *J. abnorm. soc. Psychol.,* 1957, 54, 124-126.

18. Vernon, M.D. *A further study of visual perception.* Cambridge: Cambridge Univ. Press, 1952.

19. Werner, H. *Comparative psychology of mental development.* (Rev. ed.) New York: Follet, 1948.

20. Wolff, W. *The expression of personality: experimental depth psychology.* New York: Harper, 1943.

X

Judgment and
Judging in Person
Cognition

INTRODUCTION

A PERSON REMARKS about an acquaintance: "Smith is a very sincere man." Another acquaintance remarks about the same Smith: "He is an insincere man." A clinical psychologist subjects Smith to a series of diagnostic tests and interviews and concludes that "Smith is a psychopathic personality." These varied judgments are, on the face of it, different and would probably give a different impression about Smith to different persons to whom they were communicated. The fact that, given certain qualifications and conditions, these comments may all be consistent, and even all accurate, will not concern us at the moment. In this chapter the major focus will be an attempt to analyze the determinants of variations in judgments made about the characteristics and behavior of other people.

GENERAL TRENDS AND TERMS

Although some researchers limit themselves to that aspect usually known as *perception*, the term *person-cognition* would, I believe, be much more descriptive. This is not just a semantic point; our understanding of how we know other people will be greatly augmented if we feel ourselves free to use the great body of material that has been accumulated on the cognition of objects (see below). Furthermore, the term *cognition* implies a more active process of knowing than *perception*, and it enables us to embrace an inference model of how we know other people. This model provides us with a useful way of looking at the processes involved in person-cognition, using the analogy of formal logic to describe how we proceed from the raw data to our final impression of the object-person.[7]

In recent years, there has been a great amount of literature devoted to person-cognition. Some of the work has been oriented toward problems of everyday social intercourse, while other work has concerned diagnostic judgments made by clinicians and other behavioral scientists. Both processes are probably basically the same, but we need careful analyses of the procedures used before we can say so with certainty. The question is an important one since subjective assessment is the key tool used by the clinician in his professional work. In the last few years more attention has been devoted to factors influencing the process of person-cognition than to the validity of the cognition, and in my opinion, this is the correct order of priority. The ultimate improvement of the validity of clinical judgments will depend on a clearer understanding of the cognitive processes involved, and this present analysis is submitted as a small contribution towards that endeavor.

Is person-cognition radically different from object-cognition? Much of the treatment of the former has neglected work carried out on the perception and judgment of impersonal objects. This is a mistake; our understanding of person-cognition can be greatly enhanced by the work on object-cognition, and the reverse is also the case since experiments on interpersonal judgments are mostly experiments in general cognition.

Some characteristics are operative, however, in many experiments on person-cognition that are either unimportant or non-existent in the typical study of object-cognition. For example, people tend to be more complex as cues than is the typical object in a perception experiment. Still, it would be possible to provide quite complex impersonal objects in these experiments if they were required (e.g. works of art). Also, people tend to be more variable in their behavior over a time

span than are objects, but most cognitive experiments, either
personal or impersonal, do not cover a long time span. In so
far as the judge tends to be ego-involved with the person whom
he is judging, he is likely to be affected in his judgments, but
the "new look" cognitionists have shown us that this is true also
of some impersonal judgments. The reactivity of the object is
important in some interpersonal studies, but in others, such as
judging the characteristics of persons in motion pictures, the
object does *not* provide any cues by reacting to the observer's
behavior. And yet, surely, the judging situation described in
From's chapter on the perception of the intention of persons
depicted in a movie is an interpersonal one.

The most significant special feature of the cognition of persons is that the observer frequently uses his own behavior as a
frame of reference for his judgments; thus, if he perceives the
object person to be similar to himself he will probably anticipate
that the object is having the same experiences as he would in
similar situations. If, on the other hand, he perceives the object
person as different, then he will predict different experiences
for the person than he himself would have. In other words,
person-cognition often involves an identification, or empathy,
process which is far less likely to occur in the case of impersonal
objects. It can occur in those types of object-perception which
Werner calls physiognomic, or, for example, when primitives
endow totem objects with human qualities.

All of the features of person-cognition described above are
likely sources of variation in the judgments made about other
people, and explain why individual differences are more important in the cognition of personal objects than in impersonal
objects.

There is a continuum of cognitive objects ranging from those
which have no personal qualities at all to those that savor of
full personality, including the expression of will and reciprocity
with the observer. While there could be little doubt that judgments by acquaintances about each other are interpersonal,
what about judgments of traits, movies of people, schematic
faces, observations of animals, totems, or even Card III on the

Rorschach? We see a striking contrast in respect to the degree of personality of the object in the two experiments (in the From and Tagiuri chapters) dealing with the qualities perceived in connection with human movement. In From's experiment the judges made judgments about the intentions of a person depicted in a movie. In contrast, Tagiuri's judges were confronted with a series of lines representing the path taken by a hypothetical person, and were asked to describe the characteristics of the person concerned.

The two experiments represent two different strategies in person-cognition experiments; the one taking human behavior as it may actually occur (although the situation could have been more "natural" than it was in From's experiment), while the other analyzed out the bare bones of one relevant class of variables in order to study its influence on the judgments without complications arising from other variables. Both approaches have their value to our understanding of person-cognition. By an intuitive analysis of the more full-blooded person-judgments, we can hypothesize what the relevant variables are. When we have analyzed better what the elements are that influence such judgments we can set up special experiments in which just those variables will be varied. This is virtually what Tagiuri has done. But to throw more light on the variables that influence judgments based on real human movement, we need experiments with material derived directly from human movement as it is found ecologically, rather than from mere geometrical forms.

My plea then is for both ecological studies of person-cognition and complementary analytic laboratory studies in which variables that appear to be relevant are systematically varied. The earlier analysis of the special characteristics of personal objects is intended as a contribution towards the development of experiments in which the relevant aspects of the object can be systematically varied. For example, we might ask what is the effect on the cognition of an object when that object constitutes a threat to the ego esteem of the judge. This is an area in which some work has already been done wih both personal and impersonal objects and it would be valuable to investigate whether the studies on both types of objects complement each other.

SOURCES OF VARIATION IN PERSON-COGNITION

Let us now consider briefly from what sources variations in judgments about objects arise.

Sources of variation are: the circumstances under which the judgment is made; the type of data available to the judge; the qualities of the judge; the characteristics of the object person; the type of judgment that is called for, and interactions between all these variables.* Eventually all these variables will have to be carefully considered, but in this chapter only one group of them, the judge as a source of variation, will be discussed. Four types of factors will be considered: (a) the judge's previous experience, (b) the motivation of the judge, (c) the judge's ability, and (d) interaction effects.

Factors deriving from the judge's previous experience: Like all other judgments, the judgment about the object person will depend on what the judge has learned from experience about human behavior in general and the behavior of the object person in particular. Presumably there is a learning effect in interpersonal judgments so that as a person goes through life he collects data about people. Certainly the accuracy of interpersonal judgments increases through childhood, but the evidence on the effect of age in adults is not definite.[9] Experience does not leave its mark only in cognitive processes but also becomes embedded in emotional reactions. For this reason neither experience of mankind in general nor prolonged experience with the subject himself necessarily leads to more accurate judgments. The influence of motivational and emotional factors will be dealt with further below.

The detailed study of how a person stores up his experience

---

* These sources of variation can, in turn, be related to the probabilistic relationships between the postulates with which the judge starts and also the various stages of the inference process: education of premises, utilization of cues, instantiation, and treatment of conclusions; for details see [7].

so that it can be utilized appropriately when a judgment requires it is one on which much more work is needed. The judge evidently has some relatively permanent models (or working principles) of how personality operates; these models are utilized when he draws conclusions about the cues which he perceives—including the internal cues derived from his own empathetic responses.[7] The inferences are made in a manner analogous to the operations of formal logic, excepting that the relations between general principle and instance are based on subjective probability, and the final conclusion represents a combination of probabilities. To illustrate, the judge who described Smith as "insincere" may have gone through a mental process equivalent to the following: "People who cause me to react to them with feelings like this are probably insincere; people whose friendly gestural behavior is as strong in comparison with the normal expectation under these circumstances are probably insincere. Therefore, I judge him to be insincere." The inference is made by combining probability relationships derived from general principles of human behavior which have been learned from past experience. (I am not suggesting that the judge is necessarily able to make explicit the working principles or the inferential process that he uses; the above account is simply an interpretation of what he does when he makes a judgment.)

A consideration of how the judge learns to use his experience requires a treatment of how the judge acquires the general principles; presumably partly by storing up the results of his own previous experience of similar cases, partly by postulation derived from his theoretical—even though possibly crude—analysis of human nature, and partly by enculturation. The latter mechanism is mainly responsible for the development of stereotypes; thus our culture may indoctrinate us that members of a certain nationality are insincere. This then becomes a working principle that we may use uncritically when judging a particular member of that nationality.

We should expect, then, that a judge who has had considerable experience with the type of person whom he is judging, or even with the object person himself, would be able to make more accurate judgments since he has been able to build up appropriate models of behavior and to put some content into these principles in terms of probability expectations. There is some evidence that foreigners have more difficulty in judging members of a particular culture than do natives.[10] Familiarity with the object person would seem to lead to more accurate judgments through the effect of increased information. However, the experimental evidence on this point is equivocal due to the complications arising from similarity between the judge and object, and also from emotional factors. Motivational and emotional factors distort judgments about people with whom the judge has a close relationship, as in friendship or marriage, so that experience does not necessarily operate to improve accuracy.

Apart from the effect of long-term experience on judgments, we should also consider short-term factors that lead to a particular set or expectation. Thus the events preceding the making of the judgment may influence the particular type of judgment made. An excellent illustration of this is provided by Kelley's "warm-cold" experiment.[3] Kelley informed one half of a class that the lecturer they were about to hear was "very warm," and the other half that he was "rather cold." Although the other aspects of the lecturer were equivalent for both groups, the judgments made about the quality of his lecture differed considerably as a result of the different expectations. The context of experience in which the judgment is set acts to mediate the impression received.

Motivational factors: Perhaps most important in this respect is what the judge's purpose is in making the judgment at all; the fact that he is making a judgment indicates some motive or purpose. Maybe the motive is simply to please or to comply with the request made by an experimenter. In this case, the judgments would tend to be made in a perfunctory manner, and would be based on minimal observation of the available cues, and a minimum of consideration of the validity of the possible hypotheses. It is an incidental but paradoxical point that the first of these effects may, in fact, lead to more accurate judgments than ensue when the data are considered more carefully. This effect arises from the fact that most people are near the average on any quality, and if the judgments are made in a comparatively undifferentiated way, they are more likely to be correct than if they are greatly differentiated.

Intrinsic motives on the part of the judge, rather than the mere reflection of the experimenter's motives, may be operative. For example, the judge may have a need to dominate the person object and may achieve this by seeing him as inferior; or he may need to express hostility by deprecating the qualities of the other. Or he may wish to gain support for his own affiliation needs by perceiving the other as having appropriate characteristics, e.g. as being friendly or kind or as just being interested in the judge as a person.

An important need that is now being recognized more and more in the study of social interactions is that of cognitive symmetry or consonance and consensual validation.[5] Perceived similarity by the judge may arise from his feelings of insecurity in a comparatively unstructured situation, the effect of which is to lead the judge to see the object person as supporting his own observations, beliefs and attitudes.

There are more subtle ways in which the act of judging can serve some need. For example, the judge can avoid coming to grips with some of his own characteristics which he dislikes by projecting them onto the other. Thus Sears' well-known experiment[8] demonstrates that judges may attribute "reprehensible" traits which they themselves have, but repress, to other persons, more than do judges who either do not have these traits or who are aware of these weaknesses in themselves. This is the paradigm of *projection* as described in psychoanalysis.

One special case of motives that may be served in the act of judging is that of curiosity or need to understand. There are some people who are oriented towards trying to understand almost every person with whom they come into contact. This is usually manifested by a tendency to scrutinize or probe into the background and motives of strangers that frequently borders on the impertinent. In a more subtle form this motive may underlie the choice of personality psychology or personnel selection as an occupation since they formalize such probing into appropriate role behavior. Whether this speculation is true or not, we can expect that judges who have strong needs to understand people will search for clues from others rather than just passively receiving the cues emitted by them, and will thus have different information available to them than that available to more passive judges.

We must also briefly consider the case where the judging situation is only a means to a more long-range managerial purpose. In ordinary social relations this purpose may be simply to maintain some symbiotic relationship, perhaps a dominant-submissive one, or perhaps just a pleasant reciprocal and symmetrical association. In professional practice, the long-range purpose being served by the judgment may be job placement or rejection, or perhaps a decision about incarceration or therapy in the cases of a criminal or a patient. The long-range purpose will affect the type of information that will be sought from the object person, and also the type of inferences that will be made.

Having considered the effect of motives on judgments, let us now briefly consider the effect of different attitudes. First of all comes the judge's attitude towards the act of judging itself. Here we can distinguish between a tender-minded and tough-minded attitude; the former leads to judgments that are tainted, so to speak, by some of the motives described above, while the latter is directed more towards accuracy. There is evidence, for example, that judges who are oriented towards people tend to rate them more favorably than do the more socially detached thing-oriented people.[9] Experiments are needed to investigate whether these differences are deep-lying personality qualities only, or whether they can also be experimentally manipulated in the judging situation by manipulating motivation.

The judge's attitude towards the object person is obviously another important attitude that affects the judgment, and this is referred to later in the "Interaction" section. But the judge also may have an attitude towards the type of person involved, perhaps to his ethnic, geographical or occupational background. This is the way in which social stereotypes influence judgments; the members of the stereotyped groups are judged to possess characteristics that are attributed to all the members. In some cases these stereotypes are held fairly commonly by most judges; in some other cases, judges each have their own idiosyncratic stereotypes. These latter stereotypes may be specific to certain traits that are taken to dominate all others; for example, if the judge perceives the object person as having bad manners he may also attribute certain characteristics, such as being unkind, to him. This attribution of unkindness reflects either a general negative halo which pertains to all people perceived by this judge to have bad manners, or it reflects an aspect of the judge's implicit personality theory about what characteristics go together. Thus we see that stereotypes represent the judge's preconceptions about what traits are related to other characteristics which he regards as dominant.

A statistical analysis of social judgments would reveal that they are almost entirely based on only two or three variables; this is demonstrated, for example, in Sarbin's study.[6] The characteristics about which the judge feels most strongly are the ones that form the basis of his judgments, so much so that an analysis of the judgment may even be used as a projective test.

Ability to judge others: Apart from differences in accuracy that derive from the judge's motivation to be accurate, there are also differences in skill to be considered. Most studies of this ability find a positive correlation with scores on intelligence tests. This is the case especially in judgments of a non-analytic type; that is, when the judge has to make an exact application of a described dimension to the subjects. Not many of the reported studies of judgments employ subjects who are widely dispersed on intelligence, and I suspect that if more judges with below average intelligence were used, the effect of intelligence would be revealed more markedly.

Intelligence is quite a complex function, and it is difficult to pin-point which aspects are related to the making of judgments; some relevant aspects are probably reasoning ability, concept formation, flexibility of thinking and, possibly, fluency. Recently one important intellectual function, cognitive complexity, has been shown to be related to judging people. For example, Bieri[1] measured cognitive complexity in terms of the richness of categories used by the judge in describing acquaintances.

He found that the more "complex" judges were less likely to rely on an assumption that the object person was like themselves than were "simpler" judges. In other words, the possession of rich cognitive organization aids a judge in differentiating his objects.

There may also be an "intuitive" ability which enables some people to make accurate judgments of others, or at least of certain sorts of other people, especially when global or non-analytic judgments are called for; for example, when judging emotions that another person is expressing. Much has been made of this alleged intuitive or "psychological" ability, but the evidence concerning it is as yet very slim. In Britain, Wedeck,[12] by using a factor analysis technique, found a factor that could be interpreted as "social intuition," but this has not been confirmed by any other studies, nor have its components been analyzed.

Interaction effects: Apart from the previously described sources of variation there are also important interaction effects between the judge and the object, and the judge and the types of material available. These will not be treated in detail here; the intricacies are immense and there is very little literature on the latter aspect. For instance, clinical psychologists very often have their favorite diagnostic device for extracting the cues that form the basis of their judgments; some prefer the interview, others the Rorschach, others *ad hoc* projective devices, and so on. It would be interesting to get some evidence on the correlation between the actual value of any of these instruments in clinical assessments and the clinician's opinion of their value. Apart from judgments based on tests, there are differences in judgments that derive from preferences for different types of cues, or tendencies to emphasize different cues. For example, Levine[4] demonstrates that when experienced clinicians judge a person whom they regard as maladjusted, they overemphasize the person's "negative" behavior and reject "positive" behavior as compared with judges who are not clinicians. This experiment is one of the few that has studied the interaction effects at the complex level at which they actually operate.

Different judges, because of motivational and experiential

factors, will react differently to an object person. One important variable in this respect is the similarity between the judge and the object. Here we may distinguish between actual and assumed similarity; where judge and object are similar in social background or in their traits, the judgments are likely to be more accurate than when they are dissimilar. There are two reasons for this; one, that the judge is more likely to be familiar with the meaning of the other's behavior in the particular situation and its likely implications for his future behavior; the other is that if the judge projects his own responses onto the object person—and most judges do—he will as an incidental consequence make accurate judgments.

There are many other important interactive factors; for example, the influence of an affectionate bond between the judge and his object. Tagiuri, Blake and Bruner[11] have demonstrated that judges tend to perceive others as liking or disliking them according to whether they, the judges, like the other. This "congruency" is independent of the accuracy of their judgments. In turn, we may expect that the judge will attribute traits to the other that are consonant with both the judge's attitude towards him and the other's perceived attitude towards the judge. Many such subtle interaction effects operate in interpersonal cognition.

SUMMARY AND CONCLUDING REMARKS

In studying person-cognition we note that while some experiments deal with face-to-face contacts, others use as their data judgments about highly abstract representations of persons, such as trait names or even the human-like motion of geometrical figures. This chapter has considered some aspects relating to why different persons differ in the judgments that they make about others. It has been concerned primarily with the judge as a source of variation, rather than the object person or circumstantial factors. We have discussed factors deriving from the judge's previous experience, his motives and attitudes, his abilities and interactions between these sources of variation and the material made available, the traits on which the judgments are made, similarity between judge and object and emotional ties between them.

Although only an outline sketch of the variables operating in judgments has been provided, the complexities in this area are evident. Future experiments should emanate from more clearly analyzed theoretical expectations than they have in the past, and for this purpose a model of person-cognition based on inference is recommended. If person judgments are treated as inferences, we can then apply experimental techniques to the analysis of processes occurring at the various stages of the inference. In this respect, the design proposed by the late Egon Brunswik[2] is especially promising for future experimentation. It will be a slow process to establish reliable findings in the complex area of person-cognition, but progress made in the past few years is encouraging. Once some model of the process of judging others is accepted, it should be possible to obtain integrated research findings from all along the continuum, ranging from person objects who are "real" people to objects that remotely symbolize some aspect of people.

References

1. Bieri, J. Cognitive complexity-simplicity and predictive behavior. *J. abnorm. soc. Psychol.*, 1955, 51, 263-268.

2. Brunswik, E. *Systematic and representative design of psychological experiments.* Berkeley: Univ. of California Press, 1947.

3. Kelley, H. H. The warm-cold variables in first impressions of persons. *J. Personal.*, 1950, 18, 431-439.

4. Levine, M. S. Some factors associated with clinical prediction. Unpubl. Ph.D. Thesis. Univ. of California.

5. Newcomb, T. M. The prediction of interpersonal attraction. *Amer. Psychologist*, 1956, 11, 575-576.

6. Sarbin, T. R. A contribution to the study of actuarial and individual methods of prediction. *Amer. J. Sociol.*, 1942, 48, 593-602.

7. Sarbin, T. R., Taft, R., and Bailey, D. *Clinical inference and cognitive theory.* New York: Rinehart, 1960.

8. Sears, R. R. Experimental studies of projection: I. Attribution of traits. *J. soc. Psychol.*, 1937, 7, 151-163.

9. Taft, R. The ability to judge people. *Psychol. Bull.*, 1955, 51, 1-23.

10. Taft, R. Some characteristics of good judges of others. *Brit. J. Psychol.*, 1956, 47, 19-29.

11. Tagiuri, R., Blake, R. R., and Bruner, J. S. Some determinants of the perception of positive and negative feeling to others. *J. abnorm. soc. Psychol.*, 1953, 48, 585-592.

12. Wedeck, J. The relationship between personality and "psychological ability." *Brit. J. Psychol.*, 1947, 37, 133-151.

E. P. Hollander

XI

Reconsidering the Issue of Conformity in Personality*

INTRODUCTION

QUITE OBLIVIOUS TO THE NOTIONS we may have about the categorization of behavior, people nonetheless persist in behaving. So it is that we observe some manner of behavior and call it "conformity," and so it is that we may at times attribute this to something we choose to call "personality."

By my comments here, I hope to examine this latter conception in light of certain points adduced from social psychology. Thus, in anticipation of what is to come, I mean to suggest that, whatever else it may be, conformity represents a problem of person perception, and for a set of reasons which I shall dwell upon later. But, by way of beginning, we might now give some brief consideration to personality as a construct.

THE MANIFEST AND THE UNDERLYING IN PERSONALITY

The issue of whether to deal with the manifest or the underlying strikes deeply at the roots of modern psychology. Far from

* This chapter was completed at Istanbul while the author was on leave from the Carnegie Institute of Technology as Fulbright Professor. The aid and stimulation provided by Prof. Dr. Mümtaz Turhan, Mr. Yilmaz Özakpinar, and Miss Iffet Dinç are much appreciated.

withering, this dualism is more full-bodied than ever, and no-where more so than in our conception of personality. Reflecting this, we have the recent ranging presentation of Nevitt Sanford,[11] as an example. He offers a not unorthodox view of personality with levels of "depth" such that some attributes of the individual are more basic than others, and hence accessible only through the most penetrating study.

What continues to perplex, however, is the linkage between these underlying features and the overt behaviors which are observed. Are these related? And, if so, by what mechanisms do the former mediate their influence to the latter? What of behaviors at the "surface" which appear to have little relevance to the "core"? May we accept these as in some way indicative of the nature of that core? Granted that this is possible, when are we entitled to make such inferences? Taking Sanford literally, it would seem that we can't be sure, for he suggests that the "core" be given over to study by "personologists" and that the "surface" be delivered up to further study by the social psychologist.

To the social psychologist this can only serve to compound confusion. If he is to be concerned with the individual, it must be in terms of those attributes—or "things about an individual"—which may be stably related to some palpable social behaviors. As matters now stand, there *is* precisely such a line of interest which has given rise to a multitude of attitudinally-based trait scales geared to the measurement of dispositions (e.g. authoritarianism, rigidity, empathy) presumed to be generators of characteristic social behavior. In fact, this represents a concern with that which is underlying, call it core or what you will.

But side by side with this stream of activity in social psychology, and flourishing with astonishing independence, is yet another stream. This is represented in the work of the situational determinists who focus particular attention upon the immediate situation, particularly group influences, in eliciting social behavior. Here individual characteristics are mainly taken as parameters which are given; there is, therefore, no singular handling of the individual *qua* individual.

Accordingly, we are in the first place beset with a two-fold view of personality: as an underlying individual attribute bringing about behavior, and as a literal set of behaviors typically displayed by the individual, other things being equal. We are committed, furthermore, to a conception of behavior as having some relevance to the nature of situational forces acting upon the individual. There is no royal road to understanding in either of these approaches alone. It seems reasonable to suppose that there are not only individual differences in disposition toward certain behaviors, but that there also exist situationally determined variants of behavior among individuals. How these two lines of influence may interact to yield some vector of behavior remains a focal point of concern, and one that will occupy our attention at greater length later. For the logic of what is to come, it is worthwhile to briefly draw an anology with the experience of chemistry.

The behavior of matter has a tradition of speculation which may even antedate that of primitive psychology. In the antiquity of chemistry, phenomena were noted and accounted for with reference to certain essences presumed to inhere in the substance; a given manifest property carried the imputation of its essence to the bit of matter being observed. Essences were catalogued at length in an attempt to establish causal relationships. But rather static qualities (like hardness, coldness, or dampness) were typically fixed upon and these proved quite inadequate as a foundation for a science of chemistry.

Substantial breakthroughs did not occur until the age of Boyle, Lavoisier, and Dalton, among others, when the relevant properties of a substance were recognized to be those which were affected by combination with other substances under varying conditions of exposure. The consequences of this then new view require no embellishment. Close upon the realization that *interactive* attributes were critical, rather than static features, there evolved the law of conservation of mass, the kinetic theory of gases, 19th century atomic theory, and ultimately the periodic table of elements.

Analogies may be overdrawn, and I too share a disdain for invidious comparisons with the physical sciences, as though what suits them must necessarily suit us. Yet, I have set down this particular parallel because, rough as it may be, it affords a fresh opportunity to consider some of the rubrics to which we are beholden. Thus, I submit that even with our sophistication in measurement, we are still inclined to search for those characteristics of the individual—his essences—which might account for behavior and hence be worthy of heroic feats of dimensionalization. Largely through the instrumentality of the personality test—or the F scale, the Water Jar Problem, the Test of Empathy, and so forth—we have hopefully tapped some of these already.

In this process, though, I believe that we have failed to recognize the two-pronged conception of personality we hold. And, more to the point, we may gloss over the likely fact that both prongs obscure or subsume interactive properties of the individual which require for their elicitation certain catalytic situational elements. Too often, on the contrary, we choose to deal with them as static attributes, having a level of consistency over time which is probably quite unrealistic.

Thus it is not surprising that in a recent literature coverage McClelland[9] has commented that "the best conclusion one can draw seems to be that the status of rigidity as a trait variable is, to say the least, uncertain!" We may note, as another case in point, that the F scale bears a highly varying relationship to behaviors as the situational context is varied. This is not to be taken as a dismissal of this approach, however. Rather, I would suggest that we recognize its limitations as regards prediction over many situations; its fulfillment rests on a study of those relevant situational catalysts noted earlier.

SOCIAL CONFORMITY AS PRODUCT

How the foregoing points bear upon contemporary concerns in social psychology may be better discerned through consideration of social conformity which, to my mind, constitutes the central process of social psychology—and my particular use of the word "process" is not a matter of indifference. Our interest will cover both illustrative empirical works and some related operational problems.

It is hardly news to suggest that conformity involves an individual in a situation; that is to say, it emerges from interaction. On his own terms, virtually everyone concerned with the problem will grant this as a commonplace truth. But, this widespread acknowledgement notwithstanding, we are still confronted with a persisting treatment of conformity as if it were a function of either the individual or the situation operating unilaterally.

To illuminate this issue, it is convenient to begin with reference to the well-known work on conformity by Crutchfield,[6] taking it as illustrative of a class. The features of the experimental arrangement are by now quite familiar and grow out of some earlier work by Asch[2] reported latterly. In this experimentally induced group atmosphere, the findings indicate that some subjects will characteristically conform to the norm of the group—that is, give the same response that four other subjects have given—even in the face of rather clear evidence of the group's error. From this the point is adduced that such individuals have an essentially conformist personality, and Crutchfield provides personality assessment data which appear to demonstrate the presence of correlates of conformity in other personality trait dimensions.

There are several points we might now pose about the intended sense in which the term "personality" is used here. Are these *behaviors* personality? Or does personality *determine* the behaviors? If typical behaviors are meant, clearly the sample of situations studied is exceedingly small. Hence, it would seem that the "essence" definition is implied: presumably, people have been identified who are programmed, in some underlying sense, to conform; or are they?

Let it be noted hastily that the Asch-Crutchfield studies are not being indicted, but rather the particular construction put upon their meaning. The confounding element in this picture is that conformity has been imputed to the individual from manifest behavior in this particular situational field; to then speak of conformity as an underlying attribute of the individual himself is questionable since situations vary in their properties, e.g. groups differ in their demands upon individuals, and individuals are variously motivated to respond to these demands. Moreover, we may wonder whether this ostensible conformity response was indeed prompted by motivation to comply with group demands. One might argue with reason that another motive might have been a desire to please the experimenter who, after all, represented an authority figure. Or, perhaps, subjects who "conformed" possessed a low frustration threshold and were negatively motivated, in the sense of wishing to get on with the task so as to escape from the field to some other activity. We may not be sure of their actual impact, but these factors are certainly within the realm of possible effectiveness.

There is yet another point at stake; it is dubious for us to invoke conformity as an individually-centered variable (much as pleasure or selfishness were invoked in the days of philosophical conjecture) for the simple reason that it is too gross. Thus, if we say that an individual is a "conformist," in the pervasive, personality "core" sense, we run the risk, other issues aside, of obscuring the dynamic aspects of interaction yielding this evident outcome.

We have a particularly pointed case of the pitfalls of this conception of conformity in Bernberg's[4] "test of social conformity." His rationale is as follows: people who are non-conformists will get into difficulty with social conventions; those who are conformists will comply with these conventions, as for example in the matter of religious observance. Consequently, he has taken a set of attitude items and validated them as indices of conformity vs. non-conformity by noting their discrimination between church-goers and prisoners, respectively. We are then asked to accept his ultimate scale as a measure of tendencies toward conformity. I, for one, should not be at all surprised to find that jailed prisoners are, shall we say, more antagonistic to social conventions than are church-goers—even though they might themselves have been avid church-goers at one time. But I doubt that this necessarily demonstrates any profound personality disposition toward non-conformity, unless we define conformity as an absence of overtly hostile attitudes toward the very broadest social forms. Again, the omission of a manageable situational referent is damaging to the validity of the claim advanced.

SOME POINTS OF DEFINITION

Rather than prolong this critique, I should now like to lay the groundwork for another approach to conformity through some quite general observations. For the sake of emphasis, let me say that I at once reject the view that conformity is a persisting personal attribute, like being lame, or even a passing state, like having a rash. Instead, I urge a view of conformity as a process leading somewhere; I mean to say that conformity is a set of behaviors, displayed in a given situation, evidently in keeping with certain demands of the social situation, but nevertheless related at bottom to individual motivations and perceptions.

Consider the oft-noted case of young executives in gray flannel suits. Granted that this appears to be conformity to a socially prescribed pattern of dress, I would still wish to know what motivates a given person to manifest this fashion. Is it, as we are perhaps too hastily given to conclude, just a desire for social approval? Or is it perhaps a convenient device for being readily accepted, at least superficially, so that then other, more important kinds of behavior become acceptable? Would a young executive, hoping to put across a new advertising campaign, approach his superiors or clients with a boldly checked suit so as to engender a likely perceptual block to the more important commodity he wishes to market, namely an idea? I doubt it.

Nor do I think that the political demagogue who goes into the farm country and snaps his suspenders, chews tobacco, and speaks with the tones of a farm hand, behaves as he does because he is a "conformist personality" desiring social approbation. This is patently absurd. The man wishes to create an impression, an aura, which will smooth the way for his attainment of more important personal goals such as political power. Every successful demagogue must know this implicitly.

There are some other intricacies of definition which should not escape attention. Most basic is the matter of determining *when* an individual may be said to be conforming; and this is a highly relative, rather than absolute, matter. To really distinguish conformity from non-conformity, we ought to be able to distinguish between an individual's very own dispositions and the social demands to which he is subject, something we cannot too readily accomplish now. But suppose, illustratively, we happen to know these are quite in accord. This would suggest that the *appearance* of acquiescing to social demands is not by any means a sure index of conformity. It is also true that without the individual's awareness of social demands, even his apparent acquiescence to them is really not conformity at all; he may be responding quite randomly to a situation he understands only meagerly, yet his behavior, by chance, fits the prescribed pattern.

Perceptual and motivational components: In briefest terms, then, we may say that a two-fold assumption tends to pervade our usual conception of conformity: that the individual is aware of the existence of a given group norm, and that his manifest behavior in concordance with this norm is evidence of conformity. It is doubtful that both features of this assumption necessarily hold simultaneously. And this being so, difficulties of interpretation of behavior must necessarily arise.

Therefore, if an individual were to be insensitive to some norm, he could hardly be said to be conforming to it, whatever his behavior *seemed* to betray; correspondingly, a kind of inverse "conformity" might prevail all around us in the form of adherence to a faultily perceived norm. Thus an evident failure to conform might or might not be "non-conformity" depending upon the accuracy of the individual's perception of the norm in the first place.

Returning to the matter of motivation, we would be remiss, I believe, to accept non-conformity at its face value without seeking some motive for its manifestation. Leaving aside the perceptual point noted, we must surely recognize that some individuals might quite freely non-conform because they are motivated to achieve some goal of singular importance, and— what is more significant perhaps—because they know that their status in the particular group context will permit this degree of non-conformity. I do not mean to suggest that all such behavior is reasoned, in the cognitive sense, but I do propose that some individuals may rationally weigh their acceptable range of non-conformity and balance this with the strength of their motive to personally achieve something.

This suggests, as well, the likelihood that conformity is only approximately measured, at best, by the kind of fixed-norm baseline we normally employ. It is possible, indeed highly probable, that conforming behavior for one individual may be non-conforming for another, in terms of the perceptions of group members in the situation. The question of who defines conformity should not be lightly dismissed; I think it matters a great deal whether this is done by the actor himself, by an external observer, or by a fellow group member. The differential expectations in a group, regarding the behavior of individuals in that group, are of more importance than the attention they have received would indicate.

Person perceptions from interaction: Interaction between an individual and other individuals consists of a good deal more than manifest behaviors. There is a rich current of countervailing perceptions which evolve over time and constitute a past history affecting future interactions. Thus, as I have pointed out at much greater length elsewhere,[8] the individual in a group setting reacts not only in terms of immediate reality, but also in terms of his previously determined perception of the "group expectancies" relevant to his behaviors. These may be in the nature of what we usually think of as "norms" and "roles." And it is also correspondingly the case that his manifest behavior is appraised by other group members in terms of the past history of interaction and their perception of what is appropriate behavior for him.

Consequently, in the case of leadership as representative of a high status in a group, I have argued that a greater latitude is provided for non-conformity in certain realms of behavior since, through past interaction, the leader has accumulated a reservoir of positively-disposed impressions among his group members. I call these "idiosyncrasy credits," and take the view that, while an individual may find it necessary to conform to common group expectancies as he rises to the status of leadership, he may be expected to innovate (and thus, in some sense, non-conform) as a function of his achieved status. Early in interaction, then, conformity serves to maintain or increase status, in combination with some manifest contributions to the group; later, however, status allows a greater degree of latitude for non-conformity.

Interaction does not stand still. There are time-linked variations in the requirements of leadership, at least partly, because perceptions are altered as an individual displays behavior to relevant others over time. Moreover, whether an individual conforms has some anchorage in whether he has previously conformed, and what effects this had elicited from relevant others. Conformity therefore becomes an inextricable part of the pattern of past interactions and accompanying shifts in perception. A "standard of behavior" must therefore be a highly transitory, relative affair.

INDIVIDUAL MOTIVATION IN CONFORMITY

So much for the arena of conformity, and its dynamic, viewed broadly. Let us now consider the particulars of the dynamic. While I have taken exception to any conception of conformity as an individual attribute, I have nonetheless noted the significant role of individual motivation and perception. Thus, the entire position presented here is predicated on the assumption that some impelling force, presumably motivational, operates upon the individual so that he remains in the group; that is to say, the assumption that he is attracted to the group and that he proposes to persist in "playing the game." It is rare indeed to have the argument advanced that this is a linear dimension, although Bovard[5] has taken precisely this stand in group research which yielded no relationship between conformity and attraction to the group, measured linearly. If for no other reason, this grossness leaves his findings open to question. It is not that these variables need necessarily be related in every corner of the universe of group situations, but rather that at least two kinds of things seem to be involved in attraction to the group.

In the first place, an individual may be motivated to take part in group activity for its own sake, something akin to what Festinger[7] has suggested as the "instrumental" use of the group.

But, as the second point, it is possible for an individual to be motivated by a desire to gain or sustain social approval. These categories are not offered as mutually exclusive. Viewed at the extremes, however, it may be that an individual has interests which require group activity for their satisfaction, with no great concern on his part to secure social approval from the group, along the way; alternatively, another individual might be cast into a group with little positive activity valence for him, yet he may be motivated to do his part out of a desire for social approval.*

Whether these variables, illustrative of two likely dimensions of attraction to the group, will be related positively, negatively, or not at all, will of course depend upon the unique features of the individual and group setting involved. The key point, though, is that the motive for gaining social approval is probably relatively less subject to situational variations than the other motive, and may therefore constitute a somewhat more stable attribute in the nature of an individual parameter.

Notice that this is not an assertion that an individual with this attribute will necessarily conform, in any sense of regularity across situations; by now, hopefully, we have contributed to the rejection of such a simplex view. However, taking Sears'[12] view of personality as "a potential for activity"—and adding that it is realized in certain of a person's perceptual and motivational states—one could make a probability statement which more or less affirms this as a possibility. Some people, to a degree more than others, are reinforced by some manner of social approval; on a *ceteris paribus* basis, therefore, they will strive more than others to obtain such approval. But this does not dictate conformity, in any one-to-one fashion, because of at least one important intervening element, perceptual functioning, to which we now turn special attention.

INDIVIDUAL PERCEPTION IN CONFORMITY

In viewing perceptual functioning in relationship to conformity, rather different and oftentimes difficult problems are

---

* Another dichotomy, involving "task set" and "group set" and bearing a partial similarity, has been studied experimentally by Thibaut and Strickland.[13]

confronted. Among other things, if we conceive of this at bottom as a relatively stable attribute of the individual, we are likely to find that it bears a decidedly non-linear correspondence with behavior which we may take as indicative of conformity. The reasons for this assertion may be pointed up by pursuing this line of thought.

Consider the prospect that people are arrayed in terms of some perceptual alertness attribute which we might think of as a capacity. We need make no assumptions about the source of this capacity; it is only important for our purposes as a feature of the individual which bears upon his interaction with others. It should then follow that some individuals have an initial advantage over others in accurately perceiving group expectancies.

Holding situational characteristics and motivational influences constant, we might expect thereby that some individuals will more readily perceive the demands of the social context. Thus, it might be that an individual with a limited capacity will be given to more inaccuracies of perception, and hence may "non-conform" more than would an individual with greater capacity. But, on the other hand, with greater alertness to the group expectancies, an individual may more successfully adapt his behavior to their changing course over time. Limited capacity would imply a fixity, or rigidity, if you will, in responding. Though it would not necessarily be apparent, this kind of person might be "conforming" but, in keeping with an observation offered here earlier, to an *incorrectly* perceived expectancy.

This suggests that manifest non-conformity could arise from either a very high perceptual capacity, where the individual appropriately uses the "credits" at his disposal, or from a very low perceptual capacity, where the individual misreads the expectancies and his related availability of "credits."

Though advanced speculatively, this prospect both accounts for, and accords well with, what we know empirically of certain of the personality typologies studied of late in social psychology. The bulk of these, e.g. authoritarianism, rigidity, empathy, appear to center about some such perceptual functioning factor as a core element.[1, 3, 10] Terms like "perceptual rigidity," "perceptual defense," and "social imperceptiveness," often appear as concomitants of these broader characterizations; at least in some sense, this element evidently accounts for diversity among individuals. Therefore, while one might be reluctant to accept this as a direct well-spring of conformity behavior, it is likely—again, in probability terms—that such behavior has a linkage to relatively stable perceptual states of the individual.

Limitations in prediction: By the foregoing, I have sought to convey the view that there exist individually-based correlates of conformity behavior, operating within certain limits. These are not to be considered as giving rise to linear relationships, however. To the contrary, they must be understood to be subtly related to one another, and complexly, and oftentimes perhaps discontinuously, related to conformity. Predicting from them alone is bound to prove inadequate.

Conformity behavior does not lend itself to segmental treatment as either a feature of these individual attributes—personality, if you like—or of the situational field in which the individual is immersed. It would seem rather to be a combined function of prevailing situational conditions and stable states which are likely to yield certain behavioral outcomes, at times in accordance with more or less explicit expectancies of relevant others. The ongoing nature of this interactive process, with related perceptual changes occurring in the actor and the relevant others, has significant consequences as well.

RESEARCH IMPLICATIONS

The discontents I have pictured are not designed to encourage despair. Threading through these comments are signposts aimed at research to be done, and new relationships to be explored. And this is the essential thing.

What we appear to require basally is a more rigorous specification of both the dynamic and operational dimensions of conformity. Our criterion, repeatedly challenged here, suffers from an undue acceptance of the superficial at its face value. To observe only the manifest, and then make inferences about the underlying, is to run profound risks of misinterpretation. It is no simple task to tap the motivational and perceptual innards of the individual; but we do have, after all, reasonably effective techniques for accomplishing this. Moreover, this two-level approach is in fact demanded by the nature of the phenomenon.

Thus, several lines of research might be followed, and I mention these illustratively. We might study the behavioral consequences of individual perception of expectancies, under varying motivational conditions; the accuracy of such perception under levels of restriction of environmental cues, or as a function of individual "capacity," holding motivation constant; and, the effects of perceived conformity (or non-conformity) by various persons, serving as social stimulus objects, upon the behavior toward each of them by the perceiver. Nor should we neglect time-sequence effects.

In this latter regard, we have conducted some group studies under a grant from the Office of Naval Research. On a problem-solving task, extended over numerous trials, we manipulated the time of non-conformity from group-established procedural norms by one member; his high-level of performance was held constant, however, for all treatments. Thus we find that his influence, as a status measure, is differently altered not only by the amount of non-conformity or its sheer extension in time, but reasonably enough by its *time placement*. Early evidences of non-conformity are more damaging to influence than the same degree of non-conformity displayed later; indeed, these later manifestations, if anything, are accepted as a basis for norm shifts—but, by then, understandably, the object person has already gained a predicted following from his previous record of performance and conformity.

If nothing else, this kind of study moves a bit closer to the reality of life. Conformity behavior is elicited from most of us in a richer context than is provided by a situation where one either agrees or disagrees with a judgment made by four other people. Laboratory research has an important place, but only insofar as it transcends impoverished content variables which pitifully limit generalization to the real world.

SUMMARY

Having presented a case for conformity as a complexly-determined output of interaction, there remains only one thing more to be said: manifest conformity does not appear to be a very meaningful variable of personality.

References

1. Adorno, T. W., Frenkel-Brunswik, Else, Levinson, D. J., and Sanford, R. N. *The authoritarian personality.* New York: Harper, 1950.

2. Asch, S. E. Effects of group pressure upon the modification and distortion of judgment. In Guetzkow, H. (Ed.), *Groups, leadership and men.* Pittsburgh: Carnegie Press, 1951.

3. Bender, I. E. and Hastdorf, A. H. On measuring generalized empathic ability (social sensitivity). *J. abnorm. soc. Psychol.,* 1953, 48, 503-506.

4. Bernberg, R. E. A measure of social conformity. *J. Psychol.,* 1955, 39, 89-96.

5. Bovard, E. W. Conformity to social norms and attraction to the group. *Science,* 1953, 118, 598-599.

6. Crutchfield, R. S. Conformity and character. *Amer. Psychologist,* 1955, 10, 191-198.

7. Festinger, L. Informal social communication. *Psychol. Rev.,* 1950, 57, 271-282.

8. Hollander, E. P. Conformity, status and idiosyncrasy credit. *Psychol. Rev.,* 1958, 65, 117-127.

9. McClelland, D. C. Personality. In Farnsworth, P. R. (Ed.), *Annual review of psychology.* Stanford, California, 1956.

10. Rokeach, M. Generalized mental rigidity as a factor in ethnocentrism. *J. abnorm. soc. Psychol.,* 1948, 43, 259-278.

11. Sanford, N. Surface and depth in the individual personality. *Psychol. Rev.,* 1956, 63, 349-359.

12. Sears, R. R. A theoretical framework for personality and social behavior. *Amer. Psychologist*, 1951, 6, 476-483.

13. Thibaut, J. W. and Strickland, D. H. Psychological set and social conformity. *J. Personal.*, 1956, 25, 115-129.

14. Titus, H. E. and Hollander, E. P. The California F Scale in psychological research: 1950-55. *Psychol. Bull.*, 1957, 54, 47-64.

Robert B. MacLeod

XII

Person Perception:
A Commentary

INTRODUCTION

EACH OF THE FOUR PRECEDING CHAPTERS has approached the problems of person perception from a slightly different angle. I shall not presume to pass judgment on the merits of the papers, each of which I have found stimulating and constructive, but shall concentrate rather on a few of the theoretical issues which confront us when we attack person perception as a problem for research.

Stated in broad and commonplace language, the central problem of all psychology is that of understanding ourselves and other people. Basic to the problem of understanding is the problem of perception. How does one person perceive another person? This is our present concern. Just as soon as we use the word "perceive" we run into difficulties. What do we mean by "perceiving a person"? In the traditional textbooks the chapters on perception have dealt with space, time, form, movement, etc., never with persons. In recent years the word has been adopted by social and clinical psychologists and has been used so loosely that it has lost all precision of meaning. We need a clarification of terminology. The contributors to this section are obviously aware of this need, although none has faced it explicitly. Either we can or we cannot define perception in such a way as to make it applicable to the perception of persons; if we cannot, we should banish the word from our discussions.

My contention will be that we can, in fact, establish a meaningful relationship between the perception of persons and the perception of impersonal things and events. This is, I think, From's position; and I suspect that, in less explicit form, it is present in the thinking of Taft, Tagiuri and Hollander. At any rate, this is what I should like to focus on.

But, first, we need to clear the air. Problems commonly classified as those of person perception include: What are the objective criteria whereby we judge other people? How can we reduce these to terms of test items? By means of what procedures can one person pass a valid judgment on another? Does the successful judge of other persons possess certain special capacities or abilities, like empathic ability? If so, how can these be measured? And there are many more. In all the applied fields of psychology—in the schools, in the clinics, in industry—people are constantly judging one another; and it is tremendously important that psychologists develop and refine techniques that will enable people to react to one another sensitively and intelligently. These techniques involve far more than perception, as we customarily use the term. Implicit in all the techniques, however, is a theory of perception that ought to be based on facts, coolly appraised and logically interpreted. One of the first tasks is consequently to examine the ways in which one person actually perceives the characteristics and the behavior of another person. For this reason I shall limit most of my comments to problems of basic perceptual theory.

STRUCTURAL AND FUNCTIONAL APPROACHES

Within the tradition of empirical psychology we can distinguish broadly between structural and functional approaches to the study of perception, although the various theories might be classified in a number of other ways. The difference in approach is traditionally exemplified by the alternative psychologies of Wundt and Brentano. For Wundt a percept is a mental content, to be analyzed introspectively and related as precisely as possible to its underlying causal conditions. For Brentano perceiving is a mental act, to be differentiated from other mental acts, and its functional conditions specified. For an earlier generation of psychologists this difference in approach appeared to be so fundamental that in 1921 Titchener [24] could say, "The student of psychology . . . must still make his choice for the one or the other. There is no middle way between Brentano and Wundt." Today the choice seems to be a little less urgent than it did to Titchener; in fact, few living psychologists are likely to be aware that they have made it, and there is little in the current studies of perception that would indicate an allegiance to either Wundt or Brentano. Nevertheless, the difference, in quite another guise, is still there.

Classical structuralism is Newtonian. We find it in Locke and Berkeley, reaffirmed by the British associationists, imported into Germany by Helmholtz, and then carried to America by Titchener. In its classic form it involves the assumption of primary mental elements, analogous to Newton's material particles, which are integrated in various ways into compounds. For the Newtonian structuralist a percept is a cluster of sensations welded together with the residues of previous sensations into an experience which has the appearance of objectivity. Helmholtz referred to the welding process as unconscious inference, others were content with the traditional laws of association; all assumed the existence of a primary sense datum, coordinated to the physical stimulus, and a secondary elaborative or interpretative process which provides meaning. Perception, for the Newtonian psychologist, is sensation plus judgment.

Structuralism was Titchener's word, and for him it connoted a Newtonian type of analysis. At the risk of disturbing Titchener's ghost, and at the same time of offending some of his most ardent critics, I shall use the same label for the non-Newtonian psychologists of today, including the Gestaltists, who adopt the phenomenological approach and stress the primacy of organization. More about this later. For the moment it is important to note that, different as they might be in their methods of analysis and in their explanatory constructs, Titchener and Wertheimer were at one in their curiosity about the structuring of human experience. Theirs was a psychology of mental content. One

could trace the history of structuralism, thus loosely characterized by its preoccupation with direct human experience (German
Erlebnis) back to the days of the Greeks. The Greeks tended
to mix their logic with their psychology, but they honestly looked
at the phenomena of experience. From Socrates to Augustine to
Descartes to Husserl to the modern psychological phenomenologists we find a multitude of metaphysical and theological assumptions which in retrospect seem to have silently dictated theory;
but the fact remains that *experience as such*, as an existent, has
from time immemorial aroused the curiosity of the inquirer. And
central to the problems are those phenomena which we label as
percepts.

Functionalism must also be interpreted rather loosely. Brentano's psychology of the act was functionalist, as was Aristotle's
psychology, in the sense that it conceived of the mind (or the
soul) as having certain specifiable functions. All of faculty
psychology was in the same sense functionalist, since it explained the particular item of experience or behavior by referring it back to an inherent tendency or potentiality of the mind
(or soul). Classical functionalism usually contains an explicit or
implicit teleology. "The chief end of man," says the Shorter
Catechism, "is to glorify God and enjoy Him forever." "Thought,"
says a modern Idealist, "is that activity of mind which aims
directly at truth." [3] And we find a frank teleology in many of
the modern functionalists, notably William McDougall. The
movements of a human being, he argued,[18] are purposive, "by
which we mean that they are made for the sake of attaining their
natural end . . ." and purpose is characteristic of behavior on all
levels of organization. A structure develops only within the context of a function.

On the whole, however, modern functionalism is Darwinian
rather than Aristotelian. It has tended to reject the Aristotelian
teleology (the final cause), but it has accepted as fact the striving, adjusting character of behavior. One suspects that there
may be lurking "entelechies" in the concepts of "need" and
"drive" that have recently been supplanting the "instincts." At
any rate, for the modern functionalist, perception is perceiving;
and perceiving is one of the ways in which the organism comes

to terms with its environment. Such expressions as "coming to terms with" or "coping with" or even "responding to" betray an implicit epistemology which is no less real because it is seldom acknowledged.* The Darwinians, like the Newtonians, accept the world outside ourselves as something real. For the Newtonians, our percepts are more or less faithful representations of external reality, and our task is to determine which representations are correct and which are illusory, and why; the orientation is toward the external world. The Darwinians, beginning with the same assumption about the external world, but thinking of mind as a process of adjustment *to* reality rather than as a representation *of* reality, tend to accord more and more of perception to adjustment and less and less to representation. The result has been a psychology of perception dominated by a theory of motivation, with the percept always colored by the wishes and fears of the perceiver. Freud never wrote a psychology of perception. If he had done so, and if he had been consistent with the rest of his doctrine, he would have presented the percept as man's reluctant compromise between the world as he would like to see it and the world as it really exists. A Darwinian psychology of perception, pushed to its extreme, would leave us with a Protagorean relativism.

There are, of course, few psychologists who would attempt to explain perception from either the extreme Newtonian or the extreme Darwinian position. Titchener went as far as one could go with a Newtonian type of theory, and subsequent Newtonians, the S-R theorists, have for the most part ignored the problems. The modern Darwinians, who a few years ago spoke of the "new look" in perception, have made only very modest claims. It has been demonstrated to almost everyone's satisfaction that the wishes, anxieties, and expectations of the perceiver can influence his judgments, but there has been no suggestion that motivation alone will transform squares into circles or reds

---

* Psychologists who claim that they can divorce their science from philosophy are merely deluding themselves. No one can think or act without assumptions. There are those who try to make their philosophic assumptions explicit, and there are those who fail to recognize their assumptions. It is the latter who contribute most to our confusion.

into blues. In general, the modern Darwinians have done little more than shift the emphasis from stimulus-determination to need-determination, according slightly more to the latter but without seriously challenging the fundamental proposition that there is an independently existing reality of which our percepts are imperfect copies.

One hesitates to offer a compromise when what is needed is more rather than less debate. There is some point, however, in the elimination of debate over inconsequential issues, and I suggest that many of the theoretical issues which today divide students of perception are inconsequential. The structuralist-functionalist controversy has resolved itself into an idle debate over the relative weights to be attached to external and internal determinants of our percepts, as idle as the debate over the relative importance of heredity and environment. The problem is meaningful only if we make the metaphysical assumption of a dualism of matter and mind, with the mental regarded as a distorted representation of the non-mental. If, however, we follow Husserl's procedure and "bracket" (*in Klammern setzen*) our metaphysical assumptions about mind and matter and look first at the data of experience, we may find ourselves liberated for the attack on more interesting problems.

This, I suggest, is what we ought to be doing. Experience (*Erlebnis*), however defined, is what we observed immediately; and psychology should begin with the scrutiny of immediate experience. Our first question should always be: what is phenomenally present? We may later search for causes and correlates, but it will be a fruitless search if we are not first clear as to the phenomena we are trying to explain. The word "immediate" has in the past created a good deal of confusion because of its double meaning. In colloquial English "immediate" suggests "almost instantaneous," and immediate experience becomes consequently the hypothetical raw sense-datum which is directly produced by stimulation and which has not yet been tarnished by the residues of previous stimulation. This is, of course, unsatisfactory. Sensation is always a process-in-time, and a merely temporal definition leaves unspecified the particular point in time at which a sense-datum ceases to be a sensation and becomes something else. Equally unsatisfactory, however, is the slightly more sophisticated interpretation of immediacy as "not mediated," for it leaves unanswered the question: what mediates what? Traditional faculty psychology, and even certain of the modern functionalists,* could dispose of the question readily by assigning sensation to one faculty and interpretation to certain others; and the best of the Newtonian structuralists, Titchener,[23] could argue that a properly trained introspector can so arrange experimental conditions that "one process and one process only is presented for observation." For Titchener a percept is by definition a mediated phenomenon, the mediating data being the primary sensations revealed by introspection. Percepts as such can consequently never be immediate.

Can we straighten out the confusion? I think we can, if we are willing provisionally to bracket the distinctions between what is primary and what is secondary, what is sensation and what is interpretation, what is unlearned and what is learned, and simply look at experience as it exists. This is the phenomenological approach. It is infinitely sloppier than that of the neat Newtonian, and it possesses its own quota of internal contradictions, but it at least frees us from a number of conceptual constraints and it legitimizes a scientific interest in a great array of intrinsically fascinating human phenomena which traditional approaches have excluded. Among these are our percepts of people as people.

PHENOMENOLOGICAL APPROACH

The psychological phenomenologist is a structuralist in the sense that he is interested in the structure and organization of the whole world of experience. All experience that is faithfully observed *as experience* is immediate. He may eventually embed the results of his analysis in a functional scheme, but what inter-

---

* Madison Bentley, for instance, distinguished between the apprehensive functions (perception, memory, imagination) and the elaborative functions (understanding, thinking).[2]

ests him initially is not the explanatory constructs of functionalism but the phenomena of experience which invite a functional explanation. The phenomenologist, *qua* phenomenologist, brackets all the traditional categories of classification, but he cannot refrain from asking what characteristics of experience have established these categories so firmly in psychological thinking. He may reject sensation, discrimination, emotion, and reason as faculties of a substantive mind or as functions of a biological organism, but he cannot deny the fact that thoughtful people have found these categories plausible. What are the phenomenal facts which lead us to think of sensation and reason as pure, and emotion as muddy? What is there about a color or a tone which makes it seem more primary than a relation of "brighter than" or "louder than"? What phenomenal content invites the distinction between "interpretation" and "that which is interpreted"? It would be interesting to pursue such questions further, but this is not the appropriate occasion. Suffice it to say that under scrutiny some of these distinctions break down, some are sustained, and usually there emerge a number of new dimensions which suggest further inquiry.

Let us now return to the central question. May we legitimately talk about the perception of a person? A definition of perception which I have frequently defended runs somewhat as follows: Perception is the process whereby things, events, and their qualities and relations become present to a self as here, now, and real. This is a strictly phenomenological definition, except for the word "process," which implies something functional. The phenomenologist must transcend his phenomenology, however, if he is to make his contribution to science; and, provisionally at any rate, I find the Darwinian constructs more congenial than the Newtonian. The other terms may need some elaboration. "Things" and "events" should cause no trouble. A thing is segregated, bounded, resilient, existing in space; it persists in time, but its persistence is irrelevant to its identity. An event is likewise segregated, bounded and resilient, and exists in space, but its salient dimension is temporal rather than spatial; the key to its identity is its beginning and its ending. A thing is likely to be visual or tactual-kinaesthetic; an event is likely to be auditory.

But even casual observation makes it clear that things and events do not fit neatly into the traditional categories of sense-modality.

The status of relations in the theory of perception has always been a source of confusion. For the Newtonian a relation, like "brighter than" or "equal to," must inevitably be a second-order phenomenon because it implies logically the prior existence of the data about which a relational judgment is made. Relations are deduced or, to use Spearman's term,[21] educed from fundaments. This, it seems to me, reflects the common confusion of logical with psychological analysis. It is true that if we assume that the primary existents are Newtonian particles, or their mental analogues, and if we accept Aristotelian logic as final, then we are forced to demote relations to a secondary status. If, however, we bracket the notion of primary elements, and accord primacy to every experience, we find with William James[9] that relations between and among things and events are just as truly "there" as are the hypothetical elements:

> "If there be such things as feelings at all, then so surely as relations between objects exist *in rerum natura*, so surely, and more surely, do feelings exist to which these relations are known. . . . We ought to say a feeling of *and*, a feeling of *if*, a feeling of *but*, and a feeling of *by*, quite as readily as we say a feeling of *blue* or a feeling of *cold*."

I am inclined to use the term "relations" very broadly to include much of what have traditionally been called the products of judgment, e.g. not only relations of size, shape, intensity, duration, etc., but also attributes like attractiveness and repulsiveness, and states like tension and calm, which involve the self as well as the thing or event. All of these can be phenomenally present, i.e. they can be data of immediate perception.

How about the self, to which things, events and relations are present? Is there a structure in the psychological field which is not a thing, not an event, and not a relation, to which percepts are "given"? In the good old days people believed that they had souls; but these were banished by the empiricists, and with them the concept of self. Perhaps the most brutal blows were aimed by David Hume.[8] The self, he insisted, is a complete illusion, nothing but an erroneous inference from a lot of perceptions which have nothing truly in common; and for nearly two centuries psychologists have been reluctant to readmit the self to psychology. During recent decades, however, the self has been gradually recovering respectability, partly as a direct consequence of the clinical movement but more basically as a reflection of the growing discontent with an exclusively reductive psychology. Quite intelligibly the emphasis has tended to be on the self as a variable in motivation. With the distinction between perception and motivation steadily losing its traditional significance, however, it becomes evident that the self must also be accepted as a problem of perception.[15]

My definition suggests that the self should be accorded a unique status in the perceptual field, distinct from things, events, and relations. I should hesitate to defend this position very vigorously, but I find the distinction convenient. True, many of the phenomenal properties which differentiate self from not-self, such as animation, freedom, and emotion, can be compellingly present in phenomenal things and events,[7] and the self is often phenomenally present as little more than a silent and passive anchorage point for a vastly complicated objective world. It could be argued that phenomenological analysis reveals only a set of dimensions of variation—light-dark, long-short, rough-smooth, etc.—and that subjective-objective, voluntary-involuntary, etc., are merely additional dimensions of the same order. This would be in accord with a modernized David Hume, and the argument has considerable appeal. It would be an incomplete phenomenology, however. As the Gestaltists and many others have pointed out,[12, 13, 19, 20, 25] the phenomenal world is never—except possibly in earliest infancy or in certain abnormal states—present as merely a set of dimensions. It is characteristically structured and, once the structures have become established, they defend their integrity. A sound phenomenology must recognize what Köhler[11] has called "organized entities." The self is such an organized entity, and as such is a phenomenal fact. Whether or not in transcending the phenomenal world we are prepared, with Lundholm,[14] to accord to transphenomenal selves the same status as we do to transphenomenal things and events is a problem for the metaphysician and not for the psychologist.

Communication would be simplified if we had a common name for a superordinate category that would include phenomenal things, events and selves, which are tough and resilient entities, and differentiate them from the welter of properties, attributes, states, and other relational characteristics of the phenomenal world. Language, for the phenomenologist, is always a source of insight; but it is also his most persistent source of frustration. At any rate, if we grant that the self is a valid datum of perception, "something there" analogous to but not identical with things and events, then we must accept it as a proper object of perceptual study. Let us suspend for the moment the question as to whether the "other self" can be perceived.

The definition specifies "here, now, and real" as essential to a percept. "Here" is self-explanatory; the thing or event has a more or less clear spatial location with reference to the self. I see it, I hear it, I feel it. "Now" is equally self-explanatory. The act of remembering or imagining may be now, but the object of memory or imagination is phenomenally in the past or undated. To conceive of "reality" as phenomenal is more difficult; the term is much too closely bound up with metaphysics and epistemology. Nevertheless, even a superficial inspection of phenomena makes it clear that the reality-character of a thing or an event bears no necessary relation to our sophisticated judgment as to its independent existence. The psychological dimension is reality-irreality. The floor I am standing on is here and now and real, although I may concede the hypothetical possibility that it may disintegrate beneath my feet. The stream of cold water pouring on my hand encased in a rubber glove "really" feels wet, although I know that the hand within the glove is perfectly dry. When I squint my eyes at the lamp, the shooting rays I see are visibly there, but they have an aspect of irreality; and so does the after-image of a bright light or the wispy memory of a dream. Along the reality-irreality dimension we can plot not only that which we see and hear and feel, but also that which we remember, imagine, believe, and doubt.

PERSON PERCEPTION

If we maintain a consistently phenomenological orientation, the lines which have traditionally separated perception from memory and imagination become quite blurred, as do the lines which separate these from the various levels of abstract thought. There are things which are here and now but not real, and then and there but real, and so forth; and there are experiences devoid of thing-character which, at least according to the mystics, can be here and now and real. It would be good if we could banish the traditional terminology, with its implication of separable faculties or functions, and consider in a global way a single world of experience with its salient structures, relations and dimensions. This is manifestly impossible. I suggest, as a compromise, that we at least provisionally bracket questions of veridicality and attempt to complete our descriptive analysis, all the while trying to specify the conditions which make our descriptive data predictable and intelligible.

Viewed in this way the perception of other persons becomes both a simpler and a more complex problem. It is simpler because we are temporarily freed from a clutter of epistemological assumptions about what is "really" there and what is a product of interpretation. If for us the other person is here, now, and real, then we have perceived him. Whether or not we have perceived him "correctly," we can at least try to determine why we perceive him as we do. But it is also a more complex problem because, thus liberated, we cannot in good conscience overlook any of the phenomena which make a person appear as a person. We are required accordingly to investigate not only the formal properties of a presented object, like color, size, shape, and movement, which make it perceptible as a person and identifiable as a particular person, but also the less tangible (expressive, physiognomic, dynamic) properties which perhaps bring us closer to the essence of person perception.

As a possible contribution to clarity, may I suggest a set of distinctions, borrowed from Stern,[22] which I have often found useful.[16] The person may be conceived as a non-phenomenal entity, analogous to the physical object, only some of whose properties are revealed in perception. We assume that the person, with its attributes, "really" exists and can be known. We derive our knowledge of the person by inference from a wide variety of observations and measurements, only some of which rest directly on phenomenological analysis. Our concern in the study of persons is with veridicality, and our test is the consistency with which our various indices can make predictions. The "self" and the "personality," on the other hand, are phenomenal data, structures of the phenomenal field. I have referred above to the self as an inescapable perceptual fact. The personality is the "other self," and it is apprehended likewise a perceptual fact. Neither self nor personality is likely to be a true representation of the underlying person. Nevertheless, just as our knowledge of the physical world is derived in part from our study of phenomenal things and events, so our knowledge of persons must rest in part on the phenomenology of self and personality.

The problem of person-perception, as conceived in this section, seems to be partly that of 1) the veridicality of our judgments of persons, as above defined, with consistency accepted as the test, and partly that of 2) the phenomenal properties of persons, i.e. personality as above defined, and of behavior. The first of these emphases has been characteristic of the British-American tradition, and is ably represented by Taft and by Hollander. The second, the phenomenological, is typically Continental European, and From's studies are good examples. Tagiuri's chapter reflects both types of interest. If he has not fully succeeded in integrating the two approaches, it is at least to his credit that he has tried. I shall not comment in detail on the Taft and Hollander papers. Taft makes what I think is a regrettable distinction between cognition and perception. Perception as a process, it seems to me, is a logically but not psychologically subordinate category within a more general category of cognizing, or knowing. But, having identified his problem as that of determining the conditions of veridical judgment of persons, Taft gives an admirable analysis of its dimensions, with excellent empirical support. With similar skill and honesty, Hollander has challenged the hypothesis that "conformity" can be considered as a trait of a person. There will probably be some vigorous counterattacks; but the result will be good. We now have experimental and statistical tools which will in due course enable us to specify the intra- and extra-organismic determinants of interpersonal judgments; and both Taft and Hollander have made substantial contributions. The next few decades of research should be quite exciting.

Of more pressing importance, it seems to me, is the challenge from phenomenology, represented by From and, in part, by Tagiuri. American psychology is efficiently quantitative. It is functional and practical; it loves to measure, to predict, and to control; and it has proved its usefulness in medicine, in education, and in industry. European psychology has traditionally made more use of descriptive methods and has tended to stress as its goal understanding rather than prediction and control. That the two approaches are not irreconcilable, can, I think, be easily demonstrated. The phenomenologist would argue, however, that in a relatively new field like the perception of personality it is particularly important that elaborate quantification be preceded by careful description. One could cite numerous examples from the history of psychology which show how premature attempts at quantification have not only resulted in vast amounts of fruitless research but have actually led to serious theoretical confusion. Let me touch quite briefly on two of the most challenging questions discussed in this section.

The first of these has to do with *human actions as perceptual phenomena*, presented so brilliantly by From. Classical perceptual theory has been overwhelmingly concerned with things (objects) and their properties rather than with events. This is intelligible, since thing-percepts lend themselves more readily to laboratory investigation. The classical psychology of time, with its tedious experiments on the comparison of intervals of varying length, has not yielded an adequate picture of the temporal structuring of perception. That such a structuring exists, that it is fully as complex as is the structuring of space, and that it contains unique phenomenal relations like causation and purpose, have long since been pointed out by both philosophers and psychologists. That event-structures have not been generally included in perceptual theory is due only in part to technical experimental difficulties; behind their rejection lies a silent assumption that the immediate data of experience are non-temporal, that the complex properties of events are second-order phenomena. Even Lewin, who was a good phenomenologist, tended to think of life-space in terms of successive cross-sections. Only recently have investigators begun to suspend the anti-temporal bias and explore event-structures as phenomena. Barker and Wright,[1] for instance, have patiently recorded the day by day activities of children in terms of "natural" units of behavior, and Michotte[20] and Johannson[10] have systematically explored the temporal configurations which give rise to the various impressions of causality.

That event-structures are legitimate perceptual phenomena —indeed that all percepts, including thing-structures, are temporally configured—is beginning to be accepted. What psychologists almost universally resist, however, is the notion that purpose may also be a perceptual datum. "Purpose," to our Newtonian ears, sounds altogether too Aristotelian. Nevertheless, if purposes, in line with the above definition, are here, now, and real, then purposes can be perceived. But let us keep reminding ourselves that phenomenology and metaphysics are not the same. If purpose is a phenomenal fact, as From so convincingly argues, we are not for this reason required to accept an Aristotelian teleology; we may still entertain widely different conceptions of nature. As I have suggested elsewhere, however, we cannot in our psychological analysis deny the phenomena which invite a teleological theory.[17]

The second problem which impresses me as particularly important is posed in Tagiuri's chapter. This has to do with the possibility of a *psychophysics of the personality percept*. Granted that a personality can be perceptually present as here, now, and real, is it possible to specify the conditions of stimulation which are responsible for the unique characteristics of the percept? Classical psychophysics developed as an attempt to state with mathematical precision the relation between the introspectively isolated elements and dimensions of experience and correspondingly elementary conditions of proximal stimulation. The methods of classical psychophysics may still be accepted as valid for certain appropriate problems, and their application continues to yield substantial results. The modern reaction against psychophysics has not been against the methods as such, but rather against the reductive-atomistic theory which they traditionally implied.

Psychophysics, broadly conceived, is the search for correspondences between the phenomenal and the physical. "Phenomenal" need not necessarily be limited to the hypothetical elements; nor need "physical" necessarily be limited to proximal stimulation. A complete psychophysics would find physical counterparts for all the structures and properties of the phenomenal world. Whether or not this can be done is obviously at present a matter of faith, but to a growing number of psychologists it seems to be worth trying. We find a good beginning, for instance, in the early studies of movement, form, and constancy, which yielded crude but promising correlations between properties of phenomenal organization and correspondingly complex conditions in the physical world. The question is whether or not these "global" relations can be restated in precise mathematical language, possibly in a mathematics radically different from that of traditional psychophysics.

The best case for a global psychophysics is presented by Gibson.[6] Drawing his evidence primarily from vision, and particularly from space perception, Gibson has shown how many phenomenal properties, traditionally explained in terms of secondary interpretative processes, can now be coordinated to specifiable external stimuli. Johannson's[10] studies of temporally configured perception provide supporting evidence, and the case will become stronger as we learn to deal more adequately with the temporal characteristics of stimulation. To explore the possibilities now would lead us too far astray, since our concern is with the perception of personality. Tagiuri's experiments on various types of movement as cues are, however, promising; and these can be meaningfully related to those of Heider and Simmel, of Johannson, and even of Michotte. His suggested mathematical analysis of relations among successive points in a path obviously needs support from many more experiments. As such it is extremely promising, and will undoubtedly help to blaze new trails of research. He is, I think, on the brink of a major contribution to global psychophysics.

My one adverse comment is that Tagiuri has been altogether too ready to slip from the language of perception to the older, logic-bound language of interpretation and inference. In his mathematical discussion, for instance, he suggests "some kind of unconscious integration of the meaning of the successive points constituting the path." This one would not quarrel with, were it not so reminiscent of the "unconscious inferences" of the Helmholtzian era. It is true that organisms behave as though they possessed unconsciously more mathematical skills than the average human ever consciously masters; in fact, the implied mathematical competence of von Frisch's bees[5] commands the respect of some of our better mathematicians, and, as we know from Brunswik's work,[4] even a rat can be made to behave as though he understood probability theory. There is a difference, however, between behaving in accordance with mathematical or physical law and making inferences. We have no reason to assume that the rat or the bee or the nervous system can understand mathematics or logic merely because its behavior conforms to our conception of a natural order, or even if its behavior can be replicated by rationally designed machines. Making inferences is a psychological process, as is perceiving, which it is the psychologist's duty to describe and analyze; there can be a psychology of logic and mathematics just as there is a psychology of perception. For the psychologist, a reference to interpretation or inference provides no explanation; it merely shifts the problem to another level. A good phenomenology of inference would help us bridge the chasm between perception and other cognitive processes.

My point is not that we should disparage the "central" processes (motivation, attitudes, past experience, etc.) which affect perception, but rather that we should try to specify as many as possible of the stimulus conditions which give shape to the growing percept. It is idle to say that a percept is "learned" or "interpreted" without specifying upon what the learning or interpretation is based. I dislike the term "cue," which Tagiuri uses and which has been traditional in the psychology of space perception, but I welcome his attempt to identify the stimulus cues to the perception of personality.

SUMMARY

The chapters in this section have raised many systematic issues, only a few of which I have been able to touch upon. The paramount issue may seem at first glance to be merely one of terminology, the definition of perception; but I do not think it is superficial. Our understanding of people depends in large part on what we perceive. My contention is that an inadequate theory of perception has muddied our thinking. I have proposed a definition which, I think, may liberate us from some crippling assumptions and enable us to integrate the classical psychology of perception with the current attempts to explain the perception of persons.

References

1. Barker, R. C. and Wright, H. P. *Midwest and its children*. Evanston, Ill.: Row, Peterson, 1954.

2. Bentley, M. *The field of psychology*. New York: Appleton, 1924.

3. Blanshard, B. *The nature of thought*. London: Allen & Unwin, 1939.

4. Brunswik, E. Probability as a determiner of rat behavior. *J. exper. Psychol.*, 1939, 25, 175-197.

5. von Frisch, K. *Bees: their vision, chemical senses and language*. Ithaca, N. Y.: Cornell Univ. Press, 1950.

6. Gibson, J. J. Perception as a function of stimulation. In Koch, S. (Ed.), *Psychology: a study of a science*. Vol. I. New York: McGraw-Hill, 1959.

7. Heider, F. and Simmel, M. An experimental study of apparent behavior. *Amer. J. Psychol.*, 1944, 57, 243-259.

8. Hume, D. *A treatise of human nature.* 1740.

9. James, W. *Principles of psychology.* New York: Holt, 1890.

10. Johannson, G. *Configurations in event perception.* Uppsala, 1950.

11. Köhler, W. *Gestalt psychology.* Rev. ed. New York: Liveright, 1947.

12. Köhler, W. *The place of value in a world of facts.* New York: Liveright, 1938.

13. Koffka, K. *Principles of Gestalt psychology.* New York: Harcourt, 1935.

14. Lundholm, H. The psychological self in the philosophies of Köhler and Sherrington. *Psychol. Rev.*, 1946, 53, 119-131.

15. MacLeod, R. B. Perceptual constancy and the problem of motivation. *Can. J. Psychol.*, 1949, 3, 57-66.

16. MacLeod, R. B. The place of phenomenological analysis in social psychological theory. In Rohrer, J. H. and Sherif, M. (Eds.), *Social psychology at the crossroads.* New York: Harper, 1951.

17. MacLeod, R. B. Teleology and theory of human behavior. *Science*, 1957, 125, 447-480.

18. McDougall, W. *Outline of psychology.* London: Methuen, 1929.

19. Merleau-Ponty, M. *Phénomenologie de la perception.* Paris: Gallimard, 1945.

20. Michotte, A. *La perception de la causalité.* Louvain, 1946.

21. Spearman, C. *The nature of intelligence and the principles of cognition.* New York: Macmillan, 1927.

22. Stern, W. *Allgemeine Psychologie vom personalistischen Standpunkt.* Nijhoff, 1935. Eng. trans., *General psychology from the personalistic standpoint.* New York: Macmillan, 1938.

23. Titchener, E. B. *A textbook of psychology.* New York: Macmillan, 1910.

24. Titchener, E. B. Brentano and Wundt: empirical and experimental psychology. *Amer. J. Psychol.*, 1921, 32, 108 ff.; reprinted in *Systematic Psychology: Prolegomena*, Weld, H. P. (Ed.) New York: Macmillan, 1929.

25. Werner, H. *Einführung in die Entwicklungspsychologie.* (1st. ed.), Leipzig, 1925; Eng. trans., *Comparative psychology of mental development* (Rev. ed.). New York: International Universities Press, 1948.

PART FOUR

Resources

Aase Gruda Skard
with
Bärbel Inhelder
Gerald Noelting
Lois B. Murphy
and Hans Thomae

XIII

Longitudinal Research in Personality Development

INTRODUCTION

As so well stated by Gordon Allport,[1] questions related to the formation and development of the human personality are among those least touched by psychological research. In an effort to consider recent research studies, a symposium was organized by Bärbel Inhelder at the Brussels International Congress. Under the chairmanship of Aase Gruda Skard a lively discussion ensued, summary highlights of which are presented in this chapter.

OBSERVATIONS (*Skard*)

Some recent research efforts explicitly aim at being first attempts to put bits of information into the vast empty gulf of knowledge about human personality and its formation. We might think of the problems as a large puzzle where a great number of related pieces must be joined to form an understandable structure. The initial small pieces must be both numerous and diverse if we are ever to perceive the total pattern or infer from the beginning structure hypotheses for the still unknown parts.

"Personality is less a finished product than a transitive process," says Allport, and evidently the study of personality formation must be a study of *change*. It must also be an attempt

to distinguish the sources of change; that is, the change originating in maturation of inborn potentialities, or the change
basically formed by a learning process, the change that comes
by way of modification of tendencies through the influence of
surroundings, and that which emerges from the incorporation
of cultural and personal behavior patterns. But, every single
piece of the puzzle does not have to contain *all* the various
ingredients necessary for the total picture. To grasp the framework we shall need observations of change from age level to
age level (Gesell and his co-workers), cultural anthropological
investigations of human development and syntheses of such
work,[27] and intensive studies of both individual growth[5, 26] and
large groups.[24]

Longitudinal methods have been valuable in the study of
physical growth. However, individual growth curves provided
important corrections for general statistical studies of large
population groups and may still have something to contribute
to the study of body types, both in regard to their development
in individuals and their relation to personality traits. Similarly,
Olson's[16] studies of motor behavior have been conducive to the
formulation of growth theories and for hypotheses on training
readiness and possible vulnerability to specific influences. Of
equal importance are Bailey's[3] longitudinal studies of mental
development, following Terman's pioneering.

The rhythm of maturational changes and sequences of
behavior (as emphasized by Gesell and Piaget in their different
fields of investigation) may be further illuminated by intensive
longitudinal studies of individual cases, as reported by Inhelder
and Noelting.

Other problem areas are similarly open to further investigation. Stages of growth may be saturated with experiences, modifying agents, conflict-creating situations, and emotional reactions.
How is an individual changed by these, if at all? Thomae,[24] has
well formulated the problem: "It would be important to note
how objectivity turns into sterility, activity into overactivity and
restlessness, caution into carelessness, intensity of emotional life
to extensity, or vice versa." Psychoanalytic hypotheses also cry
for verification. What are the effects of parents' attitudes toward

pregnancy on their later treatment of the child, and consequently on its development? What is the impact of feeding situations on later orality, or on other personality traits? Is there an "anal character" and are the roots of it to be found in the specific attitudes of parents to toilet training?

To quote Allport[1] once more: "What is the relative importance of earlier and later stages of development? We know that there are layers in each person that are archaic and composed of relatively isolated earlier systems. Yet there are also layers in which man is fully adult, his psychological maturity corresponding to his age. The drama of human life can be written largely in terms of the friction engendered between earlier stages and later stages of development. *Becoming* is the process of incorporating earlier stages into later; or when this is impossible, of handling the conflict between early and late stages as well as one can." What is the nature of this relationship between older and newer personality layers in presumably "normal" persons? How will "traumata" or "stress" during one period influence later development? How do "defense mechanisms" function in the long run, and how do children "cope with" or get rid of difficulties encountered at specific periods?

Lois Murphy has worked with such problems in child guidance centers. Her material may raise new, parallel questions in longitudinal studies of children *not* referred for examination due to deviant behavior. For example, we may ask which problems usually appear at various developmental levels, and whether they will or will not disappear again (as indicated in studies by Jean Macfarlane[11]). Why can some children "cope" with their difficulties while others cannot? How do problems of various kinds at different stages affect later development (such as maternal deprivation during early childhood which may have lasting effect on emotional development, according to Bowlby[4] and others)?

Through the cobweb of problems on influences and their possible effects runs the basic problem of *consistency of personality* or the persistency of certain traits. The consistency of a person's intelligence has already been widely discussed and thoroughly examined. It may be that careful longitudinal observation will tell us more about the constancy of other traits. Will we find, at least, certain established *relations* persisting within a certain culture? In other words, if individual differences do remain constant, then even if we cannot predict a specific IQ or reaction time, we should at least be able to indicate which of two or more individuals will consistently have a higher IQ, faster reactions, etc. Will we be able to localize *syndromes* of certain traits that tend to go together, in a fashion similar to Terman's theory of positive correlation between body size and intelligence? Thomae[24] has tackled this problem with tests and questionnaires to find possible maturational patterns, the covariance of specific traits.

While children grow and change they live *in a milieu,* surrounded by things and people, adults and other children. These surroundings are far from constant. Not only do families move to new neighborhoods (and what is the effect of such a move at various stages of maturation?), but also people move in and out of the immediate family surrounding the child. A grandmother arrives to stay, a tubercular mother is sent to a convalescent home, a new baby is born, a father dies, a cousin is killed in an accident, a seafaring uncle is home for some months, or a mother takes a part- or full-time job. The character of the parents' marriage may change as they gradually move from the happiness of establishing a new household to the monotony of household chores or the lasting security of an "old" relationship.

Parental roles also change with time. It is not the same to be the parent of a baby, a toddler, a four-year-old, or a school-goer. The child's growth has its effect on the parents; there are different expectations, fresh demands, and new ways of dealing with behavior. Parents expect the child not only to become more mature, but also to modify his role in society and his position in the family and among his peers. Moreover, the changing role should be different for the two sexes. Such changes can be recorded in retrospect through anamnestic interviews or questionnaires[19] or in observations and interviews at definite intervals during the child's development so as to avoid the hazards of memory. In Oslo an attempt is made to follow not only the changes in the child but also the simultaneous changes in the family and the child's widening world.

The following brief reports may be considered as first pieces for the large puzzle, with each researcher beginning at a different corner and pointing to more problems in his area. "To ask questions in the midst of our confusion may focus the effort to explore." [13]

A PILOT STUDY OF COGNITIVE FUNCTIONS
(*Inhelder and Noelting*)

Our pilot study qualifies as a longitudinal project on several counts: 1) its *purpose*—to trace changes occurring in the reasoning of children and adolescents as a function of experimentally introduced experiences; 2) its *method*—the validation of the Piaget-Inhelder experiments, which have been developed and standardized with the help of our collaborators during the past fifteen years; and 3) its *limited duration*—following the cognitive development of 4 groups of 5 children, aged 5, 7, 9, and 12 years at the beginning of the study, for a period of from 3 to 5 years.

Definition of the concept of stage and a working hypothesis: Our previous studies, based on groups of children of different ages, examined by the cross-sectional method, have led us to the formulation of certain hypotheses concerning the meaning of the stages of cognitive development; these hypotheses call for verification and an attempted explanation that only the longitudinal method can provide.

It is in the field of intellectual operations that it seems easiest to give a certain number of criteria of experimentally verifiable stages.

With Piaget we tried to define the stages as follows: 1) each stage involves a period of formation (genesis) and a period of attainment; the latter is characterized by the progressive organization of a composite structure of mental operations; 2) each structure constitutes at the same time the attainment of one stage and the starting point of a new evolutionary process; 3) the order of succession of the stages is constant; and 4) the stages form points of integration, preceding structures becoming a part of later structures.

The aim of our segmented longitudinal research is thus to study in detail the qualitative changes of reasoning in order to identify some of the evolutionary processes.

A theory of stages remains incomplete, however, as long as it does not clarify, by new facts, the contradiction between two concepts of developments, one stressing the complete continuity and the other the absolute discontinuity of stages. It seems to us, however, that this contradiction is more apparent than real. Our first investigations lead us to surmise (as a hypothesis) a third notion; namely, that in the development of intellectual operations, phases of continuity alternate with phases of discontinuity. Continuity and discontinuity would have to be defined by the relative dependence or independence of new behavior with respect to previously established behavior. Indeed, it seems as if during the formation of a structure of reasoning (characteristic of stage A) each new procedure depended on those that the child had just acquired. Once achieved, this structure would serve as a starting point for new acquisitions (characteristic of stage B). The latter would then be relatively independent of the formative process of the former. It is only in this sense that there would be discontinuity in passing from one stage to another.

Method: We chose about forty tests bearing on the formation of some invariants and mental operations in the fields of space, time, causality, numbers and probabilities. The tests are designed to tap the processes involved in the formation of concrete and abstract operations. The "operative" mechanisms in questions have primarily been analyzed by Piaget by means of models of symbolic logic. The frequency and hierarchy of the types of solutions have been established for the majority of the tests according to the principle of ordinal methods.

Since changes in reasoning can be fully understood only when imbedded in the context of the child's behavior, we are making use of sound recordings and films.

First results: Though it may appear bold to present results after only 18 months of longitudinal investigation (3 of the 4 groups of children are seen 3 times a year; a total of 5 times up to now), we would like to submit some provisional data for discussion.

Some of the hypotheses advanced in connection with our previous research find confirmation in the present study. The different types of reasoning, previously outlined (on the basis of having seen each child for only one testing and at a definite moment of its development), seem to recur in a stable, logical order of developmental stages.

In other respects we observe certain differences between the results obtained by former methods and the longitudinal one, without being able to discern in detail what role can be attributed to the method and what to the evolutionary process itself: the elaboration of certain notions and of methods of reasoning is slightly accelerated in our subjects as compared to the control groups. This acceleration, due to general or specific practice, does not seem the same at all levels. When the child is given a series of reasoning tests, we notice a tendency to homogeneity and generalization of behavior which, though slight in the course of the formation of a structure, manifests itself more clearly when the structure has been achieved.

In certain areas, it seems already possible to separate some relatively constant evolutionary processes. For example, at regular intervals a child is brought to grips with the problem of the conservation of a given physical quantity. A liquid (juice) is poured from one container into another of a different size. In early trials the child is impressed by the change in one of the dimensions of the liquid, neglecting others. With naive belief it contests any conservation of the liquid quantity. Some months later, the same child, beginning to doubt, tries to put the different changes into perspective, without, however, attaining an understanding of their compensation or inversion. A whole series of attempts to establish relationships, from the simplest to the most complex, can frequently be observed. Still later, the child finally affirms the constancy of the liquid quantity. "There is the same amount of juice to drink." The arguments become more and more coherent and indicate that it now understands the changes in the liquid as a reversible system of operations, the modifications of which compensate each other. Strangely enough, not only does the child seem to have forgotten its own trials and errors, but it considers them absurd. The events seem to suggest that a mental structure is prepared by a continuous series of trials, but that once established it becomes relatively independent of the process involved in its formation.

It is to be hoped that a longitudinal study of the process of acquisition of mental operations will one day make possible a clarification of some of the internal mechanisms of cognitive learning.

COPING METHODS (*Murphy*)

Everything we know about specific cognitive and motor functions is important in its own right for what each process contributes to the individual's grasp upon and control of his environment, and also as factors in more complex functions of creativity, restructuring the environment, and management of stress through selection, dilution, fragmenting, distancing, cushioning, delay, alternation of attention between stressful and neutral or gratifying stimuli, and other devices. Conscious and unconscious efforts collaborate in the harnessing of defense mechanisms with other active coping efforts for management of stress and for growth. We have to develop new ways of studying these dynamic processes of healthy development and integration; we have to look differently, to observe differently. We have to learn to observe the dynamics of each situation: how the child copes with a variety of everyday challenges, tasks, stresses, and, when these occur, more serious challenges or stresses. Second, we have to seek ways for formulating or conceptualizing what we find, without burdening ourselves with unnecessary new terms or clumsy, heavy phrases. A third step is to formulate the generalizations which this kind of evidence can provide. In studying behavior, we need new alertness to its changes, sequences, patterns visible through time.

To study the child's resources and their use in patterns of

coping, including the resultants of interactions or transactions between different aspects of the child's equipment and between the child and his environment, we decided to utilize standard psychiatric, pediatric, and psychological procedures which would permit us to compare the children with other children, and to use in addition "natural history" descriptive records of the total behavior seen as the child coped with the examiners and their procedures.[7, 9, 14, 15]

Subjects: 31 children in the Coping Study had been observed in detail as infants, at some time between the ages of 4 and 32 weeks, in the Infancy Study which was carried on (also under the joint auspices of the USPH Services and the Menninger Foundation) in Topeka and directed by Dr. Sibylle Escalona and Dr. Mary Leitch. From 2 or 3 years of age up to the ages of 8 or 10, we shall have seen each of them in 15 or 20 different sessions. We saw them coping with a wide variety of experiences, e.g. separation from mother, new situations structured and unstructured with more and with less permissive adult authorities, etc. We can, as a matter of fact, speak of an "expectable average" of coping problems, such as childhood diseases, traumata of separation, sibling rivalry or displacement, competition with the parent of the same or opposite sex, illness or death of loved ones, moving from one house to another, periods of parental anxiety about one or another common marital problem or problem with relatives, external hazard such as thunder, floods, and tornadoes. The failures and pressures of intelligence tests also provided one of our best sources of data.

Examples of findings: While we have some tentative general findings on the group, we are mainly interested in the development of coping style in children of different equipment and experience. Briefly, we find that *many children at the pre-school stage use a wider variety of defenses, more flexibly,* than is true in the latency period. Many of the individual children tend, however, to maintain the same general coping style from one year to another, sustained by dominant functions (rooted in their basic equipment) which have been reinforced or deeply imbedded in gratifications reinforced in the interpersonal experience of the child in his environment.

For instance, Rachel Hall, one of the "quiet" babies to begin with, passively accepted the drastic treatment of severe eczema to which she was exposed, without protest. She was confined to bed from the age of 12 months to 22 months, the last 3 months of this being in the hospital when the family was away from a flooded home. Her mother put on salves and ointments and did everything she could to get the severe eczema under control. Rachel enjoys most her sessions with the pediatrician or the Witkin tilting chair experiment, both of which demand chiefly a compliant cooperation with very structured requirements. She concentrates well and gets obvious satisfaction from her ability to meet the requirements of the situation and also from the manipulations involved. She seems to think of the world as a place where things are done to you. In keeping with her extreme passivity, she has never developed active defenses and coping devices. She is quite at a loss when confronted with an unstructured situation which can only be handled by spontaneous efforts of her own, such as to describe what she sees on a Rorschach ink blot, or to respond spontaneously at a party.

Rachel's pattern of development is in marked contrast to that of Ronald Holt, who has been a sensitive and somewhat suspicious baby and who still has low thresholds for startle. He approaches each new situation hesitantly and from behind the sheltering figure of some adult. Sensitive as Ronald is, and vulnerable to impacts from the environment, he still has a strong active drive to master his fear and anxiety. In one experiment, while he jumped and blinked every time he pulled the trigger of a large toy gun, he persisted in shooting over thirty times until gradually the startle reaction to the loud noise almost disappeared. He has never refused to come and participate in the experimental session, although over and over again he has been very hesitant to move in at the beginning or even to leave home in order to attend. In other words, here is a pattern of great sensitivity combined with a strong drive toward mastery which has persisted from infancy to the present.

A striking illustration of a child's continued use of a coping device which appeared in infancy is that of Susan. As a 28 weeks old baby she would laugh to make herself stop crying. She was desperately ill from polio when 3 years old. At this time she was very responsive to the efforts of the nurses to help her bear the painful treatments which she had to have by carrying on gay fantasies with her. At the age of 5 she was strongly denying anxiety about her physical condition and her future. Instead of worrying, she used all her energy to mobilize her forces to get well. Fantasy continued to play a large part in this. She still had a pattern of gayly denying any uneasiness about anxiety-provoking experiences. Her strong drive to conquer stress, anxiety, and difficulties is also extended to a general trend toward mastery.

While persistent characteristics are extremely important, we also find dramatic changes in overt coping style in certain children who blossom with new developmental resources or new environmental opportunities or supports, and in children who fade or lose their grip under new environmental stress or external intensification of inner problems they managed comfortably before the new stress.

Focusing on the strengths and vulnerabilities of the child together with stresses and supports from the environment, and studying the range of methods developed by children to manage their limitations in relation to environmental pressures, provides a necessary supplement to the study of "problems" and of patterns of growth.

DEVELOPMENT AND PARENTAL ATTITUDES (*Skard*)

A longitudinal research program has been conducted in Oslo since 1951. It includes 21 families from a certain socio-economic and geographical milieu, and focuses on the first or second child and parental attitudes.

Purpose: The investigation was started to test several current hypotheses in clinical psychology and child guidance, to obtain a first impression of children's development in a Norwegian milieu, and to gain some insight into common ways of treating children in this setting. More specifically, it seemed useful 1) to determine whether a group of Norwegian children would develop in the same way as reported in the literature of other countries; 2) to make an attempt to describe the parents' attitudes and treatment of the children so as to develop some initial hypotheses for the influence of various factors in the milieu of the Norwegian children that may differ from other settings; and 3) to determine whether supposedly important factors causing difficulties in problem children were absent in the lives of presumably "normal" children.

The plan was to follow the individual development of a limited number of children for whom the changing attitudes and factors in their surroundings could also be observed. To find deviations, we first had to determine common traits of child development. It was equally important to note common parental attitudes and treatment to discern specific traits in each family.

The parental traits on which we concentrated were: attitude towards authoritarian/liberal treatment of children; positive/negative desire for the specific child in question; emphasis on the needs of the child/the needs of the adults in the family; and gradual training of the child in dependence/independence. In the children we tried to observe: their general developmental level as measured by standard tests; attitude towards parents and siblings; handling of frustrating situations by aggression, withdrawal, problem-solving, magic or realistic reactions; initiative, fantasy, free activity (or passivity); and degree of dependency/independency in play and emotional expression.

Methodology: To get manageable but not surface-limited data, it was decided to follow a small number of children and their parents, to administer a variety of developmental and projective tests, to use an open but focused interview method, and to observe the child not only in standard test situations but also in the home and later in a peer group. In studying the interaction of children and parents it is of importance to include both father and mother, and whenever feasible to observe the home situation with both parents present. Because we wanted to know pre-natal home circumstances, we had our first interviews with each parent about a month before the child was expected. Since changes are more rapid during the first part of life, tests and observations were planned to be less frequent as the child grew older.

In selecting tests and situations for observation, and items for parent interviews, we kept in mind the possibility of comparing our data to those from similar investigations in other countries. As we worked we had to change and modify our plans because of shortage of time, limits of our working capacity, considerations of the family circumstances, and for other practical reasons. Some families have dropped out through the years, but fewer than expected. Of 21 families with whom the study was started, 18 are still participating; none, however, has completed the study.

Examinations and observations: During the *first year* of life Gesell and Cattell tests were given at 4, 8, 12, 20, 24, 28, 36, 40 44, and 52 weeks. Home visits centered on observations of mother-child relations and on general routine in child care at 16-week intervals. Parental interviews were held every 6 months. During the *second year* Gesell-Cattell tests were administered at 3-month periods and an interview with the parents held at year's end. Thereafter there were annual interviews with the parents, home visits at 25 and 42 months, and play observations in peer groups at 3½ and 6 years. Littman's parent questionnaire was administered at age 4. Gesell tests were repeated at 2½; the Terman-Merrill at 3 and 5. Projective techniques included the Twitchell-Allen at 3; World tests annually from 3 through 7; Rorschach at 4 and 5; Lerner Blocking Technique No. 2 at 4, 5, and 6; Free Drawings at 4 and 6; Sears' Doll House and other structured doll situations at 5 and 6; Zazzo's Bestiaire test at 5 and 6; Stone's Balloons at 6; and the Family Relation Test, Rosenzweig's PF, Jackson's Family Attitude, Goddard's Formboards, C.A.T., and Draw Your Family at 7. Physical and medical examinations, school readiness test, and observations of the child in the tested group were made at 6½ and 7 years.

Data analysis: In our investigation we encountered the same difficulty as in most longitudinal research; namely, lack of time and personnel to keep material analyzed concurrently with data collection. We are planning two approaches. First, there will be a group analysis of each developmental stage. (For example, what are parents like when their children are 6 months or 1 year, or older? And, similarly, what are children like at 1 or 2 or more years?) Secondly, as longitudinal case studies, we plan to compare each youngster relative to the group on various points, trying to find possible causes for the development of specific personality traits, particularly independence and aggression and their possible relationship.

In the prenatal interviews, now analyzed, emphasis was placed on the attitudes of the parents in respect to authoritarianism versus liberalism, in acceptance versus rejection of pregnancy and baby, and on the experience of the needs of the expected child as conflicting with their own. For the 6-month interviews, almost analyzed, we were interested in registering the routine and practice of child care as seen by the parents, their attitude towards their role, the problems encountered during the first half-year, their pleasure or disappointment in the child, and other specific concerns.

The analysis of the test results and home observations during the first year has been started, but more difficulties appeared than were initially anticipated. It now seems as if these data will be better for longitudinal rather than for group analysis.

Our analyzed data reflect more of an *absence of correlations* than definite patterns. Wanted or unwanted pregnancy shows no correlation with discomfort during pregnancy or degree of pain at delivery or duration of breast-feeding. Strict treatment of some kinds of child behavior may be combined with tolerance in other respects. Child rearing technique has practically no correlation with parents' adjustment to their parental role, their marital relations, or their emotional attitude to the child. This may indicate that our group is rather homogeneous, and that all differences are small. Formulation of theoretical hypotheses, however, will have to await further data analysis.

PSYCHO-PHYSICAL RELATIONSHIPS (*Thomae*)

Sponsored by the German Public Health Administration, the study here reported was initiated in 1952 with about 3000 children born between 1944 and 1946. Since such a large number is quite an obstacle to the real evaluation of a child's personality in annual examinations, we restricted our testing program to a small sample of intelligence, psychomotor, and personality tests, plus intensive use of behavior ratings within the testing situation as well as within school and family. Although there are many other aspects to our study[6, 8, 10, 12, 17, 18, 22, 25] I will concentrate in this chapter on preliminary findings on the relationship between physical and psychological development.[21, 23]

Our data permit application of the two forms of longitudinal approaches used so far, the comparison of cross-sectional measures of the same population from several years and the standardized study of individuals.

The *cross-sectional* analysis of our data refers to a group of around 230 boys and girls assessed as accelerated in somatic development in 1952 (when they were about 6 years old), and a group of around 250 boys and girls assessed as physically retarded in the same year. The first group will be referred to as the A-group, the second one as the R-group.

Our cross-sectional results show a low but generally significant correlation between physical and psychological developmental status. Whereas these correlations were, to some extent, extremely low in the first years of our study, they became more persuasive in some directions within the second and third year, when our children were 7 to 9 years old.

In addition to mental measurements, we tried to rate a child's behavior in the whole situation studied on eight different aspects. These included: activity, mood, general reactiveness, emotional reactiveness, adjustment, control, differentiation, and stability of behavior. Each of these aspects was assessed on a nine-point scale.

For the general activity score we found, in the first year, no clear difference in the amount of low or high scores within both groups. In the two following years we found a larger proportion of children with inactive or moderately active characteristics in the R-group; a larger proportion of very active or hyperactive children in the A-group (significant at the 1 percent level). But, in the third year of our study the percentage of very active or hyperactive children in both groups is already the same, although the A-group has far fewer cases with low activity than does the R-group. In the fourth year conditions seem to have changed even more. Whereas low activity seems to be represented in both groups to the same degree, high scores in activity are now more prevalent in the R-group.

We might explain this result as a shift in developmental impulses happening within the R-group at a later time than within the A-group.

A somewhat similar tendency is found with regard to general reactiveness, or readiness for response. In the first year of our study there were no significant differences between the A- and the R-group. In the two following years the percentage of children with a low score for readiness in the A-group is about one-half that in the R-group. Forms of reactiveness, such as "intensive responsiveness," are now more prevalent in the A-group. In the fourth year differences between both groups are again non-significant.

A constantly increasing difference between the two groups appears in relation to the differentiation of perceptiveness and reactiveness, with the fourth year showing only a slight drop.

Preliminary interpretation: Methodological factors in evaluating the physical and psychological aspects of a child's personality may be responsible for the results obtained. But changes in developmental pattern, which do not happen simultaneously within all dimensions of personality, may be equally responsible. At least, a single-factor developmental model, based on the notion that all developmental changes are regulated by one growth or maturation factor, is an evident oversimplification. The results show a certain variability of developmental speed during an individual's life and within different personality dimensions.

This statement receives some support from the *genuine longitudinal approach* to our problem; that is, the longitudinal somatic or psychological assessment of children of the A- and R-groups. So far we have completed the longitudinal assessment of 109 children characterized in the first year of our study as belonging to the A-group, and of 151 children in the R-group. Of these, one-third of both the A-group and the R-group were assessed as physically average in at least two of the following years, with a minority of cases returning to the previous somatic growth pattern. The same seems to be true for the "speed" of psychological development, as assessed on a special rating system evaluating test measures, general level of adjustment, degree of behavioral control, and stability of behavior.

In terms of personality development (as defined by our criteria) 79 were rated average every year and 82 changed from scores above average to average or from average to below average. This means that around 70 percent of our cases remained constant in personality development pattern, whereas 30 percent showed more or less definite changes during the years of observation.

Analysis of the correlations between the somatic and personality developmental scores of these 261 cases throughout the first 4 years of observation shows that a complete covariance exists in 92 (36.1 percent) of all cases. The number of cases with a temporary or moderate covariance is 64 (24.6 percent). Thus, a complete or partial degree of longitudinal covariance is present in 60.7 percent. Complete divergence of somatic and personality development is represented in 26, or 10 percent, of the 261 cases. The remaining 29.3 percent are those with constantly average personality development.

Conclusions: The over-all picture of our longitudinal findings shows a greater degree of covariance between the physical and psychological aspects of individual development than do the cross-sectional correlations. On the other hand, there appears to be no need for a single-factor developmental model.[2] It would be impossible to explain at least 40 percent of our cases if we would look on child development as a function of one biological force determining developmental pattern. Even the concept of a developmental pattern expressing itself in every somatic and personality dimension seems to require reconsideration. What becomes evident in the significant correlation between different annual cross-sectional comparisons of extreme variants of somatic development is the integrative character of personality. This integrative nature of the processes we call personality is indicated also in the genuine longitudinal covariance between physical and psychological development. Integration does not mean the patterning of all developmental processes according to one speed or form or intensity. Rather, it means a tendency towards optimal inner adjustment of a variety of processes which in themselves can have different styles or speeds or intensities.

This same finding could also be demonstrated by comparing partially asynchronous somatic development with partially asynchronous psychological development.[20]

COMMENTARY (*Skard*)

It is self-evident that the methods used in personality research will differ widely depending upon the aspect of the problem considered. Very different symptoms will be sought if the investigation is aimed chiefly at the intellectual, conscious level of the personality rather than at the more unconscious, motivational, or conflicting tendencies. Thus, developmental studies of *thinking* and problem-solving, as noted by Inhelder, will demand a more experimental setting. And, isn't it natural that "coping" with *emotional* problems, as observed by Murphy, should require projective methods combined with detailed observations of involuntary, personal reactions? Then, too, investigations of somatic changes, intellectual development, and attitude, as undertaken by Thomae in a school class, can utilize other tools than those tried in Oslo, where parent interviews, home observations, and a battery of projective techniques are used to discover more of the unconscious trends of aggression/ withdrawal and dependence/independence in the growing personality.

The general danger involved in any investigation of character formation is, first, that more material is collected than can ever be properly analyzed; and second, that the factors in the game of cause and effect are sometimes too numerous to be isolated. (It is often impossible to separate all the variables.) In addition, in these studies as in all others, there is the further difficulty of using interviews, projective techniques, and so on, which do not yield unequivocal answers to definite questions, thus rendering analysis even more difficult. Moreover, projective methods are vague and their interpretations frequently too dependent on the interpreting adult.

This is all true, and we must agree with Allport[1] that our methods are "not fully adequate." However, since the formation of personality seems more or less similar to that described by Bühler[5] and White,[26] at least during the first part of the lifespan, we can probably not obtain *full* results much more easily. We shall have to struggle with the continuous conflict between using too many methods for data collection and not managing to analyze them, or singling out a few data and taking the risk of letting the most important ones slip through our fingers. We shall have to cope with the problem of whether to follow a few cases carefully and in detail, or to use a large number of cases examined with more superficial methods. Remembering the vast lack of knowledge in this field we shall probably all along have to be grateful for whatever approaches prove helpful. Perhaps only half a century from now, when psychologists attempt to pull together what has been gathered, will we be in a position to discern the main structure of the larger puzzle.

It is impossible to claim that great new insights into the formative processes of personality were presented. The problem was approached from widely divergent angles with varying methodologies. The numerically strong German study, the ingenious individual American investigation, the systematic and well-planned Swiss experiments, and the socially-tinted Norwegian observations could not be combined to make any kind of total picture. However, in the words of Gardner Murphy,[13] they did "help in clarifying the little that we know and show its possible relations to the vast and confused domain that we do not yet understand."

It is tempting to try to pull together some points in the various studies presented in order to formulate some definite questions, and to compare facts from different studies that may be combined.

Thus, in Lois Murphy's work we find that some children maintain the same coping style over time, while others change their method of coping "with new developmental resources or

new environmental opportunities or supports" or "under new
environmental stress or external intensification of inner problems." And, in Thomae's study of somatic and psychological
matters we note that "around*70 percent of the children remained
constant in their personality developmental pattern, whereas 30
percent showed more or less definite changes." We may wonder
whether these two observations are perhaps related. Would
changes in developmental patterns also appear as new coping
styles? It is also tempting to ask whether the "new developmental resources" have something in common with the development of "cognitive functions," described by Inhelder and Noelting as similarly appearing in spurts. (Though not mentioned
explicitly, there are probably individual variations in their
cases.) Would closer analysis of the cognitive development in
individual children disclose some cases spurting more and others
less, some keeping a steadier rhythm of transition from one level
of thinking to the next, while others are more uneven in their
development? And, would the latter be the same sort of cases
as those observed by Murphy as changing in their coping style?

One may further ask about possible reasons for changes in
coping style. Would they be found in changes of physical appearance (sudden growth giving a better position in the peer
group, etc.), in varying environmental conditions (as the Oslo
study tries to reveal), or in maturing ability to grasp a problem?

Perhaps it might help if we turn the questions around. How
will the experience of successful or unsuccessful coping with
everyday problems (as studied by Murphy) affect a child's
ability to solve the cognitive questions posed in the Inhelder-
Noelting experiments? Will such success or failure in coping
experience provide a clue to the cases of lacking-co-variance in
the Thomae group? And, will the various ways of coping, their
constancy or variability, in any way be connected with different
child-rearing practices, variations in parents' attitudes to their
children, or differences in family constellations?

Further investigations may indeed show that our different
pieces of research are, after all, parts of the same puzzle. However, only through a great many different approaches will it be
really possible to distinguish cause and effect, or to find the

"hen and the egg" relationship in the interplay of child and milieu.

We need to understand more fully the language of projective tests and their relationship to the actual life of a child at a certain age. Only through research in many different cultures and subcultures will we be able to distinguish the acting forces of a milieu and its meaning for growing children faced with the features of one particular culture at one particular age. What are the positive stages for the learning of specific skills and the acquisition of knowledge, or the negative stages of vulnerability towards specific forms of stress and deprivation? Much work is still needed before we will know how to combine individual investigations so as to map trends in personality growth in interplay with its surroundings, consistent constitutional tendencies, or acquired reactive behavior.

If we agree that the child is not a consistent personality unfolding only from within, we shall have to handle practically a Gulf Stream of cultural and personal influential factors coming in response to the age changes in the child itself. The formation of human personality will have to be studied in human beings, though experiments with animals may provide valuable ideas, hunches, or general principles for further testing. Since the possibility of long-term effects, or even hidden effects appearing at later stages in human development, has to be considered, research will of necessity be long-lasting, too (with the risk that the investigator may die before the effect has appeared in his long-living subject).

SUMMARY

A series of brief reports dealing with continuing longitudinal research studies in personality development have been presented as illustrative of current approaches in varied centers and countries. Some of the problems and vicissitudes encountered were discussed in the Commentary. Cross-cultural research, international congresses, one piece of work added to that of others, and planned comparative studies are all important steps on the long road ahead before we can safely say that we know the *becoming* of an adult personality.

References

1. Allport, G. W. *Becoming.* New Haven: Yale Univ. Press, 1955.

2. Anderson, J. E. A developmental model for aging. *Vita Humana*, 1958, 1, 5-18.

3. Bayley, Nancy. On the growth of intelligence. *Amer. Psychologist*, 1955, 10, 805-818.

4. Bowlby, J. *Maternal care and mental health.* Geneva: World Health Org., 1951.

5. Bühler, Charlotte. *Der menschliche Lebenslauf als psychologisches Problem.* Leipzig: Hirzel, 1933.

6. Coerper, C., Hagen, W., and Thomae, H. (Eds.) *Deutsche Nachkriegskinder;* Methoden und erste Ergebnisse der deutschen Längsschnittuntersuchungen über die körperliche und seelische Entwicklung im Schulkindalter. Stuttgart: Thieme, 1954.

7. Escalona, Sybille and Heider, Grace. *Prediction and outcome;* a study in child development. New York: Basic Books, 1959.

8. Hagen, W., Tomae, H., Mansfeld, E., and Mathey, F. J. *Jugendliche in der Berufsbewährung.* Stuttgart: Thieme, 1958.

9. Heider, Grace. A *longitudinal study of vulnerability from infancy to latency.* (In process)

10. Kern, H. Verlaufsformen der Entwicklung bei antriebsarmen und antriebsgehemmten Kindern. Unpubl. Diploma Thesis. University of Erlangen, 1959.

11. Macfarlane, Jean W., Allen, Lucille, and Honzik, Marjorie P. A *developmental study of the behavior problems of normal children between 21 months and 14 years.* Berkeley: Univ. of California Press, 1954.

12. Mathey, F. J. Die Entwicklung des Grundschulkindes im Lichte einer Längsschnittuntersuchung. *Psychol. Rundsch.*, 1956, 7, 163-173.

13. Murphy, G. *Personality.* New York: Harper, 1947.

14. Murphy, Lois B. Psychoanalysis and child development. *Bull. Menninger Clinic*, 1957, 21.

15. Murphy, Lois B., Moriarity, A., Raine, W., and Heider, G. *Able to cope.* (To be published)

16. Olson, W. C. *Child development.* Boston: Heath, 1949.

17. Salber, W. Verlaufsformen der zeichnerischen Entwicklung. *Z. diagn. Psychol.*, 1958, 6, 48-63.

18. Schadendorf, B. Verlaufsformen der Entwicklung bei antriebsreichen Kindern. Unpubl. Diploma Thesis. University of Erlangen, 1959.

19. Sears, R. R., Maccoby, Eleanor E., and Levin, H. *Patterns of child rearing*. Evanston: Row, Peterson, 1957.

20. Steinwachs, F. Das Verhältnis von körperlicher und seelischer Entwicklung in der Reifezeit. Unpubl. Habilitation Thesis. University of Erlangen, 1959.

21. Strickmann, R. *Untersuchungen zur Frage der Beziehung von somatischer und psychologischer Entwicklung; ein Beitrag zum Accelerations-Problem*. Bonn: Bouvier, 1957.

22. Thomae, H. Probleme der schulischen Entwicklung in der Sicht einer Längsschnittuntersuchung. *Intern. Rev. Educ.*, 1957, 3, 143-154.

23. Thomae, H. Längsschnittuntersuchungen zum Problem der Beziehung zwischen körperlicher und seelischer Entwicklung. *Z. exp. angew. Psychol.*, 1957, 3, 437-450.

24. Thomae, H. Problems of character change. In David, H. P. and von Bracken, H. (Eds.), *Perspectives in personality theory*. New York: Basic Books, 1957.

25. Thomae, H. Die Bedeutung der Längsschnittuntersuchungen für die Entwicklungspsychologie und Pädagogik. In Roth, H. (Ed.), *Pädagogik und Psychologie*. Heidelberg: Quelle und Meyer, 1959.

26. White, R. W. *Lives in progress*. New York: Dryden, 1952.

27. Whiting, J. W. M. and Child, I. L. *Child training and personality*. New Haven: Yale Univ. Press, 1953.

Edwin S. Shneidman

and

Norman L. Farberow

XIV

A Socio-Psychological
Investigation of Suicide

INTRODUCTION

THERE ARE SEVERAL rather distinct approaches to the investiga-
gation of the phenomena of suicide. The ecologic, anthropologic,
psychiatric, and psychoanalytic points of view immediately come
to mind. Of these, perhaps the best known approach to the
analysis of suicidal data is that generally called "sociological."
It has, by now, a time-honored tradition and includes what is
probably the best-known single work on the topic, Durkheim's
Le Suicide.[4] Published in 1897 in France, it established a model
for sociological investigations of committed suicide, and also
delineated an essentially psychological classification of types
(anomic, altruistic, and egoistic). There have been many subsequent studies of this genre, e.g. the monographs and books
by Cavan on suicide in Chicago;[2] Schmid on suicide in Seattle[15]
and Minneapolis;[16] Sainsbury on suicide in London;[14] Dublin
and Bunzel,[3] and Henry and Short[6] on suicide in the United
States. All fall within the sociological tradition of taking a plot
of ground—a city or a country—and figuratively or literally re-
producing its map several times to show its socially shady (and
topographically shaded) areas and their multifarious relationships to suicide rates. This kind of study certainly has the merit
of employing the available sociological and suicidal data, but
it also has the characteristic of being focused in its conclusions
on generalizations about suicide which are necessarily couched

in socio-economic terminology. One result of this outcome is that the individual who has aspirations for effecting any kind of reduction in suicide rates is limited in his range of possible actions by virtue of the fact that he is given little information about the highly individual and personal *psychological* aspects of the suicidal behaviors.

It was in an effort to fill this lack that the present project was undertaken. In essence, the purpose of the study reported in this chapter is to juxtapose psychological and sociological suicidal data (for the same community and for the same temporal interval) so that congruencies between the two sets of data—the data of the individual and the data of the social structure—might be indicated and their relationships to suicidal data explored. The phenomena of suicide are obviously complicated and demand a multi-faceted approach. Practically everyone agrees that suicide is not that kind of disorder for which the researcher, no matter how diligent, can discover an etiological coccus or germ, but rather, that the phenomena of suicide are reflections of the total mental health of the individual as he lives (and dies) within the context of the mental health of the community.

SOCIOLOGICAL AND SUICIDAL INFORMATION

This study utilizes data from a specific, large metropolitan area—Los Angeles County*—and, except where specifically noted, one time—calendar year 1957.

Sociological information: After an extensive analysis of 1950 U.S. Census data, the Los Angeles Welfare Planning Council divided Los Angeles County into 100 relatively stable and homogeneous study areas (based on such factors as average economic income, average educational level, percentage of home ownership, occupational levels, etc.) Subsequently these 100 study

---

* Los Angeles County has an area of 4,083 square miles and a population of over 5 million people. A comprehensive overview of the characteristics of the Los Angeles County population is presented in *Background for Planning*.[21]

TABLE 1—*Population data for nine area types and suicide information,*

Sociological Information

Area type	Area name	Number of areas	Popula- tion	% of pop.	% youth	% 20-65	% aged	% minority	% change
Most advantaged									
I	Suburbs	4	265,180	5	35	61	4	1	49
II	Residential communities	14	828,884	16	24	68	8	3	23
III	Apartment areas	5	200,279	4	21	65	4	3	3
Moderately advantaged									
IV	Suburbs	13	1,097,822	21	40	56	4	9	124
V	Natural communities	34	1,673,977	31	31	62	7	6	24
VI	Apartment areas	8	392,863	7	18	68	14	13	—4
Least advantaged									
VII	Rural areas	1	119,000	2	42	56	2	9	177
VIII	Industrial communities	14	529,354	10	36	58	6	34	3
IX	Apartment areas	7	192,989	4	28	61	11	59	—20
Area unknown									
Total or average		100	5,300,348	100	31	61	8	15	42

areas were distributed (on the basis of an analysis of "urbaniza-
tion" and "social rank") among nine area types, as follows: I.
most advantaged suburbs, II. most advantaged residential communities, III. most advantaged apartment house areas, IV. moderately advantaged suburbs, V. moderately advantaged natural
communities, VI. moderately advantaged multiple-dwelling
areas, VII. least advantaged rural areas, VIII. least advantaged
industrial communities, and IX. least advantaged rooming-house
and apartment areas. Information on these nine area types, which

Los Angeles County, 1957

	Suicide Information			Psychological Information		
Number suicides	% of total suicides	Suicide rate	Sex Marital	Stated reason for suicide	Affect or emotion in suicide note	
31	4	12		Hi: tired of life Hi: reasons given		I
132	17	16		Low: ill health Low: rejection		II
44	6	22	Hi: females Hi: wid, div Low: married	Hi: ill health	Hi: absolution	III
93	12	8		Low: ill health	Hi: affection Low: self-depreciation Hi: general affect	IV
236	31	14	Hi: married Low: wid, div	Hi: rejection Hi: reasons given	Low: affection and love	V
84	11	21	Hi: wid, div Low: married	Low: rejection		VI
4	1	3				VII
68	9	13	Hi: males Low: singles		Low: general affect Low: affection and love	VIII
37	5	19	Low: males Hi: singles	Low: reasons given	Low: general affect Low: affection and love	IX
39	5					
768	100	14				

constitute the basic sociological data for this study, has been fully reported in the Council's publications.[21, 22, 23]

Some population figures have been collated in Table 1. It should be noted that: "Population, % of total" refers to the number of people in each area type compared to the total population of Los Angeles County; "% youth" refers to the people under 20 years of age, and "% aged" refers to the people over 65 years of age in that area; "% minority" is defined by the Planning Council as "Negroes, other races, and whites with

Spanish surnames"; and "% change" refers to the increase or decrease in population in that specific area since the 1950 Census.

Suicidal information: The Coroner's files were searched and each of the 768 cases certified during 1957 as "suicide" (of a total of 9770 cases processed by the Coroner) was examined.* The following items were abstracted for each case: sex, race, age, marital status, occupation, length of time in Los Angeles County, presence or absence of suicide note, and street address. The victim's street address was coded for study area and then for area type.

The distribution of 768 suicides in Los Angeles County in 1957 among the nine area types is also indicated in Table 1. The reader will note that the percentages of suicides within each area type (keeping in mind that 5 percent of the suicides could not be located by area type) are remarkably similar to the percentages of the total population contained within each area type, with the possible exceptions of area types IV and VI. More significant are the suicide rates for the nine area types. The range here is from 3 to 22 per 100,000 population, with an average rate of 14—somewhat higher than the national average of 9.8. Statistically, the differences among the ratios of the nine area types were significant.† The major differences were that

---

* In discussing the statistics on suicide, at least three specific cautions should be kept in mind: (a) it is generally agreed by experts in the field that the known statistics on suicide are, at best, *minimum* statistics. The reasons for this have to do with inaccuracies of reporting, suppression of data (usually listing a self-inflicted death as accidental or natural), and the absence of standardization of definitions of suicide. Our own work with Dr. Theodore Curphey, the Los Angeles County Coroner, has shown us that there are many cases of equivocal accident-suicide which can be seen accurately only after adequate empirical investigation; (b) the statistics on suicide usually relate entirely to committed suicide and do not include the much more extensive problem of *attempted* suicide. The results of a comprehensive survey completed in the Los Angeles area have led us to believe that the ratio of attempted suicides to committed suicides is at least as high as 8:1. The publications on attempted suicide by Ringel [13] and Stengel and Cook [19] are of especial interest; (c) one must distinguish between suicide *number* and suicide *rate*. For this context, rate refers to deaths by suicide per 100,000 population for whatever specific group is being discussed. Whereas the number of suicides generally decreases with advancing age, the rate of suicide increases markedly.

† The standard error of proportion was significant beyond the .01 level.

area type IV was low in suicide rate, and area types III and VI (both of them apartment house areas) were relatively high.

The suicidal data were examined for statistically significant differences within the total suicidal population among the nine area types for four items: race, sex, age, and marital status.

There were no statistically significant differences for *race* of suicidal individuals among the nine area types. Over 90 percent of all individuals who committed suicide in Los Angeles County in 1957 were Caucasian. No single area type contained more than two percent other-than-Caucasians among the suicide population. Comparison within the "% minority" column, especially for area types VII and IX, indicates that minority groups are not proportionately represented in the suicide statistics. One partial explanation is that the Planning Council data for the area types includes individuals with Spanish surnames (ostensibly to include the Los Angeles Mexican population) within the minority figures, whereas the Coroner's Office automatically classifies a Mexican-American as a Caucasian. Even so, the percentage of Negroes in area types VII and IX is many times higher than the one per cent of Negro suicides in those areas of Los Angeles County. These findings are extremely interesting in themselves.

For *sex*, there were statistically significant differences in male-female ratio within some of the area types.* These differences occurred in two area types. Area type III had a greater number of female suicides than would be expected and a smaller number of male suicides than would be expected; and area type VIII had a smaller number of female suicides than would be expected.

There were no statistically significant sociological differences for *age* groups among the area types, but we know that, in the United States, the suicide rates† generally increase in each age group, ranging from 0.2 for 10-14 year old females to 60.7 for 80-84 year old males. The differences between the suicide rates of the two sexes is a datum which needs to be kept in mind in any planning for prevention. Further, in relation to age, some

---

* The Chi square value was at the .05 level of significance.

† Published by the National Office of Vital Statistics, U.S. Department of Health, Education and Welfare—*Special Reports, National Summaries*, Volume 50, No. 5, April 24, 1959—and reproduced in Table 2.

TABLE 2—*Death rate (per 100,000 population) for
suicide by age and sex: United States, 1957
(From National Office of Vital Statistics)*

Age group	Total	Male	Female
5 - 9	0.	0.	0.
10-14	0.5	0.7	0.2
15-19	2.5	3.9	1.0
20-24	5.7	9.1	2.6
25-29	7.6	11.0	4.3
30-34	9.6	14.3	5.2
35-39	11.1	16.4	6.1
40-44	14.5	22.4	7.0
45-49	16.2	25.4	7.4
50-54	20.0	32.0	8.5
55-59	22.0	34.9	9.7
60-64	22.9	37.5	9.4
65-69	24.6	41.1	9.6
70-74	25.5	47.6	6.6
75-79	25.6	49.7	6.5
80-84	29.1	60.7	5.0
85+	26.3	56.9	4.3
Total	9.8	15.4	4.3

items of psychological interest were found, as indicated in a later section.

For *marital status* of suicidal individuals, there were statistically significant differences.* These differences occurred in six of the area types. In area type I there were fewer widowed and divorced; in III there were fewer married and more widowed and divorced; in V there were more married and fewer widowed and divorced; in VI the pattern was the same as in III; in VIII

---

* The Chi square value was at the .02 level of significance.

there were fewer single; and in IX there were more single and fewer married.

PSYCHOLOGICAL INFORMATION

One might ask, rhetorically, what are the sources from which one ordinarily obtains psychological information about an individual? The conventional answers would include such sources as anamneses, psychological test protocols, psychotherapy notes, interview records, etc. An unconventional response—but one most relevant when dealing with a population of individuals each of whom has committed suicide—would be *suicide notes*. On the face of it, genuine suicide notes (written, typically, within a few minutes before the individual kills himself, and sometimes actually written as he is dying) constitute an unusual opportunity to obtain data concerning the ideation and the affect of the suicidal person. Following Allport's[1] concept of the use of personal documents, one can make a strong case for the position that if the psychology of the suicidal individual appears in any sort of record, it might, on a common-sense basis, be expected to be found in the document the individual composed directly within the context of the suicidal act.

It is of interest that an exhaustive survey of the bibliography on suicide since 1897 (prepared by the present writers) reveals that the literature on suicide *notes* is, by and large, a very recent one. With the exception of a monograph on suicide notes by Morgenthaler and Steinberg[11] (which reproduces 47 suicide notes obtained in Berne, Switzerland, during the period 1928 to 1935) published in 1945, the remaining few references to studies involving notes are all within the past three years: an article and some book chapters by Shneidman and Farberow;[17, 18] an article by Tuckman, Kleiner, and Lavell;[20] and an article by Osgood and Walker.[12] Shneidman and Farberow selected 33 genuine suicide notes (from their ten-year sample of 721 notes), matched them man-for-man with 33 simulated suicide notes which they elicited from non-suicidal individuals, and then conducted a number of analyses with their 33 pairs of suicidal-pseudocidal notes, including an analysis of the implied logical syllogisms contained within the notes and an analysis in terms of Mowrer's Discomfort-Relief Quotient (DRQ). In addition, they attempted to test Menninger's theory of suicide[10]—to kill, to be killed, to die—by analyzing 489 male suicide notes-and 130 female suicide notes by age categories (20-39, 40-59, and 60 plus). Tuckman, Kleiner, and Lavell, "following the approach employed by Shneidman and Farberow," analyzed the emotional content of suicide notes left by 165 (of a total of 742) suicides in Philadelphia over a five-year period, 1951-1955. Osgood and Walker also used Shneidman and Farberow's 33 pairs of matched notes, as well as their own set of 100 ordinary letters-to-relatives, and analyzed aspects of the language in the notes from the point of view of hypotheses derived from motivation theory. The outline employed to analyze suicide notes in the present study (as indicated in Table 3) includes the "content categories" used by Osgood and Walker.

In all, we analyzed 948 genuine suicide notes (obtained from the Los Angeles County Coroner's Office) for the three-year period, 1956-1957-1958. All the analyses were performed by one rater, a psychologist, who had no knowledge of the race, address, etc., of the note-writer—as a matter of record, had no information about the purpose of the study at all. In addition, 100 (of the 948) suicide notes were rated independently of the initial rating by another rater.

Psychological variables were educed by analyzing each suicidal note in terms of the following scheme:

1) To whom the suicide note was addressed (e.g. spouse, parent, child). This rubric was intended to yield the interpersonal involvements, the directions of diadic relationships, etc.

2) Reasons for suicide explicitly stated in the note (e.g. ill health, rejection, finances). This category described the victim's stated conscious "reasons" for killing himself. The question was whether the reasons were different among the nine area types.

3) Affect indicated (or implied) in the suicide note (e.g. anger, sorrow, affection). Our interest here was to see whether emotional expressions varied among the area types.

4) Content other than affect (e.g. did the note include references to money and insurance, material possessions, disposition of remains). The purpose was to get at the victim's main concerns at the time—whether these concerns were with himself, with others, with material possessions, with death, etc.

5) The general focus of the suicide note (i.e. did the note focus on the reason, on affect, or on instructions). The purpose was to obtain an indication of the over-all tenor of the individual's last communication.

A listing of all the scoring categories is given in Table 3.

TABLE 3—*Outline for analysis of suicide notes*

A. *Addressee of suicide note*

1. No address
2. To Whom it may concern
3. Police
4. Spouse
5. Parent
6. Child
7. Sibling
8. Friend
9. Specific, but not able to ascertain
10. Other: (Specify)

B. *Reasons stated in suicide note*

11. No reason stated
12. Ill health, illness, physical disability, symptoms, pain
13. Rejection by another; jilted; unloved; not understood; can't live without you
14. Finances, money, bills, debts
15. Job, occupation, unemployment
16. Ennui, tired of life
17. No point in living; not worth trying
18. Interest in death, other world, hereafter
19. To "join" a (deceased) loved one
20. As a "way out," reached end, couldn't go on

21. Isolation, loneliness
22. Love triangle (other man, woman)
23. Confusion, depression, fear, anxiety
24. Being persecuted; hearing voices; losing mind
25. Sex
26. Other: (Specify)

C. *Affect indicated in suicide note*

31. No affect
32. Hostility, criticism, blame, revenge
33. Absolution of other, giving forgiveness (to specific persons)
34. Sorrow, seeking forgiveness (from specific persons)
35. Seeking forgiveness from deity
36. Self-depreciation, self-derogation, self-criticism, guilt, self-blame (fault) better off without me
37. Love, idealization, praise, defense
38. Other: (Specify)

D. *Specific content other than affect*

51. No specific content other than affect
52. Mention of religion, fate, life, world, death (abstraction)
53. Goodbye, farewell
54. Reference to suicidal act, no one responsible
55. Reference to suicide note
56. Instructions re money, business, power of attorney, funeral expenses
57. Instructions re insurance
58. Instructions re material possessions
59. Instructions re children
60. Instructions re own remains
61. Instructions re notification of others
62. Instructions re message to others
63. Other: (Specify)

E. *General focus of the suicide note*

71. Primarily *reason* for suicide
72. Primarily *affect*

73. Primarily *instructions*
74. Primarily *abstractions*
75. Primarily *content other than affect*
76. Primarily *reflecting own confusion*
77. Extremely short; cryptic; enigmatic
78. Other: (Specify) No content

Two methodological questions concerning the suicide notes need to be mentioned. They are: a) Are the results obtained by the present scoring system replicable with another rater? And: b) Are the suicide note writers representative of the total population of individuals who committed suicide? We shall discuss these two issues, briefly.

a) *Inter-judge reliability.* As a check upon the reliability of the categorizing, 100 of the suicide notes were re-analyzed by another judge. All but nine were categorized as they had been previously, yielding a reliability figure which indicated that the two analyzers scored the notes in essentially the same manner.*

b) *Representativeness of suicide note writers.* A statistical comparison of distribution by sex, age categories, and marital status between the 1957 suicide note writers, on the one hand, and the 1957 suicides minus the note-writers, on the other, indicated that the two groups were similar; there were no statistically significant differences between the two groups in any of these three categories. These results concerning the representativeness of suicide notes are consistent with the findings previously reported by Shneidman and Farberow[18] in which they state, in relation to the 721 suicide notes collected over a ten-year period, that "the socio-economic statistics of the note-writing group have been compared with the similar data from the non-note-writing group and the two groups have been found to be essentially the same." Similarly, Tuckman, Kleiner, and

---

* Reference to the figures published by Guetzkow[5] gives the least value that p—the probability that an item has been consistently categorized—might take 99 times out of 100 as .90; the probability that an item has been incorrectly categorized would be as high as .10 only once in 100. Such a figure may be considered as indicative of adequate reliability.

Lavell[20] report, in relation to 165 suicide notes collected over
a five-year period, that "a comparison of those who left notes
with those who did not showed no significant difference between
the two groups with respect to age, race, sex, employment,
marital status, physical condition, mental condition, history of
mental illness, place of suicide, reported causes of unusual circumstances preceding the suicide, medical care and supervision,
and history of previous attempts or threats."

ANALYSIS OF SUICIDE NOTES

The heart of the psychological data is in the analysis of the
suicide notes. What did the statistical analyses of the scorings of
the notes yield? Were there any indications of statistically significant differences in "psychology," as revealed in note content,
among the nine different sociological area types? The results
indicated that in two of the five aspects of suicide note analysis
—2) reasons for suicide and 3) affect—there were significant
differences.*

Area type I—most advantaged suburbs: 5 percent of the population; 4 percent of the suicides; suicide rate 12; minority groups
less than 1 percent; small proportion of widowed and divorced.

In their suicide notes, members of this wealthy group more
often than other area types give reasons for their suicide, and
these reasons are not concerned with ill health or rejection or
finances, but rather with such reasons as "tired of life," "as a way
out," "no point in living," "can't go on"—almost as though they
were surfeited with life itself. (Without commenting on the
reported differences in the national suicide rates between two
countries with obviously different standards of living, e.g. Spain
and Sweden, it would be a most interesting study—apropos the
findings reported in this paragraph—to analyze the differences in
the content of the suicide notes left in the two countries.) One

---

* The Chi square for the difference among the nine area types for
"reasons" was significant at the .01 level of significance (indicating that
these results could have occurred by chance only one time in 100) and
the Chi square for "affect" was significant at the .05 level.

implication of this finding is that thorough-going suicide prevention not only will have to concern itself with intra-psychic and sociological factors, but, eventually, will have to deal with the basic cultural values as well. Two area type I suicide notes, with identifying data changed, read as follows:

> No funeral. Please leave the body to science. William Smith
>
> *
>
> I'm sorry. Don't bother with a post. It's sodium cyanide. At 11:12

Area type II—most advantaged residential communities: 16 percent of the population; 17 percent of the suicides; suicide rate 16; almost no minorities.

The suicide notes of this group give little indication of the psychology of the note writers. The notes show no particular affect or lack of it and the focus of the notes is rather general in nature. Reasons for suicide are not often given, and when given they are conspicuously lacking in any reference to ill health or feelings of rejection or loneliness. Area type II contains a large percentage of 40 to 49 year olds who are relatively financially independent and successful, and their notes may reflect this quality in the apparent lack of any special need for communicating the reasons, instructions or emotions relative to the suicidal act. Two area type II notes follows:

> Don't take life too seriously. You'll never get out of it alive anyway. Mary Smith
>
> *
>
> [On Bevery Hilton Hotel stationary]
> Nobody to blame. Call YO 12345

Area type III—most advantaged apartment house areas: 4 percent of the population, 6 percent of the suicides; suicide rate 12; low minority percentage; larger proportion of female suicides; larger proportion of widowed and divorced; smaller proportion of married.

The outstanding characteristic of the suicide notes from area type III is that they are conspicuously filled with reasons of ill

health (physical disability, symptoms, pain)—as though much
of the writer's existence depended on his body and its functioning. The affect expressed is focussed, more than in any other
area type, on absolution (giving forgiveness, etc.). One gets the
picture of self-centered, pontifical people assuaging their deep
intrapsychic conflicts with ready assumption of guilt and blame
and with rationalizations of physical pain. These people have, in
many ways, more in common with some moderately and least
advantaged area types than with the other two most advantaged
area types. A typical area type III suicide note is reproduced
verbatim:

> To All My Friends:
>
> Please forgive me and thanks for all your kindness.
> My courage has run out. In the face of poor health, deserted
> by my sisters, and persistent cruelty of my husband I have no
> further reason to keep fighting.
> All my life I have tried to be decent. I have worked hard to
> make a marriage out of puny material. To be deserted at such a
> time of my life is too disillusioning and too harsh. It is more than
> I can bear. I just feel that those who should be close to me are
> like "rats deserting a sinking ship." Therefore I do not want any
> of them (my sisters or my husband) near me in death or to have
> any part of my possessions.
> But I do appreciate the goodness and the kindness of my
> friends, my doctors and my lawyer—it kept me going up to this
> point.

Area type IV—moderately advantaged suburbs: 21 percent of
the population; 12 percent of the suicides; suicide rate 8; almost
no minority population.

Suicide notes of people from this area type differ in many
ways from those of area type I, the most advantaged suburbans.
The suicide notes indicate many reasons for suicide but they are
conspicuously low in listing ill health as a reason for suicide.
Their notes contain a great deal of feeling—there is rarely a note
with no affect—but the affect infrequently includes self-depreciation (self-derogation, self-criticism, guilt, self-blame). Most
often they include such emotions as affection (love, idealization
of others, praise, defense of the other). The over-all impression

is that these note-writers are individuals in their thirties who are very much involved in the feelings of interpersonal relationships. Their suicides are not for health or money, but rather have to do with love—and the converse of love, hostility, although this is more by inference than from actual content of the notes. These people manifest the conflicts of love and hate and, along with the individuals in area type V, could probably be most helped by psychotherapeutic intervention. An area type IV suicide note follows:

Mary:

Here is the note you wanted giving you power of attorney for the house and everything else (including all of *your* bills.)

I hope that my insurance will get you out of the whole mess that you got us both in.

This isn't hard for me to do because it's probably the only way I'll ever get rid of you, we both know how the California courts only see the women's side.

My only hope is that you can raise Junior to be as honest and as good as he is right now.

I think that Junior and Betty and George are really the only things in the world that I'll miss. Please take good care of them.

Good luck, Bill

P.S. I love you Junior, and thank you Betty for all you've done for me and Junior. Love Daddy.

Area type V—moderately advantaged natural communities: 31 percent of the population; 31 percent of the suicides; suicide rate 14; low minority percentage; high proportion of married, and low proportion of widowed and divorced. The communities in this area type are the "little cities" within the greater Los Angeles community.

These people very often give reasons for the suicide in their notes, and the reasons mentioned often have to do with feelings of rejection by another (not being understood, feelings of isolation, loneliness, loss of love). Curiously enough, the notes of these people also contain a conspicuously low percentage of affection toward the note recipient, even though many of them are married. They have been rejected and they are very angry

—it would appear, angry at themselves. Here again, as with the individuals in area IV, the possibilities for psychotherapeutic help through insight, resolution of feelings, etc., are important. Two notes written by the same individual follow:

Dear Mary:

   Be sure you hold fast to what you think you have now. I go with no bitterness toward you only pity and love.

   I pray this example will be the means of you going forward in life in the right way. Take good care of Junior and love him, do not vent your spite out on him when things do not go your way. Here are my car keys. If Dad will grant my one wish this car is yours.   Mother

   This Ten dollars is from what I earned last week, part of it I mean. Nothing to do with Dad's money. I've left him $70 more than he would have done for me if the shoe had been on the other foot.

                                                       ✿

Dear Bill:

   Please do not have a lot of hypocrisy such as burial etc. Give my carcass to a hospital or cremate it.

   If you have a spark of honesty in you and you love our son try and arrange for him to live with George and Mary, where he will be happy and raised in a decent home. He will never be happy with you.

   Here's what money I've left. I've sent Henrys to him and I've left Mary ten dollars out of it what I earned last week.

   Goodbye and God bless you.   Betty

Area type VI—moderately advantaged apartment areas: 7 percent of the population; 11 percent of the suicides; suicide rate 21; small minority population; low proportion of married and high proportion of widowed and divorced. This suicidal group is weighted primarily in the non-married direction.

   In terms of the reasons given in the suicide notes, rejection is indicated less often than in any other area type except type II. Area type VI has the next to the highest percentage of suicide of any area type in Los Angeles County (type III which is also an apartment house area has a rate of 22). It is interesting that the third highest rate, 19, occurs in the remaining apartment house area, area type IX. However, the psychology of the suicide notes obtained from these three area types does not seem to be similar in emphasis. Two sample suicide notes of area type VI follow:

> Dear Mary. I am so sick and disgusted cant get well so do the best you can. So sorry cant take it no longer. Cremate my body no flowers no minister. Just cremate me the least expense. My all my love to all of you.   Bill

*

> Bill. Im sorry but I had this all made out and decided when you called. A hell of a day today. Thanks for the call. But call George.   Henry

Area type VII—least advantaged rural areas: 2 percent of the population; 1 percent of the suicides; suicide rate 3; small minority population.

The psychological characteristics of the suicide notes for area type VII were not subjected to statistical analysis (and not included in the over-all statistical analyses) inasmuch as this area type includes only one study area, and has only 2 percent of the population.

Area type VIII—least advantaged industrial communities: 10 percent of the population; 9 percent of the suicides; suicide rate 13; fairly large minority population; low proportion of single individuals. Affect is indicated in the notes less often than in any other area, except type IX, and, along with area type IV, there is a conspicuous absence of affection. The suicide notes focus primarily on instructions, in this case, to the relatives. These instructions have to do mainly with material possessions, the notification of others, and the disposition of the victim's remains. The notes give the impression of matter-of-fact directives having to do with the mundane and material aspects of a hard existence. Two notes from area type VIII follow:

> To Whom It May Concern: I live at 100 Main Street, Los Angeles, California. In case of extreme emergency, please notify my daughter, Mary B. Jones, Box 100, San Diego, California. In my apartment there is a letter to her giving all necessary in-

structions about what do do with my affairs. I have a checking account with the National Bank, 1st Street Branch, Los Angeles. It is my wish that all of my friends listed in my address book be notified. I am a Protestant. Belong to no lodges now. My apartment rent is paid to the 15th of next month.   William B. Smith

*

Robert:

BE ALERT . . . CLOSE THE DOOR . . . NOW HEAR THIS . . . BE ALERT. By the time you read this, I shall have *disposed* of *myself*. (I can only guess your reaction. If its bad, massage your crotch and breathe deeply) FINISH READING:
I felt better when I decided, several weeks ago. Too many adjustments to make. Ten years ago may have been able to do it. Too rigid now. Too many crystallizations. Too late to utilize the recently acquired revelation that many years ago, fear of world obstructed and stunted natural drives and imagination. Just the one fear was enough. World as total. Not individuals as such. What complete jerks make up this world.

First, check in my room. I may have goofed. If I did, I'll kill myself. That's a joke. Come on relax. You have things to do.

If you want to avoid Mom knowing (boy, am I burdening you) . . .get hold of the police—and tell them to co-operate, to *quietly* come and take me to city facility. I should have passed out from strangulation about five hours ago, so only necessary to cart me away.

Pull this off! To ease your mind, tell Pop. Then both of you tell Momm I took off and you don't know where—say Merchant Marine—

The V.A. can bury me. Pop has my papers. they ship me out of town don't bother to go. In fact don't bother anyway. It's incredibly stupid the way people mourn the dead. My only regret is that I didn't have the world by the balls. If you don't, *you* suffer. Remember that.

You may doubt this letter, Robert. Satisfy your curiosity . . . but don't immediately hate me for imposing on you. Get things done. You can even stay home from work. I could have gone away and done it. But· for once, let this ass hole family be practical. I would have taken my car.—but now you have it.

If (I hate that word) I am dead, pull yourself together and do the things I said.

So help me if you go into the bathroom during the night and read this before you are supposed to, I'll kill you. Two cars and all.

Area type IX—least advantaged apartment areas: 4 percent of the population; 5 percent of the suicides; suicide rate 19; very high minority population; high proportion of single persons; and low proportion of married.

The suicide notes written in this area type are conspicuously low in the reasons for suicide given and in affect shown. The only exception to this is that where affect is shown at all, the emotion of affection is noticeably absent. As in area type VIII, the notes are concerned largely with instructions having to do with the workaday details: things for people to do, things to get, things to fix, things to put aright. These notes—unaddressed as they are in many cases—seem to be directed to the world at large, a world which, from the victim's point of view, has probably been harsh and unrewarding. A sample suicide note from area type IX is reproduced:

My name is William B. Smith. In case of my death I am leaving everything I have in this room to Mr. Henry B. Jones. His address is 100 Main Street, Los Angeles, California. YO 12345. W. B. S.

Suicide and aging: In relation to chronological age generally, a psychological analysis of the 42 suicide notes found in Los Angeles in 1957 written by individuals over age 65—combined with our previous analyses of suicide notes of individuals in various age brackets (20-39, 40-59, and 60 plus) and in various socio-economic strata—led us to the following tentative formulations about suicide and aging. Suicide among the higher aged is neither primarily the rich man's disease nor the poor man's curse; it is both. Our analyses of the socio-psychological factors in suicide indicate that, among the over-65-year-olds, many come from high social rank areas as well as from low social rank areas, and that, further, individuals (primarily men) from both these groups show concern with physical health and with the financial problems of paying for prolonged illness. They differ in that the well-to-do speak of being "tired of life" (even though they obviously have the material advantages of existence), and their poorer brethren speak, in their suicide notes, of the many mundane details of existence which crowd in on them and make up their perception of what "life" is like. The environmental difference between a mansion and a slum is not only in what one "sees," but, perhaps more importantly, in what one is forced to think about and be concerned with. There is another group of suicidal oldsters (although their suicide rate is not especially high) from the middle social ranks. Their suicide notes seem to have to do much more with interpersonal conflicts, with the emotions of love and of hate, and even, at their more advanced age, with difficulties with the spouse, often reflecting the re-orientation of their own unfulfilled dependency needs as they have grown older and found themselves less self-sufficient.

Some of the salient sociological, suicidal, and psychological items for each of the nine area types are summarized in Table I.

IMPLICATIONS AND SUMMARY

If a light touch is not inappropriate, we may state that when Ralph Rackstraw says, in *H.M.S. Pinafore*, that "love burns as brightly in the fo'c'sle as it does on the quarterdeck," he perhaps misled his mess-mates by limiting their attentions to the quantitative variations in brightness. It may be, that love (and other emotions as well) burns *differently* in different areas. There can be no doubt that the concerns with everyday living, the details of existence that press for obsessive rumination, the pervasive milieu which the individual sees as "life" are indeed different in many important qualitative respects in the areas type I and type IX. Recent comprehensive studies cutting across social strata, such as the Kinsey investigations of patterns of sexual behavior,[8, 9] have made it clear that socio-economic factors play important roles in determining the patterns of demonstrations of emotion—causing either their taboo or their open acceptance. The Yale studies of alcoholism have revealed fairly specific patterns of the expressions of the alcoholic symptom at different socio-economic levels. The study by Hollingshead and Redlich[7] on social class and mental illness demonstrated that mentally ill individuals of different social classes not only fall heir to different modes of treatment, but, more importantly for the present context, also present different types of emotional maladaptation, in part related to the social class membership.

The research data here reported are in line with the studies cited in indicating that the emotions expressed by suicidal persons will vary more or less consistently within socio-economic areas, and that the patterns for expression of these emotions will be reflective of the nature of the social class position of which the victims are members. Not only are different *methods* (shooting, hanging, jumping, etc.) used in suicide, but people apparently commit suicide in different *ways*—i.e. with expression or denial of affection, with mention or avoidance of specific reasons—some of which are definitely related to the socio-economic level (or, in this study, area type) to which they belong.

What clues for prevention of suicide can be gathered from this study? It may well be that in an individual consultation with a potentially suicidal person, there must be some cognizance taken of his social class membership and some recognition given to the implications which follow such awareness. Why should area type I people—with all the material advantages—be "tired of life"? Is there really more physical sickness in area type III, or is there a large element of hypochondriasis? What is the meaning of the affection indicated by the area type IV suicides? And why are the area type V suicides conspicuously rejected, or why do they feel that they are? And area types VIII and IX: How could one hope to treat their suicidal impulses without taking into account their lack of diadic relationships and their obvious difficulties in expressing affection or finding someone to express affection to? These are some of the socio-psychological implications. Another implication from the data is that traditional psychotherapeutic techniques might be most effective (in the total population of potentially suicidal individuals) for those persons who come from the *moderately* advantaged area types (IV, V, and VI) and who are concerned with affection and rejection (and apparently with the resolution of conflicts of feelings) rather than for individuals in either the most advantaged or least advantaged area types.

But if there is any single implication from this study it is that the occurrences of suicide, those enigmatic acts of complete self-destruction, are events neither exclusively of the psyche nor of the society, but events which can be understood best in terms of the admixture of both—as socio-psychological phenomena.

References

1. Allport, G. W. The use of personal documents in psychological science. *Soc. Sci. Res. Bull.*, 1942, No. 49.

2. Cavan, R. S. *Suicide*. Chicago: Univ. of Chicago Press, 1926.

3. Dublin, L. I. and Bunzel, B. *To be or not to be*. New York: Random House, 1933.

4. Durkheim, E. *Le Suicide*. Paris: Alcan, 1897. (Glencoe, Ill.: Free Press, 1951.)

5. Guetzkow, H. Unitizing and categorizing problems in coding qualitative data. *J. clin. Psychol.*, 1950, 6, 47-58.

6. Henry, A. F. and Short, J. F., Jr. *Suicide and homicide*. Glencoe, Ill.: Free Press, 1954.

7. Hollingshead, A. B. and Redlich, F. C. *Social class and mental illness*. New York: Wiley, 1958.

8. Kinsey, A. C., Pomeroy, W. B., and Martin, C. E. *Sexual behavior in the human male*. Philadelphia: Saunders, 1948.

9. Kinsey, A. C., Pomeroy, W. B., Martin, C. E., and Gebhard, P. H. *Sexual behavior in the human female*. Philadelphia: Saunders, 1953.

10. Menninger, K. A. *Man against himself*. New York: Harcourt, 1938.

11. Morgenthaler, W. and Steinberg, M. Letzte Aufzeichnungen von Selbstmördern. *Beih. Schweiz. Z. Psychol. Anwend.*, 1945, No. 1.

12. Osgood, C. E. and Walker, E. G. Motivation and language behavior; a content analysis of suicide notes. *J. abnorm. soc. Psychol.*, 1959, 57, 58-67.

13. Ringel, E. *Der Selbstmord*. Vienna: Maudrich, 1953.

14. Sainsbury, P. *Suicide in London: an ecological study*. New York: Basic Books, 1955.

15. Schmid, C. F. Suicide in Seattle, 1914-1925; an ecological and behaviorist study. *Univ. Washington Publ. Soc. Sci.*, 1928.

16. Schmid, C. F. Suicide in Minneapolis, 1928-1932. *Amer. J. Sociol.*, 1933, 39, 30-48.

17. Shneidman, E. S. and Farberow, N. L. Some comparisons between genuine and simulated suicide notes. *J. gen. Psychol.*, 1957, 56, 251-256.

18. Shneidman, E. S. and Farberow, N. L. (Eds.) *Clues to suicide.* New York: McGraw-Hill, 1957.

19. Stengel, E. and Cook, N. G. *Attempted suicide; its social significance and effects.* London: Chapman and Hall, 1958.

20. Tuckman, J., Kleiner, R. J., and Lavell, M. Emotional content of suicide notes. *Amer. J. Psychiat.*, 1959, 116, 59-63.

21. Welfare Planning Council. *Background for planning.* No. 15. Los Angeles: Welfare Planning Council, 1955.

22. Welfare Planning Council. *Differentiating communities in Los Angeles County.* No. 51. Los Angeles: Welfare Planning Council, 1957.

23. Welfare Planning Council. *Fact sheets on 100 study areas, Los Angeles County, 1957.* Los Angeles: Welfare Planning Council, 1957.

Acknowledgments

This investigation was supported by Project Grant #OM-128 from the National Institute of Mental Health, National Institutes of Health, U.S. Public Health Service. In addition, grateful acknowledgment is made to Theodore J. Curphey, M.D., Coroner, Los Angeles County, for his stimulation and for his active cooperation; to Mr. Sederio Roldan, of the Los Angeles Welfare Planning Council, for helping us obtain the sociological data for Los Angeles County; to Mr. Charles Q. Forslund for analyzing the suicide notes; to Mrs. Calista V. Leonard for her over-all contribution to this study; to Mrs. Eunice Pierce, Miss Jacqueline Bailey, and Mr. Charles Neuringer for their helpful assistance; to Mr. Alcon G. Devries for aid in making the statistical computations; and to the members of the staff of the (Los Angeles) Suicide Prevention Center—Robert E. Litman, M.D., Norman Tabachnick, M.D., Raymond E. Anderson, Ph.D., and Marvin Kaphan, M.S.W.—for their assistance and encouragement in the preparation of this chapter.

J. C. Brengelmann

XV

Problems of Measurement in Objective Personality Evaluation

INTRODUCTION

"In all sciences, the method of investigation must be adjusted to the subject matter under investigation." This statement by von Allesch[1] will sound perfectly reasonable to everyone. The short history of personality research is, in fact, full of such *attempts* of adjustments; implementation has not followed the path of a smooth learning curve but has rather resulted in a welter of frequently disagreeing methods and techniques. Quite unlike other biological sciences, personality research has not developed standard methods or instruments of investigation. Other than ability and paper-and-pencil tests, there are, presently, no objective personality measures with established norms and validity.

Concern with individual differences and multiple independent variables has led away from the analysis of restricted functions to an assessment of "total" personality. The inadequacy of some of these techniques is becoming increasingly obvious. Although, for example, the interview and related methods have proved useful, when carefully developed for specific purposes, there is still the problem of reliability or interference by biasing factors of personal or interpersonal perception.

Yet another group of global methods, projective techniques, have fared no better. These devices are beset with a variety of error sources in addition to known defects of interpretation. Attempts to develop objective scoring have generally proved too complex for the purposes served, and even formidable statistical approaches have produced little improvement. Many psychologists are now looking beyond subjective to *objective tests* (in the sense of apparatus measurement). Here, however, the problem is usually one of generating sufficient precision for adequate assessment of multi-faceted personality factors.

The present chapter will suggest ways of increasing the precision of objective personality tests, with illustrations drawn from the author's recent experiments. Discussion will focus on some experimental conditions and the purity of test scores so essential for improved precision. The choice of such concepts as extraversion, rigidity, or response set is incidental. The problem here is not to discover what traits or dimensions should be investigated, but simply how precision of measurement may be increased. For the same reason, the question of which statistical techniques should be applied to integrate measures obtained by the means advocated will not be considered.

THE ACTUAL-GENETIC OR DEVELOPMENTAL PROCESS

In earlier times behavioristic psychology treated responses as a function of the stimuli exposed to the subject. The amount of information obtained was limited, and eventually another approach evolved in Germany. It was termed the "actual-genetic process" of changing response modes, or distortions, analyzable in stages of an orderly development from vague awareness, or highly unspecific response to the stimulus, to a correct or specific response. Using actual-genetic methods of observing developmental characteristics of a percept in the visual field, it was frequently noted that, at first, individual responses deviated from the stimulus to a large and variable extent. Such deviations, or distortions, led to the introduction of a third type of variable, in addition to stimulus and response, usually referred to in German as "subjective" or "central" variables, intervening between stimulus and response. These factors are most observable when the normally rapid process of perception is studied during the various phases of its development.

In the typical actual-genetic experiment, the stimulus is represented in the initial response only very indistinctly or unspecifically. With practice the two main characteristics of such responses, high degree of distortion and great individuality in response mode, adapt gradually to the objective stimulus conditions. This process passes through several easily recognizable stages, as previously shown by the author in the case of learning.[3] A set of 8 complex designs was presented serially to 100 subjects. They were asked to draw and express verbally what they remembered after each of a maximum of 30 serial trials. Initial responses were frequently characterized by more or less vague feelings of familiarity like "I am sure there was something, but I don't know what," or "there was something geometrical," "something round in character," "something three-dimensional." Following this, drawn reproductions tended at first to be highly distorted, but with practice gradually assumed similarity to the stimulus.

It is important to know that individual differences in mode of response were highest at the beginning. Interindividual similarity and more systematic modes of response deviation occurred only after a certain amount of practice. The latter were, for example, characterized by tendencies towards symmetry, or by reverting and inverting parts of the stimulus. Such response modes, which represent only sections of the entire process, have been investigated by adherents of the Berlin Gestalt school (Wertheimer, Köhler, Koffka). Relevant Gestalt principles such as normalization, sharpening and levelling in responses have become well-known.

In contrast to the Berlin group, the Leipzig (Krüger, Sander, Wellek) and Göttingen (von Allesch) groups of *Ganzheit* psychologists use the entire range of the developmental process as a basis for discussion. Methods other than the actual-genetic kind employ, from their point of view, sections of the process or, more often, simply the final stages, or "end results." This limitation may be of serious consequence, as the mode of arriving at the end result is claimed to be more and in a different manner characteristic of the individual than the end result itself.

The fundamental stages in the process of perceiving have been described by Vernon[31] as follows:

First stage: Vague awareness or knowledge that there is something in the visual field or, according to Bartlett,[2] "having a feeling of" or "an impression of" something.

Second stage: The stage of the *generic object*, the awareness that the visual stimulation is connected with some kind of object with an existence in the visual field.

Third stage: The stage of the *specific object*, where some parts of the percept take on specific characteristics. That is to say, they are recognized as appertaining to some particular and specific object.

Fourth stage: The final stage of the perceptual process is that of *identification* and *understanding of meaning*.

All actual-genetic studies produced in the various European countries, as well as the one reported in the United States by Douglas, [22] agree on the existence of such distinct stages, leading to an objectively definable hierarchy in the emergence of response modes. The fact that such phenomena have, until recently, not been exploited for the assessment of personality, is due partly to their high degree of complexity which does not readily lend itself to direct measurement. Methods for measurement of two of the main aspects already mentioned, the degree of distortion and the individual response mode, are proposed in the following.

Measurement of the degree of response distortion is the easier problem and some progress has been made, as demonstrated by the following three test methods.

1) Complex *pictures*, such as a pair of sun glasses, an ashtray with cigarette ends, the outline of a woman's figure, with exposure times varying from 1/100 second up to 60 seconds. Responses were scored in two ways, once in terms of number of trials required for correct solution (traditional method), and then by classifying responses according to process stages (similar to those just described) and by assigning differential error weights to these stages.[12, 29] In these, as well as in a number of

other experiments performed by independent investigators in various countries, both scores discriminated with a high degree of significance between normals and abnormals (neurotics and psychotics). The important point is, however, that this result was retained even when cancelling out the effect of number of trials by using the ratio process error score divided by trial number. This indicates that individuals vary considerably with regard to the frequency of the various actual-genetic stages found in the responses.

2) *Three-dimensional objects,* as the sculpture of a person's head.[4] With brief exposure times, such objects are usually perceived as absolutely flat. With increasing exposure time, a number of stages of varying degrees of three-dimensionality from flatness through relief-like impression to full spatial perception may be distinguished. Again, singularly significant results were obtained in terms of discrimination between normals and abnormals.

3) Measurement of complex patterns drawn from memory.[7, 11, 13] Previous tests of this kind, as the Bender Gestalt Test, had to rely on complicated assessments and have yielded no appreciable results in the field of personality measurement for reasons explained elsewhere.[14] Abandoning the traditional and unsatisfactory method of scoring simply "right-wrong," as in the case of nonsense syllables, the Figure Reconstruction Test (FRT) was developed. Being an objectively scorable test—requiring drawn reproduction or recognition of visually presented patterns of geometric shapes (Figure 1)—it may be applied to stimulus materials of any degree of complexity. It is applicable to learning, recall and recognition alike, and permits detailed concurrent analysis of certainty in performance. Of the various results achieved to date, significant and consistent differentiation between neurotics and psychotics, as well as significant relationships to questionnaire scores of extraversion and rigidity, may be mentioned. Some of these results are discussed below.

Measurement of individual response modes is a much more difficult proposition than that of error degree and has not, to our knowledge, hitherto been achieved in other than broadly descriptive terms. However, the following method should prove feasible. For a particular set of complex stimuli, a sufficiently large number of different individual response modes should be collected empirically and separately for all relevant process stages. The corresponding frequency distributions along the trial axis, or practice stages, are then determined. They indicate the time order in the emergence of the various response types. Provided all relevant response types and their location in the perceptual, or memory, process are thus determined, any new response requiring assessment may then be classified by using the established reference system.

This method may prove of great advantage in all cases in which response distortion is high, as in brain damage, personality deterioration, and severe acute disturbances. It may be argued that breakdown of perceptual and other functions can be more meaningfully understood in terms of a regression along an established order of process characteristics. One important point in this connection is that subjects do not have to perceive or to learn a criterion of correct performance, which they frequently cannot attain. There are also indications that the type of material usually unsuccessfully analyzed by projective techniques will be more accessible in situations employing actual-genetic methods. Motivational factors strongly emerge during certain early stages of the actual-genetic process, apparently much stronger than in the Rorschach, TAT, or other similar techniques, where perception is in direct contact with the stimulus and little impeded. Finally, there is already sufficient evidence to expect that such methods will substantially contribute to the understanding of formative or constructive tendencies, usually referred to as gestalt principles, like preference for orthogonal positions (rotation effects), tendency towards complexity or simplicity, or others already noted. Whether these principles are of a general kind or are specific to personality is entirely unknown.

Personality test scores are, with rare exceptions, treated as if they were of a static nature, whereas, on the contrary, they represent points in an orderly hierarchy of response modes, the sequence of which is of importance. Any single response, or narrowly defined response type, represents only a section of a much wider range of responses having process character. This process is, for individuals, not of a linear nature. The writer has demonstrated, in the learning experiment already outlined,[3] that some subjects distorted only to a moderate degree but required many trials to reach the criterion of correctness, whereas others distorted excessively during early stages of learning but solved the problem more rapidly. This suggests that degree of error, in the developmental sense, may correlate relatively low with the traditional error measure of number of trials required to reach a criterion. There is, in fact, empirical evidence for this important point. Using a test similar in nature to the Figure Reconstruction Test, the author[15] found the following correlations between intelligence (Raven's Progressive Matrices) and learning in three abnormal groups: 0.564, 0.523 and 0.585. In this case the number of correct responses (traditional measure) was used as score. Since error degree (developmental measure) was introduced as a score, corresponding correlations were, as a rule, found to be considerably lower and frequently insignificant,[11] as seen in the following means of various coefficients obtained.

These correlations are probably as low as one can possibly hope to achieve in this field, and they are largely lower than

TABLE 1—*Degree of error, in contrast to the traditional measure of error frequency, lowers correlation with intelligence*

	Controls	Neurotics	Psychotics
Error level	−0.41	−0.35	−0.26
Practice effect	0.28	0.20	0.24

those obtained between FRT error and various personality questionnaires. The suggestion may be made that the developmental method of scoring provides a greater contribution of personality factors to learning variance than does intelligence. This appears reason enough for expecting actual-genetic methods to play an important role in future personality research.

VARIATIONS IN STIMULUS CONDITIONS AND PERFORMANCE VALIDITY

We now call attention to the dependency of performance variables on stimulus conditions, another neglected area in personality research. Whenever the experimental situation permitted, the author observed that significant relationships between personality criteria and performance scores emerged only under certain conditions. On a number of occasions the validity of a test score changed considerably by relatively small modifications of stimulus conditions. Some relevant examples are reported below.

First, let us describe an example of the *dependency of memory performance on exposure conditions*. In one experiment, significant differences in learning visual patterns were found between normals, neurotics, and psychotics, with errors increasing in the order stated. As no learning or memory tests of this kind have hitherto provided similar results in a consistent manner, it was believed that the conditions under which the task was executed had been accidentally favorable. For reasons of economy, a pilot experiment[17] using lysergic acid (LSD-25) and amytal in normals was performed with the result that significant differences on a recall task were found only for a long exposure time of 15 seconds and not after shorter exposure times (1 and 1/100 second). Accepting the hypothesis that LSD-effects are similar to those obtained in schizophrenics, it was then predicted that neurotics and schizophrenics differ significantly in immediate recall only when a long exposure time is used. The actual exposure conditions were 30 seconds and 2 seconds. Before presenting the results let us explain the test score, derived from the *Figure Reconstruction Test* (FRT), while inspecting Figure 1.

As shown (top left), an entire FRT set (recall version) of this level of difficulty consists of ten patterns of five geometrical

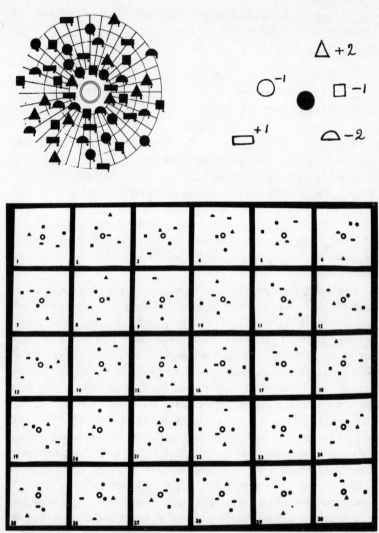

Fig. 1. Figure Reconstruction Test (FRT). *Top left:* distribution of test elements of a set of 10 patterns of 5 shapes each. *Top right:* example of drawn reproduction of the 5 shapes pertaining to each pattern, with statements of certainty in the correctness of performance. *Bottom:* Recognition card, containing the 10 patterns of the one recall set to be recognized, dispersed among 20 similar dummy patterns.

shapes each, distributed around a central reference point for scoring. A variety of individual stimulus patterns can be seen on the FRT recognition card (bottom). The score consists of the mean degree of rotation per individual shape about the central reference point, as found in the drawn reproductions (compare example of reproduction, Figure 1). The direction of rotation is disregarded and the score is named "rotation error."

As predicted, and consistent between males and females, schizophrenics scored significantly higher error only after the long exposure time.[13] Moreover, significant correlations between personality questionnaires and rotation error were obtained. All 48 neurotics completed Eysenck's questionnaire of extraversion,[24] as well as Nigniewitzky's questionnaire of rigidity.[28] The correlation between extraversion and rigidity was found to be insignificant (−0.22), whereas the correlations between the questionnaire scores and rotation error were as follows.

TABLE 2—*The size of correlation between memory and personality test scores depends significantly on experimental conditions*

Correlations (48 neurotics)	Rotation error			
	Test 1		Test 2	
Exposure secs.	30	2	30	2
Extraversion	−0.20	−0.08	−0.01	−0.44†
Rigidity	0.31*	0.28*	0.03	0.09

Significance: *=.05, †=.01 level

A significant correlation with extraversion was found only after a certain amount of practice and use of the short exposure time. An analysis of variance between the three subgroups composed of 16 extraverted, 16 introverted, and 16 ambiverts resulted in an F-ratio of 12.62, with 2/45 degrees of freedom, which is significant at the .01 level. Rigidity, on the other hand, revealed significant relationships only for the initial practice stages, regardless of exposure time. The stability of these results is demonstrated by their consistency between males and females. This specific manifestation of rigid behavior in initial stages of practice was found again, using a completely different type of task.[9] In this experiment, scores derived from tracing while wearing prismatic inversion lenses proved significantly related only on the first application of the test. These results may be considered to support the hypothesis that one type of rigid behavior is associated with initial difficulties in the adaptation to a variety of performance tasks.

Using two conditions of exposure time, a more precise test of the assumption that schizophrenics occupy an extreme position on a hypothetical continuum of rigidity becomes possible. This hypothesis had in fact received support in that a number of test scores varied with the degree of rigidity in neurotics whilst the extreme position was reserved for the schizophrenics (unpublished findings). The present results, however, are inconsistent with this assumption, for the following reasons. Recall impairment in schizophrenics, as against neurotics, was specific to a long exposure time of 30 seconds. This specificity does not obtain for the neurotic subgroups, divided according to their degree of rigidity, as the respective subgroup positions with regard to mean rotation error are similar for both the short and long exposure time of test 1. With practice from test 1 to 2, the situation remained unchanged for the comparison between neurotics and schizophrenics, and the respective discrimination remained significant only for the long exposure time. However, as seen from the correlations in Table 2, rigidity in neurotics correlated significantly with rotation error only for test 1 and not for test 2. Both exposure time effects and practice effects are, therefore, not wholly in agreement with the hypothesis discussed.

It has thus been demonstrated that the validity of recall performance in terms of its relationship to abnormal and questionnaire criteria may be considerably affected by the exposure time. used as well as by the amount of practice given. It was also shown that the severity in testing personality hypotheses may be greatly increased by considering such variations in stimulus conditions. The outcome in testing hypotheses may, in fact, depend on variations of this kind. The general conclusion to be drawn from this is that relevant environmental stimulus variables require systematic variation, if failure of validation is to be avoided or precision of measurement increased.

STIMULUS CONDITIONS AND EXTREME RESPONSE SET

Another example of the dependence of important personality characteristics on stimulus conditions is demonstrated with regard to *response set*. Again, the suggestion for this analysis was originally derived from a previous study[3] of the process character of learning. It was noted that individual differences in subjective feelings of certainty (*Evidenzgefühl*) regarding correctness of performance appeared highest in initial stages of learning when performance was extremely vague or "unstructured." The significance of this reproduction certainty has recently been analyzed by using the FRT. The reproduction example (Figure 1, top right) contains the four degrees of certainty from very certain ($+2$) to very uncertain (-2). Subjects were required to mark each test element reproduced with one of these four degrees depending on how certain they felt about the correctness of their drawings. After each of the two recall conditions of 30 seconds and 2 seconds exposure, employing a set of 10 stimulus patterns each, a larger set of 30 stimulus cards was successively exposed twice (Figure 1). Of these 30 cards, 20 had never been exposed before, whereas the remaining 10 were those employed during recall. Subjects had to state which of the 30 patterns they believed to have seen during recall and how certain they felt about the correctness of their statement, using the same four degrees of certainty. It was noted that with relatively small changes between tests 1 and 2 (reliability of means), differences in positive extremes between neurotics and schizophrenics increased from 30 second recall through 2 second recall to recognition. Significance increased accordingly from chance result to high level of significance. It may be concluded that successful measurement of individual differences in extreme response set and their validity depends largely on the experimental conditions under which scores are obtained.

A second and more specific effect was also observed. During recall, positive extreme certainty decreased in both the neurotics and schizophrenics with the 2 second recall condition. This may be a function of the difficulty of task involved, whereby confidence would decrease with greater difficulty. However, regardless of whether the remaining recognition conditions are more difficult or easier, level of difficulty would be inadequate to explain the results obtained. If recognition were more difficult, the schizophrenic score should have decreased; if it were easier, the neurotic score should have increased.

These inconsistencies may be simply due to differences in the functions measured, recall and recognition. Or, it is possible that "lack of structure" or "insight in task performance" is more typical for recognition of this particular kind, and that certain personality traits are manifested more easily in such a medium regardless of the difficulty of the task involved. Whatever the truth may be, it appears obvious that a suitable type of functional analysis is required to solve the problem.

To demonstrate the generality of the effects discussed, let us briefly consider the individual variation on extreme positive response set within the neurotic sample. Since the hypothesis of a continuum of rigidity through neurosis into schizophrenia has been a good starting point on several occasions, it appeared reasonable to test its tenability with regard to the variable here under discussion. It was anticipated that extreme positive certainty would vary with rigidity in neurotics, as it varied with the neurotic/schizophrenic dichotomy. When the neurotics were divided into equally large subgroups of high, medium, and low rigidity, separately for males and females, it was noted that extreme positive certainty increased consistently in the order low-medium-high rigid neurotics, with the extreme position left for the schizophrenics. Even more relevant to the present discussion, however, was the finding that this result was achieved only during recognition and not during recall, as illustrated by the correlations between rigidity and extreme positive response set for the entire neurotic sample of 48 subjects (Table 3).

TABLE 3—*Example of dependence of significant personality correlates on test conditions*

Rigidity versus extreme positive certainty

Correlations (48 neurotics)	Recall		Recognition	
Exposure secs.	30	2	30	2
Test 1	0.25	0.26	0.40†	0.43†
Test 2	0.18	0.19	0.47†	0.44†

Significance: †=.01 level

During recall no correlation is significant at the .05 level; for recognition, all correlations are significant at the .01 level. In all, the consistent picture emerges that extreme positive certainty is related to the personality criteria used only under certain specifiable conditions. With this empirically established result in mind, it now becomes possible to design more effective functional or condition analyses with the aim of gaining deeper insight into the factors governing response set. Systematic manipulation of the stimulus conditions, it may be said, appears to be a *conditio sine qua non*.

EFFECT OF COMPLEXITY OF TEST SCORES

In personality research we are often confronted with complex situations. As a result of this, the rigor exercised by many investigators in hypothesis construction is frequently deceiving. For instance, Callaghan,[20] who investigated the hypothesis that electroshock reduces "psychoticism," predicted that the size of certain *expressive movement* scores would be reduced as a result of shock, but did not allow for the fact that shock, apart from possibly reducing psychoticism, also causes (transient) brain dysfunction and hence an increase in expressive movement scores. This was, in fact, the only significant finding observed and was, wrongly, taken to contradict the hypothesis. In Ingham's[26] analysis of the relationship between neurosis and *suggestibility*, it was found, according to expectation, that the extent of arm movement of neurotics in response to suggestion was greater than that of normals. This difference, however, disappeared when groups were equated for same movement extent without suggestion. Broadbent,[19] investigating kinesthetic *figural after-effect* in its relationship to extraversion detected that the predicted correlation only appears if the apparatus is positioned in a particular way. Important as these matters are, we restrict ourselves at present to the problem of complexity of scores.

It is a common complaint that objective personality tests, though superior to subjective methods, have low validity and do not stand up to cross-validation. This may have led to two major, but rather ineffective, types of reaction. One is an excess in construction of new tests, the other an excess in theorizing. As to the former, Cattell[21] reports that some 4000 tests have been devised to explore personality; and, as to the latter, MacKinnon's[27] remark may serve as a reminder: "In personality research our theorizing and building of models have outrun activities more intimately concerned with observation and data collecting. Our greatest need for the more adequate study of personality is systematic observation and systematization of the data we collect, and this, I submit, is something more than theorizing." A systematic study of data may indeed, in view of their frequent complexity or lack of purity, be highly rewarding, as the following discussion may show.

The first example refers again to *extreme response set*, the positive $(+2)$ and negative (-2) extremes on a four point scale of certainty. This variable has for a long time been used in an undifferentiated manner, until it became known that positive and negative extremes may mean different things. We found that schizophrenics used more extreme positive certainty in judging the correctness of their recall performance, whereas neurotics scored higher on extreme negative certainty. If only extreme response set *per se*, undifferentiated for positive and negative extremes, had been analyzed, the conclusion would have been different; the decrease between the 30 second and 2 second conditions of recall was largest for schizophrenics, but between recall and recognition the decrease was largest for the neurotics. This inconsistency would have led to the assumption that maintenance of response set is not general to the tasks used. However, by dividing the score into its components of negative and positive extremes it may be concluded that schizophrenics "rigidly" maintained the highest level of positive extremes and the lowest level of negative extremes practically throughout.

The second example concerns *motor performance*. In a recent experiment, the author wanted to test the hypothesis that the increase in rate of performance was lower for extraverted than for introverted subjects. The 49 normal subjects were asked to complete an extraversion questionnaire and to trace wavy lines while wearing prismatic lenses which cause inversion of the visual field.[9]

Using as criterion for correct performance a limit of 2 mms. either side of the target line (total limits of 4 mms.), it was found that extraverts, after starting from a level similar to that of the introverts, scored lower through most of the experiment in comparison to the introverts. When, however, the criterion for correct performance was changed to 8 mms. either side of the target line (total limits of 16 mms.) extraverts scored higher than the introverts. This means that the score used to test the hypothesis was not a suitable one and that in fact a completely different type of variable, that of sideward movement extent, determined the outcome of the prediction. In the light of these results it may be suggested that the use of similar hypotheses proposed by other authors relating extraversion to motor performance (pursuit rotor) is invalid, as long as the effect of target size of the pursuit rotor is not considered.[23, 25, 30]

Further analysis of the prismatic tracing experiment revealed movement extent and variability of movement to be significantly related to both extraversion and rigidity,[9] not however, the performance scores used. Furthermore, a variable called smooth-restrained versus irregular-excessive tracings was specific to rigidity. Results for rigidity are shown in Table 4. Those of extraversion remained insignificant. (Note that in the original publication a different significance level was erroneously stated).

TABLE 4—*Relationship between mode of movement and rigidity as an example of empirical analysis*

Mode of movement	smooth-restrained	medium position	irregular-excessive	N
High rigid	3	8	13	24
Low rigid	14	8	3	25
N	17	16	16	49

$X^2 = 13.388$ (2 d.f.)   Significance: .01 level

These analyses demonstrate the difficulty often experienced in choosing the essential variables. The validity of tracing performance scores, as frequently used in personality research, should be regarded as dependent on the mode, or style of movement, at least under certain conditions. This might resolve frequent inconsistencies found between investigators using slight variations in apparatus or scoring methods, which permit the style of movement to interfere differentially with the actual performance score. Almost the entire personality work on *mirror drawing* may have remained inconsistent because of such inadequate consideration of test scores and, to a lesser degree, the same may apply to other motor performance tasks, as discussed elsewhere.[14]

The third example of reducing complexity of test scores is quoted from the field of *expressive movement*. During time-consuming attempts to validate drawing and related scores, derived from the FRT (Figure 1) and other tests, the familiar difficulties of inconsistency, large between-groups overlap, and specificity to task conditions were encountered.[5, 6, 8, 16, 18] This is consistent with the fact that the vast number of expressive movement studies, including graphology, have yielded very few results of acceptable validity,[14] though continuing to suggest that expressive movement may be a sensitive indicator of "some" aspect of personality.

Of the various successful attempts to reduce the error variance encountered with the FRT "distance" score, one is described below. *Distance* is defined as the mean distance in mms. at which the 50 individual shapes of one FRT recall set (Figure 1) are drawn by the subject; its standard deviation forms a second score (S.D.-distance). These two scores were analyzed separately for positive and negative certainty, using records of an earlier experiment with drugs.[10] It was found, with unusual regularity, that S.D.-distance was highest for items with positive confidence and lowest for those with negative confidence. This effect was subsequently investigated from the individual differences point of view. Table 5 presents the correlations, with coefficients pertaining to rigidity added to those of extraversion.

TABLE 5—*Reduction in test score complexity may considerably improve validity*

Standard deviation of distance (2 secs. exposure)

Correlations (48 neurotics)	Total score	Negative certainty	Positive certainty	Diff. neg.—pos. certainty
Extraversion	0.36°	−0.08	0.48†	0.54†
Rigidity	−0.51†	−0.47†	−0.35°	−0.06

Significance: °=.05, †=.01 level.

These correlations demonstrate a significant difference in S.D.-distance between the conditions of negative and positive certainty in the case of extraversion. For rigidity no such effect is observed. It appears that the variation in expressive movement of extraverts depends to a significant degree on their subjective states of confidence, whereas the rigid person appears little affected by varying conditions of this kind.

Reduction in score complexity may lead to a remarkable increase in efficiency, in terms of overlap between operationally defined groups. As regards the *total score* of S.D.-distance, the overlap between the most extraverted and most introverted subjects (each group containing one third of the entire, unselected sample of neurotics) was 25 percent for the males and 31.3 percent for the females. After development of the *difference score,* i.e. the difference between negative and positive certainty, the corresponding overlap was nil for the males and 6.3 percent for the females.

These analyses have shown that S.D.-distance, or the spread of items drawn on the reproduction sheet, is a complex score. Its division according to negative and positive certainty provides at least a partial solution of the three difficulties of validation stated at the beginning of this discussion.

In this section it has been shown that experimental situations and test scores are frequently of a highly complex or impure nature. This impurity is in part responsible for many inconsistent results and low validities. To overcome such difficulties, careful empirical analysis of measuring instruments and scores appears necessary. It should be remembered in this context that much of the progress in other biological sciences has depended on the development of precision instruments, which in turn provide more refined and specific hypotheses.

SUMMARY

In this chapter some of the problems encountered in the objective measurement of personality have been discussed and several experimental approaches suggested. This was attempted for several reasons: objective personality tests generally suffer from too low validities; most of the reviews in the literature report widespread inconsistencies between investigators; and, in contrast to other biological sciences, experimental methods are seldom discussed. We are all too frequently confronted with a paradoxical mixture of carefully argued theory and poor control of experimental and instrumental variables. Yet, it is quite possible that theories have remained highly vulnerable, largely because slight changes in the experimental situation or scoring procedures have frequently led to widely different results.

To achieve greater precision and stability, several experimental methods have been proposed. Study of the actual-genetic process will contribute to measurement and interpretation of a range of complex response modes. Functional analysis and condition analysis will reveal the conditions necessary for the occurrence of events. Both these methods imply that responses are not static in nature, but are part of an inherent process of development (actual-genetic approach), with a definable place in this process and intimately dependent on the changing structure of environmental conditions. This suggests that meaningful and significant information can best be attained by analyzing experimentally the effect of antecedent conditions on both behavioral and phenomenological responses. There is also a need for more extended analysis of experimental and score complexity. A satisfactory degree of uniformity of measurement, now largely absent in personality research, will not be achieved without careful purification of test scores. This was shown to affect not only precision in measurement but also the qualitative outcome in evaluating hypotheses.

Admittedly, control of all relevant independent variables is impossible in personality research. This, however, should not preclude the applicability of functional and condition analysis. The problem is one of degree of efficiency, varying from macrophysics through biology to the study of personality. Using rudimentary forms of the methods here discussed, considerable improvement was obtained in controlling a number of variables in areas where significant progress had been lacking for a long time. To have demonstrated this *ad oculos*, and not merely by way of argument, has been the main aim of the present chapter.

References

1. Allesch, J. von. Zur Methode der Psychologie. *Psychol. Rundsch.*, 1949, 1, 75-81.

2. Bartlett, F. C. An experimental study of some problems of perceiving and imaging. *Brit. J. Psychol.*, 1916, 8, 222-226.

3. Brengelmann, J. C. Der Aufbau des Gedächtnisses in Allgemeinheitsgraden. Z. exp. Psychol., 1953, 1, 422-452.

4. Brengelmann, J. C. Der visuelle Objekterkennungstest. Z. exp. angewand. Psychol., 1953, 1, 422-452.

5. Brengelmann, J. C. Grösse und Veränderung der Grösse von Reproduktionen als Mass des Bewegungsausdrucks. Z. diagn. Psychol., 1955, 3, 23-33.

6. Brengelmann, J. C. Figurrekonstruktion: Grösse und Variabilität der Grösse von Reproduktionen als Bestimmer der Extraversion-Introversion. Mschr. Psychiat. Neurol., 1955, 130, 209-233.

7. Brengelmann, J. C. Figurrekonstruktion: Rotationsfehler und Rotationsvariabilität als Indikatoren der Persönlichkeit, vorzüglich der Psychose. Fol. psychiat. neurol. neurochir. neerl., 1946, 59, 230-254.

8. Brengelmann, J. C. Complex perceptual processes. In Eysenck, H. J., Granger, G. W., and Brengelmann, J. C., Perceptual processes and mental illness. London: Chapman & Hall, 1957.

9. Brengelmann, J. C. Extraversion, neurotische Tendenz und Rigidität im Umkehrversuch (Prismenbrille). Z. exp. angewand. Psychol., 1957, 4, 339-362.

10. Brengelmann, J. C. d-amphetamine and amytal: II. Effects on certainty and adequacy of certainty in recall and recognition. J. ment. Sci., 1958, 104, 160-166.

11. Brengelmann, J. C. Learning in neurotics and psychotics. Acta psychol., 1958, 13, 371-388.

12. Brengelmann, J. C. Weitere Validierung der Bilderkennung im Gruppenversuch. Z. diagn. Psychol., 1958, 6, 3-17.

13. Brengelmann, J. C. The effects of exposure time in immediate recall on abnormal and questionnaire criteria of personality. J. ment. Sci., 1958, 104, 665-680.

14. Brengelmann, J. C. Expressive movement. In Eysenck, H. J. (Ed.), Handbook of abnormal psychology. London: Pitman, 1959.

15. Brengelmann, J. C. The effect of repeated electroshock on learning in depressives. Ph.D. Thesis. Univ. of London, 1953.

16. Brengelmann, J. C. and Pinillos, J. L. Le test de reconstruction de figures. Rev. psychol. appl., 1954, 4, 187-202.

17. Brengelmann, J. C., Laverty, S. G., and Lewis, D. J. Differential effects of lysergic acid and sodium amytal on immediate memory and expressive movement. J. ment. Sci., 1958, 104, 144-152.

18. Brengelmann, J. C. and Marconi, J. Expressive movement in abnormals, with particular reference to extraversion and psychoticism. Acta psychol., 1958, 14, 200-214.

19. Broadbent, D. E. Extraversion and the kinesthetic figural aftereffect. B.P.S. Ann. Conf., 1958.

20. Callaghan, J. E. *Effect of electro-convulsive therapy on the test performance of depressed patients.* Ph.D. Thesis. Univ. of London, 1952.

21. Cattell, R. B. *Personality: a systematic theoretical and factual study.* New York: McGraw-Hill, 1950.

22. Douglas, A. G. A tachistoscopic study of the order of emergence in the process of perception. *Psychol. Monogr.*, 1947, 61, No. 6.

23. Eysenck, H. J. Reminiscence, drive, and personality theory. *J. abnorm. soc. Psychol.*, 1956, 53, 328-333.

24. Eysenck, H. J. The questionnaire measurement of extraversion and neuroticism. *Riv. psychol.*, 1956, 50, 113-140.

25. Eysenck, H. J., Casey, S., and Trouton, D. S. Drugs and personality. II. The effect of stimulant and depressant drugs on continuous work. *J. ment. Sci.*, 1957, 103, 432, 645-649.

26. Ingham, J. G. Psychoneurosis and suggestibility, *J. abnorm. soc. Psychol.*, 1955, 51, 600-603.

27. MacKinnon, D. W. Fact and fancy in personality research. *Amer. Psychologist,* 1953, 8, 138-146.

28. Nigniewitzky, R. D. A statistical study of rigidity as a personality variable. M.A. Thesis. Univ. of London, 1955.

29. Pinillos, J. L. and Brengelmann, J. C. Bilderkennung als Persönlichkeitstest. *Z. exp. angewand. Psychol.*, 1953, 1, 422-452.

30. Star, K. An experimental study of 'reactive inhibition' and its relation to certain personality traits. Ph.D. Thesis. Univ. of London, 1957.

31. Vernon, M. D. *A further study of visual perception.* Cambridge: Cambridge Univ. Press, 1954.

Henry P. David

and

William Rabinowitz

XVI

Brief Projective Methods
in Personality Assessment

INTRODUCTION

ONE OF THE DISTINGUISHING MARKS of clinical psychology in the United States, since the war, has been the growing emphasis on the assessment of complex personality processes.[170] This development occurred, in part, through the expanding use of projective techniques which made unconscious material available to researchers.[1, 7, 13, 58, 96, 137, 143]

In recent years much has been said and written about the advantages and limitations of such methods as the Rorschach, Thematic Apperception Test, Szondi, Human Figure Drawings, Sentence Completions, etc.[3, 15, 57, 73, 93, 94, 110, 178] Not only has there been a recognition of the need for extensive training and clinical acumen, but also of the considerable technical problems of validation. Many interpretive principles and assumptions, once taken for granted, are now being seriously questioned.

This re-evaluation of projective techniques has been accompanied, on occasion, by concern over the amount of time required by the most widely used procedures,[125] the manpower problem,[4] the applicability of a routine standard battery in the absence of specifically defined purposes,[74] and "the sheer economics of hours put into testing, recording, reviewing, pondering, interpreting results and reporting conclusions."[89]

Some clinicians[62, 67, 89, 117, 178] have openly questioned whether the data and inferences obtained after 10 to 15 hours of extensive testing and detailed report writing allow more expeditious treatment or disposition of the patient. How much attention is actually paid to this costly material? Is this the best utilization of the psychologist's time? Perhaps most important, can it be justified on the basis of available research evidence?

A review of the literature suggests that the search for brief methods began when standardized psychological tests were first used. In 1883 Galton[61] described his initial work as "an experimental method of measurement . . . characterized by its brevity," as contrasted with the elaborate psychophysical procedures acclaimed at the time. Experimental studies on association began with Aschaffenburg[8] in 1896, and a year later Ebbinghaus[46] developed a crude sentence completion test to observe mental capacity and reasoning ability. By 1949 Mensh[114] could cite over 200 studies on brief measures of intelligence, an area of interest that still receives considerable attention in current psychological journals.

Historical treatises show that early clinicians used brief queries—dealing with wishes, dreams, memories, etc.—to probe the psychological forces animating their patients. Some of these procedures, with standardized directions, have survived in the form of modified mental status examinations.[172] Inkblots and other "tests of imagination" also have an ancient history.[50, 130] They were the forerunners of continuing efforts to explore an area which James[82] described in 1902 as "outside of the primary consciousness."

Enterprising researchers, whether clinical or academic, have repeatedly modified existing projective techniques and experimented with shorter, more limited, especially prepared methods, as for example, in Murray's pioneer studies at the Harvard Psychological Clinic.[123] Others designed projective stimuli almost like aptitude tests, in an effort to obtain answers to concrete diagnostic screening, descriptive, or predictive questions. It is the purpose of this chapter to survey some of the more recent clinical and nonclinical explorations with brief projective methods, their advantages and limitations, and to consider a theoretical rationale relating test data to the decision-making process.

SURVEY OF BRIEF PROJECTIVE METHODS

An attempt at definition: It is far easier to describe varieties of brief projective methods than to define their basic characteristics. Brief is, at best, a relative term, frequently dependent on the purposes for which a particular item is used. For example, in a setting that requires screening of thousands of subjects in relatively little time, a test requiring 15 minutes to administer might not be considered short. On the other hand, when thorough study of a few cases is required, a two-hour test might be regarded as brief. In defining the concept "brief," we have used an elastic temporal yardstick. Although, ideally, brief methods should take not more than 15 to 30 minutes to administer, we have included, as within the scope of this review, any projective technique which appeared to involve less testing time than is customary.

Brief projective methods may be surveyed in terms of the stimulus materials used or the purposes for which they are intended. We will cite some of the major stimuli from the literature, giving representative references wherever possible, and then devote most of this section to a consideration of the objectives for which brief methods have been specifically used.

Stimulus materials: Brief projective methods are extremely varied, ranging from condensations or elaborations of well-known techniques to unique queries. While TAT-like pictures and cartoons have stimulated considerable research effort,[14, 19, 42, 83, 98, 106, 111, 148] the use of inkblots has been far more limited.[44, 45, 71, 179] Drawing methods have been explored in many ways,[72, 131, 146, 160] as have handwriting samples[129, 176] and photographs.[65, 158, 159] Still other techniques include the completion of sentences, essays, stories, or fables,[39, 68, 77, 138, 139, 165] free association,[30, 63, 84, 90, 135, 145] early memories,[152] and proverbs.[11, 17, 65]

Perhaps most unusual are brief verbal items, usually posed in single-question form or in a series.[97] For example, subjects may be asked what they would most (or least) like to be,[40] to describe how they would paint themselves,[18] or to tell their favorite joke.[180] They may also be faced with the query: "Who Are You?"[25, 26, 162, 177] At times, brief methods have been combined into short batteries,[80, 99] apparently with sufficiently good results to warrant further research.

CLINICAL SCREENING

Adults: In 1922 Marjory Bates,[10] a psychologist on the staff of the Worcester State Hospital in Massachusetts, wrote in the *American Journal of Psychiatry* that "except for the work with association tests the large majority of psychological experiments conducted with the insane have been those requiring rather complicated apparatus and feasible only in a hospital possessed of a well-equipped laboratory. Many hospitals nevertheless could use to advantage certain simple tests which had been studied with a special view towards aiding in diagnosis and in prognosis." She then went on to report her findings with only 50 of 100 Kent-Rosanoff words, several puzzles, and drawings. Today, nearly 40 years later, her suggestions are still valid.

Drawings have retained their popularity, as perhaps best exemplified by Machover's Draw-a-Person technique.[109] Its validity has been seriously questioned by Swenson,[157] but with the added comment that "some evidence supports the use of the DAP as a rough screening device, and as a gross indicator of 'level of adjustment.'" Among the more novel variations of the drawing procedure are the Inside-of-the-Body test,[160] the Geosign test,[134] Harrower's Most Unpleasant Concept,[72] War-tegg's Drawing Completions,[91] and the standardized graphomotor projection technique described by Kutash and Gehl.[95] The use of "doodling" has also been reported, as a "fever chart" of psychoanalysis, reflecting changes in character.[9]

Among picture techniques the TAT has spawned considerable offspring.[11, 14, 20, 168] Rather typical is Smith's et al.[149] use of eight cards "as a means of quickly gaining traumatic material" for the subsequent psychiatric interview. More unique are Libo's[102] four pictures vaguely illustrating patient-therapist relationships. When administered at the end of the patient's first visit, it yields an "attraction score" predicting whether or not a second appointment will be kept.

Hypothetical situations, such as the Projective Question,[40,41,55] Three Impossibilities,[43] etc., serve mainly as rapid screening devices. For example, inability to shift away from the human concept on the Projective Question is almost pathognomonic for a severe disturbance in identification, nearly always associated with paranoid thought processes. As Lehner[100] has noted, hypothetical situations remove the subject from actual and real circumstances so that the personality, ideally, can be expressed free of its usual restrictions. While it has been charged by Feifel[52] that such techniques reflect "cultural and conventional stereotypes more than personal and idiosyncratic outlook," it is difficult to arrive at definite conclusions in the absence of group reference points or base lines from which clinicians can assess individual responses or deviations. Some patients require more "inquiry" than others; highly charged personal themes may occasionally be hidden behind rather conventional choice reactions.

Sentence completion techniques combine the advantages of speedy group administration with somewhat less demand for technical skill in interpretation. They have been used in many clinical situations[108,156,164,175] and afford an excellent basis for therapeutic probing.[56] The subject is usually asked to finish a sentence of which the first word or words are given; variations are readily tailored for specific needs, such as marriage counseling[92] or work with the physically handicapped.[53] Among the more focused versions is Sacks'[140] Make-a-Sentence Test, where the subject is told to write sentences about himself. Stein's[151] Sentence Construction Test requires combining three "loaded" words into one sentence. Perhaps least structured is Michaux's[115] Sentence Composition Test, with its instructions to write 20 sentences each containing the word "because."

Children and adolescents: Among the clinical screening methods devised particularly for children is the doll play interview;[6] the examiner addresses specific questions to the doll which the child then answers. This individual technique permits a fairly rapid exploratory approach that may not be possible in direct questioning. Pigem's Wishing Test,[32, 33, 127, 128] as used by van Krevelen[166, 167] in child psychiatric diagnosis, is similar to other projective questions[40, 174] in probing for depth material. Scribbling[48] or fairly free drawing devices[16, 49] serve the same purpose. The findings obtained may be clearly indicative of severe disturbance, or its absence, and may also provide important leads for psychotherapy.

The Despert Fables[54] and the Deuss Stories[122] have also been helpful in diagnostic work with children. In both instances the examiner reads a very short story which the child is either told to complete, or about which he may be asked a penetrating question. It is not necessary to give all the fables; certain items may be combined to form brief tests of dependency, hostility, etc. The objective is to elicit depth psychological material focused on interpersonal relations. Since storytelling is so common among children, it becomes a natural approach to their fantasy lives.

Much attention has been given to the earliest memory, both in therapeutic probing and in dynamically oriented research studies.[21, 47, 59, 85, 103, 113, 144, 152, 171] Available findings suggest, however, that this approach may be more limited with children than with adults.

A number of techniques, although not specifically developed for clinical purposes, seem well suited as screening procedures. For example, Heppell and Raimy[75] produced 15 photographs portraying child-parent relationships for a study with pre-adolescent boys. As a brief diagnostic device with 5 and 6 year olds, Cummings[38] used 11 pictures of children and adults with neutral, frowning, or smiling expressions on their faces. The youngster was then asked to say what he thought of each picture. Hulse[79] requested his adolescent and post-adolescent subjects to draw their families, which provided him with possible clues about conflicts. In an attempt to identify the status of children in a group, from leaders to isolates, the Hares[70] instructed their subjects to "draw a picture of your group doing the thing you like to do best." Jackson[81] reported that normal children related more "realistic stories" than matched groups of neurotics and delinquents in response to 6 black and white drawings of family scenes. Lastly, Crandell[34] offered observations on the use of projective techniques in child development research, including especially constructed pictures to test hypotheses derived from social learning theory.

ATTITUDE ASSESSMENT

Objective attitude tests typically require the respondent to express agreement or disagreement with a series of stated propositions. As with most paper and pencil questionnaires, one of the major technical problems is that of respondent simulation—i.e. faking. Rarely are items so subtly stated as to mislead a test-sensitive subject; he can, if he chooses, reply in the manner he believes will cast him in the most favorable light.

The widely recognized limitations of conventional attitude inventories[35] induced a search for pertinent projective devices. It was hoped that indirect expression of a subject's general perceptual and cognitive functioning might be more representative of his private world of beliefs and opinions than forced reactions to specific test items.

Fromme[60] was perhaps the first psychologist to explore the use of projective methods in the study of social attitudes; his 1941 paper described especially designed cartoons and TAT-type pictures. Most of the work of the 1940's has been reviewed by Campbell.[28] Applications of projective techniques have also been noted in sociological research,[136] opinion and attitude surveys,[31, 150] action research,[132] and advertising.[107]

Racial attitudes have been investigated with modified Rosenzweig cartoons,[24] and with photographs of Anglo and Spanish cowboys.[83] Projective questions and TAT-like pictures were used in an extensive study of anti-semitism.[2,101] Brief projective questions were also employed to assess personality characteristics associated with antidemocratic beliefs,[141] attitudes held by former Soviet citizens,[12, 69] and political apathy or activity.[124]

Many attitudinal studies, including those using brief projective devices, give little attention to the problem of validity. Most frequently validity is implied or assumed on the basis of internal consistency among items or among various test measures. An outstanding example was reported by Sanford and Rosenstock[142] who used both projective and "objective" attitudinal measures in a house-to-house survey of 963 subjects; their predicted relationships among the various test measures were in virtually all cases substantiated.

Correlation with an external criterion is one of the most commonly accepted procedures for determining validity. For example, Burwen, Campbell, and Kidd[27] developed 24 incomplete sentences to assess superior/subordinate attitudes of Air Force cadets. The technique yielded satisfactory validity relative to other test measures but failed to correlate significantly with nontest reputational criteria. Walter and Jones[169] reported that the attitudes of manual arts therapy patients, as elicited by 37 sentence completions, correlated significantly at the 1 percent level with ratings independently and concurrently assigned by therapists.

In a particularly interesting study Kamenetzky, Burgess, and Rowan[88] compared the relative effectiveness of four different attitude assessment techniques in predicting willingness to sign a petition. The correlations between the tests and the criterion were all significant beyond the 1 percent level of confidence; also, the correlations did not differ significantly from one another. The single projective device (cartoons) was not only as effective a predictor as the three more conventional methods (a Likert-type scale and two scalograms), but was far richer in yielding additional qualitative information.

OTHER NONCLINICAL APPLICATIONS

Educational achievement: Prediction of educational achievement has traditionally stemmed from such cognitive measures as intelligence test scores, school grade averages, etc. In an effort to improve predictions, educational psychologists began to explore noncognitive approaches, including brief projective devices.

Chahbazi[29] found that adding two brief projective items to a battery of six cognitive measures produced a statistically significant increase in the coefficient of multiple correlation with grades: 40 percent of the variance of first term college averages was accounted for by the full battery; only 26 percent without the projective items.

Significant correlations between achievement and school grades have been reported by Morgan,[120, 121] who used a picture interpretation task and projective questions. She also observed that "achievers" tended to give far fewer egocentric references. Hadley and Kennedy[66] noted significantly more conflict in the sentence completions of underachievers compared to students whose achievement was consistent with their aptitude.

Diagnosis of learning abilities has been studied by Monroe,[119] who asked elementary school children to select a picture from among several shown and then tell a story about a youngster having difficulty in school. A series of 15 structured but incomplete stories has been developed by Mills[116] for counseling college students.

Personnel selection: The use of brief projective methods has also been extended to the area of personnel assessment.[22, 23, 154] For example, in a hospital setting a 20-item make-a-sentence test, combined with an information-achievement test, was the most effective combination in predicting the work adjustment of psychiatric aides.[155]

A cartoons situation test,[147] depicting children with teachers or parents, has been developed for selecting teachers and studying personality aspects pertinent to the teaching process. Rabinowitz and Travers[133] asked student teachers to draw a picture of a teacher with a class and found that the productions were related to stages in teacher education. According to Hessel and Travers,[76] ratings assigned to the drawings discriminated among adequate and inadequate student-teachers as rated by their supervisors. The technique was subsequently employed by Stern, Stein and Bloom[153] and reported in their personality assessment volume. An objective scoring procedure is now available.[118]

Cross-cultural studies: Responses to a single picture were used by Kaldegg to explore national differences among secondary school boys[86] and teacher-training students[87] in England and Germany. Farber[51] studied English and American middle class values with two incomplete sentences. Five brief story endings provided Hanfman and Getzels[69] with comparative material on interpersonal attitudes expressed by Americans and former Soviet citizens. Henry[7] reviewed TAT adaptations in studies of group and cultural problems. A relatively ambiguous picture of a group of people was developed by Horwitz and Cartwright[78] for studying group properties.

ADVANTAGES AND LIMITATIONS

The most obvious feature distinguishing the techniques discussed in this chapter from the more familiar projective methods is, of course, their brevity. In view of the enormity of the contemporary demand for professional psychological services,[4] brevity is a distinct advantage in evaluation. But, brevity also imposes certain restrictions. Since the instructions and stimulus materials usually provide some focus or structure, the responses elicited by brief projective techniques are often limited in length and range. Although there are opportunities for healthy or pathological originality, there is less scope for richness, variety, and subtlety. Projection is more "controlled."[142]

As with most projective techniques, it is at times difficult to decide whether a given response reflects overt conscious trends or unconscious latent tendencies. While much projective material has symbolic value, not every response necessarily reflects deep dynamics. Glib interpretive analogies and direct transposition of psychoanalytic concepts constitute a constant threat for the novice.

The limited and defined quality of the response material elicited by brief projective techniques generally permits direct, uncomplicated, and rapid scoring, a decided economic advantage. Most of the methods described use a simple content analysis involving only a few classification categories with explicit, operational rules, thus minimizing inferences or interpretations in making scoring judgments.

The frequent criticism of poor agreement among independent scorers, often voiced against traditional projective techniques, is only rarely applicable to brief methods. Perhaps even more important is the observation that high levels of agreement can be achieved in a short training time with scorers of unsophisticated psychological background.

The relatively simple and structured nature of most brief projective techniques brings additional advantages. As Sanford and Rosenstock[142] observe: "It is possible to create stimuli that elicit projective responses all of which, or almost all of which, are psychologically relevant to a prechosen variable. This means that for the testing of a specific hypothesis about personality the researcher may be able to tailor a projective device to his own specific research needs rather than having to fall back on the more omnibus devices now so widely used." Determining the validity of such tailor-made devices becomes a simpler matter —although never really a simple one. Since the techniques are developed for specific purposes, rather than as global personality measures, relevant criteria are more readily available. In many cases, the relationship between the test and criteria of interest can be established with little difficulty. The defined purpose of these techniques and the relative simplicity of scoring thus combine to make the empirical study of validity a more feasible enterprise.

The ease with which brief projective measures can be administered and scored makes it possible to collect data on large numbers of subjects. Test norms describing the response characteristics of relevant criterion groups can be developed, in that way obviating one of the more frequently cited criticisms of projective methods. Subjects can more easily be tested on several occasions over a period of time in order to study trends in the development of particular characteristics. Reliability and validity coefficients can be estimated more precisely.

It is important to note that although these advantages are real enough, they have rarely been realized by the developers of brief projective techniques. There are, for example, few studies in which truly large numbers of subjects were studied. Norms for brief projective measures are conspicuous more often by their absence than their presence. In some cases the advantages of a simple scoring system were disregarded in favor of complex scoring procedures which, as often as not, yielded relatively low scorer agreement. Data on reliability and validity, although not too difficult to obtain, were sometimes not collected or inadequately presented. All this would seem to reflect less upon the potential advantages of brief projective measures, however, than upon the failure of psychologists to capitalize on these advantages and make them manifest.

BRIEF PROJECTIVE METHODS AND TEST THEORY

At the risk of oversimplification, personality tests may be divided into two classes: measures of personality constructs and predictors of specific criteria. Although these two classes are not mutually exclusive, they are different enough to have been incorporated as types of validity in the test standards of the American Psychological Association,[5] and to be the subject of much contemporary debate on the proper function of tests.[104, 105,112,163]

Historically, projective methods have been employed primarily as measures of personality; only rarely as direct predictors of concrete future behavior. The issues raised by Meehl[112] suggest that the assets of time-consuming and costly traditional projective methods are being reconsidered in terms of their ultimate contributions to the decision-making process in which administrators, and clinicians, are constantly engaged.[36] In schools, industry and clinics, psychologists are asked to help decide whether specific pupils shall be admitted to various educational programs, whether particular applicants shall or shall not be employed in some capacity, or which patients shall receive what therapy.

Considering tests as aids in a decision-making process is both reasonable and appealing. Yet, this view was not formally developed until the recent publication of a monograph by Cronbach and Gleser[37] that foreshadows a veritable revolution in test theory.

The worth of a test can be determined by the extent to which it contributes to the improvement of decisions; that is, a useful test is one which results in better decisions than can be made without it. In making decisions about a subject, certain basic data are almost always available (e.g. age, sex, education, work history, marital status). Additional relevant information may be obtained by using simple, brief projective or nonprojective devices, whose value, however, is dependent on the extent to which they improve prediction. The frequent practice of evaluating a test by implicitly assuming that decisions made without it are no better than chance, is both deceptive and misleading, since initial information is already available.

No test has a single over-all validity coefficient. Instead, every test has a different validity for each decision problem to which it is applied. Any change in the decision problem can change the validity of the test. In the main, a test may be useful if it has (a) great *bandwidth*, i.e. the range and number of decisions to which it contributes relevant information is large; or (b) great *fidelity*, i.e. the information it provides is very accurate. Classical test theory has emphasized fidelity at the expense of bandwidth. Thus, tests containing little error variance (chiefly objective intelligence and achievement tests) have been considered better measuring devices than tests with a great deal of error variance (chiefly projective methods). Decision theory suggests that, in evaluating a test, bandwidth must be considered along with fidelity. Projective techniques are wide-band instruments; they elicit information relevant to many decisions, but the information is, in general, less accurate than that obtained from tests with a very restricted bandwidth.

Decisions are often most effectively reached by a sequential procedure. The first test administered should divide the group of subjects grossly. For some subjects, particularly those with very high and very low scores, further testing may be unnecessary. For others the decision reached would be to continue testing. A terminal decision on the more "doubtful" subjects could be deferred until much more additional information was collected. For the less doubtful subjects a terminal decision could be reached after fewer tests were administered.

Tests with different characteristics are needed at different stages in a sequential testing program. In the first stage a wide-band instrument, even one with low fidelity, seems most appropriate. At subsequent stages bandwidth should be reduced, while fidelity is increased.

Conventional projective methods and clinical interviews meet the requirements of the first stage of testing. Their merit lies in their flexibility, i.e. their ability to elicit a broad range of potentially relevant information about the subject. This very breadth means, however, that some of what is elicited will be false or misleading. To distinguish what is accurate from what is not, further testing is necessary.

One reason why projective methods and clinical interviews have not fared too well in research efforts at validation is that they have been misused to reach terminal decisions (for which they are not accurate enough). When employed sequentially, to suggest leads which further testing is to clarify, the projective methods and interviews do serve a vital function. The confidence which clinicians continue to express in them is probably the result of the sequential way in which they actually use these devices.

Some of the brief projective methods here surveyed, particularly those that are relatively unstructured, seem to have the bandwidth so desirable in an initial phase of testing. In a sequential testing program, they may prove fruitful sources of hypotheses. Additional research should determine how effectively they elicit leads worthy of further, more focused, testing. Ideally, the initial wide-band techniques will suggest many more true than false hypotheses, but even techniques with low validity, as conventionally determined, may be worth using. The significance of the decision problem must be considered along with the cost of testing, and one of the obvious merits of any brief procedure is that its cost is low.

The more structured brief projective techniques, by focusing on a limited range of personality processes, seem to be well suited to the task of separating true leads from false. As Cronbach and Gleser[37] observe: "There is a continuum from great to narrow bandwidth. The tester can spread himself too far, just as he can confine himself too narrowly. By structuring the interview or the projective technique one can reduce the bandwidth with a corresponding gain in fidelity. The fact that the bandwidth of current projective methods is almost unlimited suggests that it would be profitable to restrict them to some degree. In the TAT, for example, better information about relations with parents would presumably be obtained by increasing the proportion of plates involving parent figures. In many diagnostic problems the attendant sacrifice of information about other aspects of the person would surely be justified." Here, in their more focused forms, we find probably the strongest rationale for brief projective tests. In following up the hypotheses suggested by other, less structured procedures, the decision maker needs additional, highly relevant information. The information must often be obtained at fairly low cost, and must be related to the specific decision problem in question. At their best, brief projective methods hold great promise of providing information which meets these requirements.

In the final analysis, the question for any given decision problem is: "What is the best information-gathering procedure?" With the demand for psychological services far exceeding available supply, we can rarely afford the costly luxury of clinically analyzing the whole personality, but may have to reach the best possible decision through an intelligent distillation of limited but focused data. As Cronbach and Gleser[37] conclude so appropriately: "The problem is to find the procedure which, in the time available, offers the greatest yield of important, relevant, and interpretable information."

SUMMARY

The constantly increasing demand for professional psychological services in widespread areas of our society is fostering a reappraisal of traditional procedures of personality assessment.

It has been the purpose of this chapter to survey some of the more recent clinical and nonclinical explorations with brief projective methods, their advantages and limitations, and to consider a theoretical rationale relating test data to the decision-making process.

References

1. Abt, L. E. and Bellak, L. (Eds.) *Projective psychology.* New York: Knopf, 1950.

2. Adorno, T. W., Frenkel-Brunswik, Else, Levinson, D. T., and Sanford, R. N. *The authoritarian personality.* New York: Harper, 1950.

3. Ainsworth, Mary D. Some problems of validation of projective techniques. *Brit. J. med. Psychol.,* 1951, 24, 151-161.

4. Albee, G. W. and Dickey, Marguerite. Manpower trends in three mental health professions. *Amer. Psychologist,* 1957, 12, 57-70.

5. American Psychological Association. Committee on Test Standards. Technical recommendations for psychological tests and diagnostic techniques. *Psychol. Bull. Suppl.,* 1954, 57, (2), 1-38.

6. Ammons, Carol H. and Ammons, R. B. Research and clinical applications of the doll play interview. *J. Personal.,* 1952, 21, 85-90.

7. Anderson, H. A. and Anderson, Gladys L. (Eds.) *An introduction to projective techniques.* New York: Prentice-Hall, 1951.

8. Aschaffenburg, G. Experimentelle Studien über Assoziation. *Psychologische Arbeiten.* 1896.

9. Auerbach, J. G. Psychological observations on "doodling" in neurotics. *J. nerv. ment. Dis.,* 1950, 111, 304-332.

10. Bates, Marjory. An experiment with simple tests for the insane. *Amer. J. Psychiat.,* 1922, 2, 61-65.

11. Baumgarten, Franziska A. A proverb test for attitude measurement. *Personnel Psychol.,* 1952, 5, 249-261.

12. Beier, Helen and Hanfmann, Eugenia. Emotional attitudes of former Soviet citizens, as studied by the technique of projective questions. *J. abnorm. soc. Psychol.,* 1956, 53, 143-153.

13. Bell, J. E. (Ed.) *Projective techniques.* New York: Longmans, Green, 1948.

14. Bellak, L. *The TAT and CAT in clinical use.* New York: Grune & Stratton, 1954.

15. Bellak, L. A study of limitations and "failures": toward an ego psychology of projective techniques. *J. proj. Techn.*, 1954, 18, 279-293.

16. Bender, L. and Rapoport, J. Animal drawings of children. *Amer. J. Orthopsychiat.*, 1944, 14, 521-527.

17. Benjamin, J. D. A method for distinguishing and evaluating formal thinking disorders in schizophrenia. In Kasanin, J. S. (Ed.), *Language and thought in schizophrenia.* Berkeley: Univ. of California Press, 1944.

18. Boernstein, W. S. The verbal self-portrait test. *Psychiat. Quart. Suppl.*, 1954, 28, 15-25, 209-227.

19. Breiger, B. The use of the W-B Picture Arrangement subtest as a projective technique. *J. consult. Psychol.*, 1956, 20, 132.

20. Briggs, D. L. A modification of the TAT for naval enlisted personnel. *J. Psychol.*, 1954, 37, 233-241.

21. Brodsky, P. The diagnostic importance of early recollections. *Amer. J. Psychother.*, 1952, 6, 484-493.

22. Brower, D. and Weider, A. Projective techniques in business and industry. In Abt, L. E. and Bellak, L. (Eds.), *Projective psychology.* New York: Knopf, 1950, 437-461.

23. Brower, D. The applicability of projective techniques to personnel appraisal. *Personnel Psychol.*, 1955, 8, 235-243.

24. Brown, J. F. A modification of the Rosenzweig P-F test to study hostile interracial attitudes. *J. Psychol.*, 1947, 24, 247-272.

25. Bugental, J. F. T. and Zelen, S. L. Investigations into the self-concept: I. The W-A-Y technique. *J. Personal.*, 1950, 18, 483-498.

26. Bugental, J. F. T. and Gunning, Evelyn C. Investigations into the self-concept: stability of reported self-identifications. *J. clin. Psychol.*, 1955, 11, 41-46.

27. Burwen, L. S., Campbell, D. T., and Kidd, J. The use of a sentence completions test in measuring attitudes toward superiors and subordinates. *J. appl. Psychol.*, 1956, 40, 248-250.

28. Campbell, D. T. and Burwen, L. S. Trait judgments from photographs as a projective device. *J. clin. Psychol.*, 1956, 12, 215-221.

29. Chahbazi, P. Use of projective tests in predicting college achievement. *Educ. psychol. Measmt.*, 1956, 16, 538-542.

30. Cobb, Katherine. Measuring leadership in college women by free association. *J. abnorm. soc. Psychol.*, 1952, 47, 126-128.

31. Cobliner, W. G. On the place of projective tests in opinion and attitude surveys. *Int. J. Opin. Att. Res.*, 1951-52, 5, 480-490.

32. Cordoba, J. R. and Pigem, J. M. La expresion desiderativa como manifestacion de la personalidad. *Med. Clinica*, (Barcelona), 1946, 4, No. 3.

33. Cordoba, J. R., Pigem, J. M., and Gurria, F. J. *Estudio experimental de la vitalidad y de la angustia.* Barcelona: Acad. Ciencias Medicas, 1951.

34. Crandell, V. J. Observations on the use of projective techniques in child development research. *J. proj. Techn.*, 1956, 20, 251-255.

35. Cronbach, L. J. Response sets and test validity. *Educ. psychol. Measmt.*, 1946, 6, 475-494.

36. Cronbach, L. J. New light on test strategy from decision theory. Princeton: Educational Testing Service 1954 Conference on Test Problems, 31-36.

37. Cronbach, L. J. and Gleser, Goldine C. *Psychological tests and personnel decisions.* Urbana: Univ. of Illinois Press, 1957.

38. Cummings, Jean D. Family pictures: a projective test for children. *Brit. J. Psychol.*, 1952, 43, 53-60.

39. Curtis, J. W. *The Curtis Completion Form.* Chicago: Science Research Associates, 1953.

40. David, H. P. Brief, unstructured items: the Projective Question. *J. proj. Techn.*, 1955, 19, 292-300.

41. David, H. P. and Leach, W. The Projective Question: further exploratory studies. *J. proj. Techn.*, 1957, 21, 3-9.

42. Derner, G. F. *Aspects of the psychology of the tuberculous.* New York: Hoeber, 1953.

43. Diamond, S. Three impossibilities: a verbal projective technique. *J. Psychol.*, 1947, 24, 283-292.

44. Dörken, H., Jr. The inkblot test as a brief projective technique: a preliminary report. *Amer. J. Orthopsychiat.*, 1950, 20, 828-833.

45. Dörken, H., Jr. The inkblot test; clinical application of a brief projective test. *Rorschachiana*, 1952, 1, 196-221.

46. Ebbinghaus, H. Über eine neue Methode und Prüfung geistiger Fähigkeit und ihre Anwendung bei Schulkindern. *Z. Psychol. Physiol. Sinnesorg.*, 1897, 13, 410-457.

47. Eisenstein, V. W. and Ryerson, Rowena. Psychodynamic significance of the first conscious memory. *Bull. Menninger Clin.*, 1951, 15, 213-220.

48. Elkisch, Paula. The "scribbling game"—a projective method. *Nerv. Child*, 1948, 7, 247-256.

49. Elkisch, Paula. Children's drawings in a projective technique. *Psychol. Monogr.*, 1945, 58, No. 266.

50. Ellenberger, H. The life and work of Hermann Rorschach. *Bull. Menninger Clin.*, 1954, 18, 173-219.

51. Farber, M. L. English and Americans: a study in national character. *J. Psychol.*, 1951, 32, 241-249; 1953, 36, 243-250.

52. Feifel, H. Note on hypothetical situations in personality appraisal. *J. clin. Psychol.*, 1955, 11, 415-416.

53. Fielding, B. B. A "story completion" for use with the physically handicapped. *J. proj. Techn.*, 1951, 15, 299-306.

54. Fine, R. Use of the Despert Fables in diagnostic work with children. *J. proj. Techn.*, 1948, 12, 106-108.

55. Fitzelle, G. T. Basic needs of a selected group of widows as revealed through projective questions. *J. Amer. Geriatrics Soc.*, 1955, 3, 902-909.

56. Forer, B. R. A structured sentence completion test. *J. proj. Techn.*, 1950, 14, 15-30.

57. Forer, B. R. Research with projective techniques: some trends. *J. proj. Techn.*, 1957, 21, 358-361.

58. Frank, L. K. Projective methods for the study of personality. *J. Psychol.*, 1939, 8, 389-413.

59. Friedman, A. Early childhood memories of mental patients. *J. Child Psychiat.*, 1952, 2, 266-269.

60. Fromme, A. On the use of certain qualitative methods of attitude research. *J. soc. Psychol.*, 1941, 13, 425-459.

61. Galton, F. *Inquiries into human faculty and its development.* New York: Macmillan, 1883.

62. Garfield, S. L. *Introductory clinical psychology.* New York: Macmillan, 1957.

63. Goodenough, Florence. The use of free association in the objective measurement of personality. In *Studies in personality contributed in honor of L. M. Terman.* New York: McGraw-Hill, 1942.

64. Gorham, D. R. Use of the proverbs test for differentiating schizophrenics from normals. *J. consult. Psychol.*, 1956, 20, 435-440.

65. Graham, M. D. The effectiveness of photographs as a projective device in an international attitudes survey. *J. soc. Psychol.*, 1954, 40, 93-120.

66. Hadley, J. M. and Kennedy, Vera E. A comparison between performance on a sentence completion test and academic success. *Educ. psychol. Measmt.*, 1949, 9, 649-670.

67. Hadley, J. M. *Clinical and counseling psychology.* New York: Knopf, 1958.

68. Hanfmann, Eugenia and Getzels, J. W. Studies of the sentence completion test. *J. proj. Techn.*, 1953, 17, 280-294.

69. Hanfmann, Eugenia and Getzels, J. W. Interpersonal attitudes of former Soviet citizens as studied by a semi-projective method. *Psychol. Monogr.*, 1955, 69, No. 4.

70. Hare, A. P. and Hare, Rachel T. The draw-a-group test. *J. genet. Psychol.*, 1956, 89, 51-60.

71. Harrower, M. R. Group techniques for the Rorschach test. In Abt, L. E. and Bellak, L. (Eds.), *Projective psychology.* New York: Knopf, 1950, 146-184.

72. Harrower, Molly R. The Most Unpleasant Concept test: a graphic projective technique. *J. clin. Psychol.*, 1950, 6, 213-233.

73. Harrower, Molly R. Clinical aspects of failures in the projective techniques. *J. proj. Techn.*, 1954, 18, 294-302.

74. Harrower, Molly R. Screening—for what? *Brit. J. med. Psychol.*, 1957, 30, 19-26.

75. Heppell, H. K. and Rainy, V. C. Projective pictures as interview devices. *J. consult. Psychol.*, 1951, 15, 405-411.

76. Hessel, Martha G. and Travers, R. M. W. Use of drawings as a screening device in education. *J. educ. Res.*, 1954, 48, 145-147.

77. Holsopple, J. Q. and Miale, Florence R. *Sentence completion.* Springfield, Ill.: Thomas, 1954.

78. Horwitz, M. and Cartwright, D. A projective method for the diagnosis of group properties. *Hum. Relations*, 1953, 6, 397-410.

79. Hulse, W. C. Childhood conflict expressed through family drawings. *J. proj. Techn.*, 1952, 16, 66-79.

80. Isham, A. C. Use of brief psychological battery in psychiatric practice. *Amer. J. Psychother.*, 1957, 11, 790-802.

81. Jackson, Lydia. Emotional attitudes toward the family of normal, neurotic, and delinquent children. *Brit. J. Psychol.*, 1950, 41, 35-51.

82. James, W. *The varieties of religious experience.* London: Longmans, Green, 1902.

83. Johnson, G. B., Jr. An experimental projective technique for the analysis of racial attitudes. *J. educ. Psychol.*, 1950, 41, 257-278, 428-439; 1951, 42, 357-365.

84. Jung, C. G. *Studies in word association.* London: Heinemann, 1918.

85. Kahana, R. J., Weiland, I. H., Snyder, B., and Rosenbaum, M. The value of early memories in psychotherapy. *Psychiat. Quart.*, 1953, 27, 73-82.

86. Kaldegg, A. Responses of German and English secondary school boys to a projection test. *Brit. J. Psychol.*, 1948, 39, 30-53.

87. Kaldegg, A. A study of German and English teacher training students by means of projective techniques. *Brit. J. Psychol.*, 1951, 42, 56-113.

88. Kamenetzky, J., Burgess, G. G., and Rowan, T. The relative effectiveness of four attitude assessment techniques in predicting a criterion. *Educ. psychol. Measmt.*, 1956, 16, 187-194.

89. Kass, W. Projective techniques as research tools in studies of normal personality development. *J. proj. Techn.*, 1956, 20, 269-272.

90. Kent, G. H. and Rosanoff, A. J. A study of association in insanity. *Amer. J. Insanity*, 1910, 67, 37-96, 317-390.

91. Kinget, G. Marian. *The drawing-completion test.* (Wartegg) New York: Grune & Stratton, 1952.

92. Komisar, D. D. A marriage problem story completion test. *J. consult. Psychol.*, 1949, 13, 403-406.

93. Korner, Anneliese F. Theoretical considerations concerning the scope and limitations of projective techniques. *J. abnorm. soc. Psychol.*, 1950, 45, 619-627.

94. Korner, Anneliese F. Limitations of projective techniques: apparent and real. *J. proj. Techn.*, 1956, 20, 42-47.

95. Kutash, S. B. and Gehl, R. H. *The graphomotor projection technique: clinical use and standardization.* Springfield: Thomas, 1954.

96. Kutash, S. B. The impact of projective techniques on basic psychological science. *J. proj. Techn.*, 1954, 18, 453-469.

97. Lachman, S. J. *The self-explorations inventory.* Detroit: Wayne Univ., Author.

98. Laricchia, R. and Beretta, P. The bunch-of-grapes test of Sanguineti and Sigurta applied to 100 schizophrenics. *Neurone*, 1954, 2, 307-316.

99. Lehmann, H. and Dörken, H., Jr. The administration, scoring, and percentile standardization of the Verdun Projective Battery. *Canad. J. Psychol.*, 1953, 7, 69-80.

100. Lehner, G. F. J. and Saper, B. Use of hypothetical situation in personality assessment. *J. Personal.*, 1952, 21, 91-102.

101. Levinson, J. Projective questions in the study of personality and ideology. In Adorno et al., *The authoritarian personality.* New York: Harper, 1950.

102. Libo, L. M. The projective expression of patient-therapist attraction. *J. clin. Psychol.*, 1957, 13, 33-36.

103. Lieberman, Martha G. Childhood memories as a projective technique. *J. proj. Techn.*, 1957, 21, 32-36.

104. Loevinger, Jane. Objective tests as instruments of psychological theory. *Psychol. Rep.*, 1957, 3, 635-694.

105. Lord, F. M. Some perspectives on "the attenuation paradox in test theory." *Psychol. Bull.*, 1955, 52, 505-510.

106. Luborsky, L. R. Self-interpretation of the TAT as a clinical technique. *J. proj. Techn.*, 1953, 17, 217-233.

107. Lucas, D. B. Projective techniques in advertising research. *Trans. N. Y. Acad. Sci.*, 1954, 16, 254-260.

108. Luft, J., Wisham, W., and Moody, H. A projective technique to measure adjustment to hospital environment. *J. gen. Psychol.* 1953, 49, 209-219.

109. Machover, Karen. *Personality projection in the drawing of the human figure.* Springfield, Ill.: Thomas, 1949.

110. MacFarlane, Jean W. and Tuddenham, R. D. Problems in the validation of projective techniques. In Anderson and Anderson (Eds.), *Introduction to projective techniques.* New York: Prentice-Hall, 1951, 26-54.

111. McClelland, D., Atkinson, J., Clark, R., and Lowell, E. *The achievement motive.* New York: Appleton-Century-Crofts, 1953.

112. Meehl, P. E. *Clinical vs. statistical prediction.* Minneapolis: Univ. of Minnesota Press, 1954.

113. Meltzer, H. Memory dynamics, projective tests, and projective interviewing. *J. Personal.*, 1950, 19, 48-63.

114. Mensh, I. N. Brief psychological measures. *Nerv. Child,* 1949, 8, 349-359.

115. Michaux, W. W. The sentence completion test. *J. clin. Psychol.*, 1957, 13, 174-175.

116. Mills, E. S. A story completion test for college students. *J. clin. Psychol.*, 1954, 10, 18-22.

117. Mintz, Elizabeth E. Personal problems and diagnostic errors of clinical psychologists. *J. proj. Techn.*, 1957, 21, 123-128.

118. Mitzel, H. E., Ostreicher, L. M., and Reiter, S. R. Development of attitudinal dimensions from teachers' drawings. New York: Office of Research and Evaluation, Division of Teacher Education, College of City of New York, 1954, No. 24.

119. Monroe, Ruth L. Diagnosis of learning disabilities through a projective technique. *J. consult. Psychol.*, 1949, 13, 390-395.

120. Morgan, H. H. A psychometric comparison of achieving and nonachieving college students of high ability. *J. consult. Psychol.*, 1952, 16, 292-298.

121. Morgan, H. H. Measuring achievement motivation with "picture interpretations." *J. consult. Psychol.*, 1953, 17, 289-292.

122. Moss, Hilde L. The Deuss test. *Amer. J. Psychother.*, 1954, 8, 251-264.

123. Murray, H. *Explorations in personality.* New York: Oxford Univ. Press, 1948.

124. Mussen, P. H. and Wyszynki, A. B. Personality and political participation. *Hum. Relations*, 1952, 5, 65-82.

125. Odum, C. L. A study of the time required to do a Rorschach examination. *J. proj. Techn.*, 1950, 14, 464-468.

126. Pattie, F. A. and Cornett, S. Unpleasantness of early memories and maladjustment of children. *J. Personal.*, 1952, 20, 315-321.

127. Pigem, J. M. *La prueba de la expresion desiderativa.* Liberia de Ciencias Medicas, Barcelona, 1949.

128. Pigem, J. M. *Clinical utility of the desiderative expression test.* Paris: *Proceedings,* Congress of Psychiatry, 1950.

129. Perl, W. R. On the psychodiagnostic value of handwriting analysis. *Amer. J. Psychiat.*, 1955, 111, 595-602.

130. Piotrowski, Z. A. *Perceptanalysis.* New York: Macmillan, 1957.

131. Ponzo, E. An experimental variation of the DAP technique. *J. proj. Techn.*, 1957, 21, 278-285.

132. Proshansky, H. M. Projective techniques in action research: disguised diagnosis and measurement. In Abt, L. E., and Bellak, L. (Eds.), *Projective psychology.* New York: Knopf, 1950, 462-487.

133. Rabinowitz, W. and Travers, R. M. W. A drawing technique for studying certain outcomes of teacher education. *J. educ. Psychol.*, 1955, 46, 257-273.

134. Reichenberg-Hackett, Wally. The geosign test: a semi-structured drawing situation utilized as a screening test for adjustment. *Amer. J. Orthopsychiat.*, 1950, 20, 578-594.

135. Riklin, F. Jung's association test and dream interpretation. *J. proj. Techn.*, 1955, 19, 226-235.

136. Rose, A. W. Projective techniques in sociological research. *Soc. Forces*, 1949, 28, 175-183.

137. Rosenzweig, S. with Kogan, Kate. *Psychodiagnosis.* New York: Grune & Stratton, 1949.

138. Rotter, J. B. Word association and sentence completion methods. In Anderson and Anderson (Eds.), *An introduction to projective techniques.* New York: Prentice-Hall, 1951, 279-311.

139. Sacks, J. M. and Levy, S. The sentence completion test. In Abt, L. E. and Bellak, L. (Eds.), *Projective psychology.* New York: Knopf, 1950, 357-402.

140. Sacks, J. *Make a Sentence Test.* Author: Mimeo, 1958.

141. Sanford, F. H. The use of a projective device in attitude surveying. *Publ. Opin. Quart.*, 1950-51, 14, 697-709.

142. Sanford, F. and Rosenstock, I. M. Projective techniques on the doorstep. *J. abnorm. soc. Psychol.*, 1952, 47, 3-16.

143. Sargent, Helen. Projective techniques: origins, theory, and application in personality research. *Psychol. Bull.*, 1945, 42, 257-293.

144. Saul, L. J., Snyder, T. R., and Sheppard, Edith. On earliest memories. *Psychoanal. Quart.*, 1956, 25, 228-237.

145. Schafer, R. Word association test. In Weider, A. (Ed.), *Contributions toward medical psychology*. New York: Ronald Press, 1953, 577-589.

146. Schwartz, A. A. and Rosenberg, I. H. Observations on the significance of animal drawings. *Amer. J. Orthopsychiat.*, 1955, 25, 729-746.

147. Shapiro, Edna, Biber, Barbara, and Minuchin, Patricia. The cartoon situations test: a semi-structured technique for assessing aspects of personality pertinent to the teaching process. *J. proj. Techn.*, 1957, 21, 172-184.

148. Shneidman, E. S., Joel, W., and Little, K. B. *Thematic test analysis*. New York: Grune & Stratton, 1951.

149. Smith, J. A., Brown, W. T., and Thrower, F. L. The use of a modified TAT in a neuropsychiatric clinic in a general hospital. *Amer. J. Psychiat.*, 1951, 107, 498-500.

150. Smith, M. B., Bruner, J. S., and White, R. W. *Opinion and personality*. New York: Wiley, 1956.

151. Stein, H. *Sentence Construction Test*. Author: Mimeo, 1958.

152. Stern, E. Childhood in the adult's memory. *Arch. Psicol. Neurol. Psichiat.*, 1952, 13, 372-393.

153. Stern, G. G., Stein, M. I., and Bloom, B. S. *Methods in personality assessment*. Glencoe, Ill.: Free Press, 1956.

154. Stone, C. H. and Kendall, W. E. *Effective personnel selection procedures*. New York: Prentice-Hall, 1956.

155. Stotsky, B. A., Sacks, J. M., and Daston, P. G. Predicting the work performance of psychiatric aides by psychological tests. *J. counsel. Psychol.*, 1956, 3, 193-199.

156. Stotsky, B. A. Comparisons of normals and schizophrenics on a work-oriented projective technique. *J. clin. Psychol.*, 1957, 13, 406-408.

157. Swenson, C. H. Empirical evaluations of human figure drawings. *Psychol. Bull.*, 1957, 54, 431-466.

158. Szondi, L. *Experimental diagnostics of drives.* New York: Grune & Stratton, 1952.

159. Szondi, L. *Ichanalyse.* Bern: Hans Huber Verlag, 1956.

160. Tait, C. D., Jr. and Ascher, R. C. Inside-of-the-body test. *Psychosom. Med.,* 1955, 17, 139-148.

161. Thun, T. Versuche mit einem explorativen Phantasiegespräch nach dem Schema Zaubertraum. *Z. diagn. Psychol.,* 1954, 2, 309-321.

162. Tolor, A. Self-perception of psychoneurotic patients on the W-A-Y test. *J. clin. Psychol.,* 1957, 13, 403-406.

163. Travers, R. M. W. Rational hypotheses in the construction of tests. *Educ. psychol. Measmt.,* 1951, 11, 128-137.

164. Ullman, L. P. Selection of neuropsychiatric patients for group therapy. *J. consult. Psychol.,* 1957, 21, 277-280.

165. Ungericht, J. Der "Sohn-Aufsatz" als psychodiagnostisches Hilfsmittel. *Schweiz. Z. Psychol.,* 1955, 14, 27-45.

166. Van Krevelen, D. Arn. Die Anwendung des Pigem-Test in der Kinderpsychiatrischen Diagnostik. *Z. Kinderpsychiat.,* 1953, 20, 2-12.

167. Van Krevelen, D. Arn. The use of Pigem's test with children. *J. proj. Techn.,* 1956, 20, 235-242.

168. Van Lennep, D. J. The four picture test. In Anderson and Anderson (Eds.), *Introduction to projective techniques.* New York: Prentice-Hall, 1951, 149-180.

169. Walter, V. A. and Jones, A. W. An incomplete sentences test and the attitudes of manual arts therapy patients. *J. counsel. Psychol.,* 1956, 3, 140-144.

170. Watson, R. I. A brief history of clinical psychology. *Psychol. Bull.,* 1953, 50, 321-346.

171. Weiland, I. H. and Steisel, I. M. An analysis of manifest content of the earliest memories of children. *J. genet. Psychol.,* 1958, 92, 41-52.

172. Wells, F. L. *Mental tests in clinical practice.* Yonkers: World Book Co., 1927.

173. Wertheimer, Rita and McKinney, F. A case history blank as a projective technique. *J. consult. Psychol.,* 1952, 16, 49-60.

174. Wilde, K. *Die Wünschprobe.* Göttingen: Hogrefe, 1956.

175. Wilson, Isabelle. The use of a sentence completion test to differentiate between well-adjusted and maladjusted secondary school pupils. *J. consult. Psychol.,* 1949, 13, 400-402.

176. Wolfson, Rose. Graphology. In Anderson and Anderson (Eds.), *Introduction to projective techniques.* New York: Prentice-Hall, 1951, 416-456.

177. Zelen, S. L., Sheehan, J. G., and Bugental, J. F. T. Self-perceptions in stuttering. *J. clin. Psychol.*, 1954, 10, 70-72.

178. Zubin, J. Failures of the Rorschach technique. *J. proj. Techn.*, 1954, 18, 303-315.

179. Zulliger, H. *Der Diapositiv Z Test.* Bern: Hans Huber Verlag, 1948.

180. Zwerling, I. The favorite joke in diagnostic and therapeutic interviewing. *Psychoanal. Quart.*, 1955, 24, 104-114.

XVII

Research in
Personality Assessment:
A Commentary

INTRODUCTION

IT MAY APPEAR ALMOST pointless to write anything at all appropriate about present trends and tasks regarding methods of personality assessment. Not only is it almost impossible for any one individual to survey adequately all the work, especially if not limited to one country, but also the problems selected and the methods used are extraordinarily varied. Little would be gained from attempting to judge current trends from a complete survey and statistical analysis of pertinent problems discussed in the literature of the past several years. The most frequent characteristics may not necessarily be the most important or the most interesting. To make a diagnosis, I have to rely on the clinical method, with all its inherent uncertainties and potentials for subjective distortion.

This commentary will consider historical trends in the development of personality measures, the difficult problems of validation and prediction, the important role of intervening variables, and some research contributions of briefer methods and other experimental approaches. Effective progress in personality assessment, however, may ultimately depend on greater clarification of commonly used concepts and descriptions of personality characteristics.

HISTORICAL TRENDS

First we must ask whether the chapters in this section provide a sufficient basis to make a diagnosis. They represent only a small sample but an especially selected one. Although the selection is not statistically representative, it is nevertheless somehow characteristic of the present status of research in personality assessment. I believe that this opinion can be supported by considering the development of personality research. The moment seems to be ripe for studies such as these; they are not accidental products of external influences. When viewing any lawful development, whether that of a science or an individual, it is usually possible to determine whether a particular phenomenon is appropriate and typical for a certain stage, or whether it falls outside this realm and has been determined by external circumstances. This procedure, which I propose to follow, is also very useful in pychological diagnosis. I believe that the historical perspective to which it leads will facilitate a better understanding of the present situation in personality diagnosis and a recognition of those problems which must be considered.

In our historical approach, we will delimit the first period as beginning with the twenties and ending in the late thirties. It was characterized by the creation of the great "classical" methods: Rorschach, Wartegg, TAT, Szondi, and such major personality questionnaires as the MMPI. It was no longer essential to delineate single functions as accurately as possible; instead, enough courage was mustered to try to encompass the whole personality. This had been done previously only by graphologists. A survey of the literature of the period shows that presentations, discussions, and defenses of these new methods predominated.

A second period began roughly with the forties, lasting into the fifties. I like to designate it as the period of validation studies. With the growing dissemination of so-called projective tests, psychologists of a more psychometric tradition—at times with sharply critical intentions—submitted the new methods to vigorous control studies. Also, the proponents of projective techniques perceived the need to prove their scope or to defend them against attacks.

It is not easy to judge the results. One would have to determine not only the number of positive and negative studies, but also their importance. It seems to me that the outcome of this fight is still undecided. Only a few would wish to assert that projective tests have been proven definitely worthless, and only a few of those who have studied the results of the validation studies will deny that they show that great caution is required in the use of projective methods. These findings are probably responsible for the appearance, in the third period now beginning, of new questions and new methods of investigation.

VALIDATION AND PREDICTION

There has been no widely accepted reason for the unsatisfactory results of validation studies, and there probably is no single cause. One cannot ascribe negative results simply to faulty criteria or the essential inadequacy of statistical evaluation, as adherents of projective tests, especially in Europe, are wont to do. In some of the validation studies, this may have been so; yet, the main difficulty is usually of a more basic nature.

What is a validation study? A comparison of behavior or combination of behaviors (test result) with another behavior or combination of behaviors (criterion), or perhaps a comparison of the conclusions drawn from the former with the conclusions from the latter, etc. On one side are behavior and conclusions drawn, and on the other, the same thing. Then, comparisons are made of behavior with behavior, behavior with interpretation, interpretation (from tests) with behavior or also with interpretation from observed behavior (for example, when there is a criterion for clinical diagnosis). Since direct comparison of one form of behavior to another is usually impractical (although it, too, has been tried without success), interpretation always plays a role either through tests or the criterion. And here is the rub of validation studies. It has, of course, always been known that not the tests but the interpretations were being validated, but it has usually been conveniently forgotten. That is why low validities frequently inspired a search for better *means* of prediction and not for better interpretation. I would therefore like to generalize that in this process, leading from test behavior to predicted behavior, there arise difficulties which cause unsatisfactory validation studies, and which have to be examined more carefully.

Where does this deficiency lie? Meehl,[8] in his basic work on clinical versus statistical prediction, cited studies showing that statistically-based predictions generally produced better results than clinical ones. He explains that the statistically oriented psychologist has objectively determined the specific numerical weights of his relevant experiences and knows how to combine them, whereas the clinician does his combining on a purely intuitive basis. Meehl's remarks do not refer specifically to projective techniques, rather to the art of using the results. But, since projective techniques are usually applied clinically, his reflections are relevant.

In his interesting reply to Meehl, Holt[4] attempts to show that the demonstrated superiority of actuarial techniques does not perhaps rest on the different ways of combining test data. He first attempts to present an exact analysis of the entire prediction process, that is, the transition from behavior to behavior as formulated above. It consists of five steps, only the last of which concerns the combining of data envisioned by Meehl. It is preceded by 1) an exact analysis of the behavior to be predicted, 2) a decision on which *intervening variables* will be considered to make a prediction, 3) determining the kind of data which will facilitate the measurement or assessment of these intervening variables, and 4) collecting the data, e.g. conducting the tests.

It is of interest that the first three steps stipulate prior experimental investigation, surely in conjunction with statistical methods, and that Holt talks about intervening variables. It is his view that, after completion of the initial tasks, the fifth step —the combining of data—will also yield good results with clinical material. His own findings in selection studies of psychiatrists tend to support his assumptions. After careful execution of the first three steps, predictions were made on the basis of projective and intelligence tests administered before the start of residency training. Validation coefficients were fairly satisfactory (up to .58) and were considerably better than in an earlier effort with the same people and the same criterion but without preliminary study. This indicates that validation can be improved through exact psychological analysis of the behavior to be predicted and then basing the interpretation of test results on such findings.

Holt wanted to show that the clinical method *per se* is not inferior to the purely arithmetical one; it is handicapped only when the clinician makes blind predictions without first exploring "what" he is trying to predict and "how" he can elicit the needed information from the test results. The statistician might reply that the actuarial method demands just this sort of data and that the clinical method is dangerous because it seduces practitioners to neglect necessary preliminary tasks. If Holt had proceeded even more exactly, analyzing every step on the basis of exact statistical findings, he would have obtained even better results.

Whether all this is correct will not be considered here. I have cited this discussion only because it is among the first to offer a more pertinent answer to the question of where the difficulty lies in the transfer of behavior from one situation to another. It suggests that the problem resides in failing to analyze the several different steps involved. There is, of course, no argument about the need for statistical methods. But it would be a great illusion to hold that validation studies are unsatisfactory only due to incomplete statistical analyses of the results. What is missing is correct insight, not a method for attaining it. No method by and of itself leads to correct insight.

Other possibilities are indicated, in Holt's work, by the concept of *intervening variables*. Such intermediaries (they can also be called personality constructs, personality variables, characteristics, etc.) are necessary to go from one behavior or behavioral complex to another or *varied* others. We should know much more about them to achieve better results with tests. When one considers the complexity of projective techniques —which reflect the total personality—then it is important to know not one or another such intervening variable, but the whole inner structure of personality. Any single variable can probably only be defined in relation to the others.

BRIEF TECHNIQUES AND EXPERIMENTAL APPROACHES

The creators of important methods of personality study were psychologists who did not approach their task blindly but with definite theoretical assumptions which were well grounded at the time. No one supposed that the results of these tests would be directly translated into definite behavioral patterns. It was thought that one could discern certain basic trends, general tendencies, drives and such (that is, intervening variables), which might express themselves in manifold ways of behavior. But, as the job of validation began, it became necessary to compare certain aspects of test responses with certain more or less well defined modes of behavior. One slipped, without always being aware of it, from "constructs" to behavioral patterns, identifying one with the other. This is natural because as soon as a construct is to be verified, it is necessary to again fall back on behavior. A too narrowly behavioristic view, against which Allport and others have always cautioned, probably led to the overly simplified assumption that test results have a close direct relationship with other forms of behavior.

Even when attempts were made to first interpret results and then offer conclusions regarding behavior, findings were hardly better (for example, M responses on the Rorschach, extraversion/intraversion, aggression, etc.). This was evidently because the studies were undertaken with unsatisfactory hypotheses. All of us probably had illusions about our capacity to comprehend complex psychic processes, as represented by projective test responses or by behavior in practical life situations. Somehow, the whole preoccupation with personality tests was based on the notion that we really could perceive and characterize people very well, and that all that was necessary was to find methods with which this perception could be accomplished even faster and safer without having to observe people very long in daily behavior.

We assumed too much. This recognition is becoming more widespread and has resulted in efforts to work our way out of this impasse. We will briefly consider some examples of such efforts, beginning with those presented in this section. One of the newer trends is the increasing use of shorter projective methods, about which David and Rabinowitz have reported. The one advantage of these methods is in economy of time. This is purchased either through narrower "bandwidth" or through lessened "fidelity." Greater bandwidth and correspondingly lesser fidelity are useful for initial screening purposes, and it is in this sense that the great growth of graphology in different European countries must be understood. However, the screening aspect of shorter methods is of lesser interest to our problem; it presents no new attempt to solve the problem of interpretation, but only circumvents it. Since fidelity is waived, it is not necessary to know the exact psychological meaning of the information received; and, since measurement is not exact, it does not matter so much to know exactly what it means.

The situation is somewhat different in brief methods of narrower bandwidth. Whether they really have greater fidelity can, on the basis of currently available research, only be considered a fond hope. There is an assumption that the influence of certain factors can be eliminated—one does not expect to see everything in one test—and this makes interpretation easier. The simplification is twofold: first, only a special part of the total field of psychic tendencies or needs is encompassed, e.g. only those concerning behavior with the opposite sex, or with the family, etc.; secondly, *interpretation* is simplified, e.g. when the influence of intelligence is eliminated from a test. I believe that tests which simplify interpretation represent an advance. However, it seems to me that their main characteristic is not brevity, but their analytic nature. Among the most elucidating contributions in this area are those of Bialick and Hamlin[3] who showed how simplification of material in Rorschach protocols can produce rather reliable interpretations of certain variables.

Perhaps one danger of simplification connected with "analytic" short methods should be noted. The global techniques were developed, in part, as a reaction against too isolated observation of single characteristics, and it would surely not be desirable to fall back into the earlier methods. Professional practice has repeatedly shown that a single observation, no matter how accurate, rarely yields a conclusion regarding some definite behavior; one has to say afterwards: "Well, if I had only known that too, then I would have expected something else." Kornreich[6] showed that interpretation of certain test results is different in varied groups of somatic illness, and other studies, such as Lesser's,[7] indicated that the relationship between aggression in TAT stories and manifest aggression is of different proportion, dependent on the attitude of the subjects' mothers to open aggression. Such results support the known hypothesis that a certain test result must be differently interpreted, dependent on the variables characterizing a given subject. Hörmann[5] found this in the relationship between rigidity and interference. It simply means that, as the global test constructors postulated, one must "see" the total personality if partial behavior is to be interpreted correctly.

It seems to me that one should not be content with using any single brief test, but should combine several which encompass various partial samples of the "total band," thus joining the advantages of greater reliability of analytic methods with those of the global technique.

The approach Brengelmann suggests also involves a narrowing of "bandwidth" as a means of increasing reliability. But, his methods go much further in this direction, since he shows the necessity of determining very exactly the conditions under which an experiment is executed. The outcome can indeed depend on experimental variables. That this must be pointed out is perhaps quite characteristic for personality studies since it is so generally accepted in experimental research on perception, motor functions, etc., that all experimental conditions must be controlled. On the other hand, experimental research has rarely paid attention to the fact that changes in psychic reaction, which depend on changes in an experimental condition, are not equal for all subjects.

The research orientations of experimental and differential psychology have remained far too independent of each other. The former has been concerned only with the variables of the experimental situation, neglecting the influence of individual differences, whereas differential psychology has considered variations of reactions only as a function of personality variables. Progress in both areas will probably greatly depend on agreement to consider both kinds of variables simultaneously.

While it is relatively easy to control the external variables of the experimental situation, it is exceedingly difficult to do the same with the variables of personality. One possible way to do this, the one used most often, consists in comparing different psychopathological groups. But this is a rather rough procedure. If, for example, normals and neurotics are compared, then much more than one personality variable is varied. For just this reason, such comparisons have mostly led to unproductive results. When one succeeds, as Brengelmann apparently did, in finding characteristic, different results in exactly defined groups on simple procedures under closely controlled conditions, then this is surely an important first step. It is, however, necessary to offer hypotheses for the reasons for the differences of psychic processes in the groups compared, and such hypotheses must be confirmed in further experiments. This brings us to the fundamental difficulty of such studies, which often induces failure. There are two unknowns that condition each other: the process and the personality variables determining the process. A hypothesis about either one implicates the other, and, strictly speaking, no verification of one hypothesis alone is possible. That is why one can progress only by slow approximation.

In a similar sense, it may be desirable to pursue experiments, as recently initiated in large number, in which changes of reaction in a specific situation can be obtained by placing the same person in another state, e.g. through psychic pressure, excitement, fatigue, etc. Note for example, the work of Shakow[12] and Burdock et al.[1] Perhaps one can offer the rule (following the principle of general experimental methodology) that the simpler the experiment and the better defined the situational change, the more clear-cut the results.

CONCEPTS AND CHARACTERISTICS

A deeper and more exact understanding of personality variables is necessary, and it is probably true that it can be won only through briefer methods and the simplification of the test situation afforded by experimental approaches. However, there is another point which must be considered in the current development of theoretical bases for personality diagnosis.

I believe it is necessary to seek more clarity about concepts used in personality research. We speak about attributes, character traits, personality variables, intervening variables, "constructs," factors, behavior patterns, and many other concepts, which are used more or less frequently, depending on country and the need to keep up with the times. These varied concepts are relatively interchangeable, simply because the same term can also be applied in a different sense.

One only has to consider "rigidity," which has given rise to so many studies. Even before it entered personality psychology, rigidity, or its opposite "plasticity," was used by Gestalt psychologists to characterize certain thought structures (Lewin, Duncker). Cattel and Luchins, among others, applied the concept in the sense of a personality variable of more or less wide generality. But, in many studies it has become a behavior attribute; for example, we talk about stiffness and/or inability to change from one attitude to another. When we then compare several behavioral patterns to which the concept "rigidity" can be applied (because all are characterized by more or less stiffness), we usually find low correlations.[2]

From these low correlations it is often concluded that rigidity is not a general trait. However, all that can actually be conjectured is that behavioral patterns which outwardly appear stiff do not stem from a single personality variable. This does not exclude the possibility that there can be a "general" personality variable or a general rigidity factor which may be expressed in many different behavioral patterns. Misunderstandings arise when the same concept is used both as behavior description and as a personality variable.

Similar conceptual confusion is frequently noted in connection with such expressions as aggression, frustration, anxiety, extra/introversion, etc. Perhaps a little more clarity could be gained by adopting a rule that each expression should be followed by, respectively, (b), (p), or (c) to indicate its use as pure *b*ehavior description, a *p*ersonality variable, or a *c*onstruct.

One problem inherent in behavioral concepts is often overlooked and may be the reason for some of the lack of clarity and the difficulties arising in the evaluation of test results and their confrontation with manifest behavior. A concept is lucid when it refers to concrete behavior. For example, behavioral criteria of aggressive acts or inhibition reactions can be developed. In proceeding purely behavioristically, one must first determine whether a person acts in a certain way frequently or rarely, and then judge him accordingly as more or less aggressive. Strictly speaking, it could only be said that he is frequently or less frequently aggressive. We proceed, however, from a behavioral attribute to an attribute of the person himself. We say something about *him,* even if the report refers to behavior. A behavioral attribute is therefore, in one instance, an attribute of the behavior itself and, in another, that of the person, referring to his behavior.

This is the first of the distinctions to be considered, which becomes unimportant only if personality is defined in strictly behavioristic terms as the sum of behaviors, which no one does in practice.

A report about an attribute based on behavior usually has a double meaning in still another sense. Because in a certain behavior different degrees of intensity can usually be distinguished, the gradation of an attribute can be undertaken not only according to the frequency of its appearance, but also according to its intensity. But we are usually satisfied to name simply the degree of the attribute, without stating which of the dimensions is meant. There are many indications, however, that the psychological conditions, leading to frequent or to intensive reactions, are not identical. Obviously, the use of seemingly simple behavioral concepts is loaded with ambiguity.

So far we have discussed the instance where one goes from observation of behavior to behaviorally based personality attributes. If one works in the realm of expressive psychology, whether with projective tests or through direct observations, one again uses concepts which refer to behavior. On the basis of expressive data, a person may be judged as more or less aggressive, kind, passive, extraverted, etc. We are not interested here how such judgments are reached, or how well they are founded, but only in what they mean in general.

This mode of judgment is always present when, without explicit logical or empirical foundation, observations (for example, facial expression or drawing) which have nothing to do with the discussed behavior yield a judgment that does refer to behavior. What such a personality attribute means is often not very clear, apparently even to those who use it. Actually, it can refer to frequency or to intensity or to both of the behaviors in question. This would be transfer in a purely behavioristic interpretation. However, if a validity study then shows that the real behavior does not correspond with the given attribute, the answer would probably be: "Well, I did not mean it that way. The person *has* the given attribute; only, it does not manifest itself, or it does so very differently."

Here the attribute, which seems to refer to behavior, is considered a personality variable in the real sense. Most often the term "personality variable" refers to an intervening variable, a personality construct; that is, a condition underlying both behavior and expression or test results. From the point of view of many *Ausdruckspsychologen* these personality variables can be perceived directly from the expression, which itself is a form of behavior. Whether or not this concept is correct, it is a mistake to use terms, originally applied to behavior patterns, to designate such personality constructs, an error inherited from pre-scientific psychology.

This interpretation can be contrasted with another, which must be mentioned, if all possible interpretations and different applications of the same concepts are to be surveyed. From everything that can be learned, seen, or heard from or about a person, a pertinent portrait can be developed. In every perception of the object "personality" we comprehend an aspect of it, just as we look at a building from different standpoints, judging it in aesthetic, economic, technical terms. These perceptions of personality are psychologically similar to other perceptions and can be correctly comprehended only in Gestalt psychological terms. They develop, just as any Gestalt perception, from a dynamic, Gestalt-determined interpretation of a multitude of specific data and are therefore something other than their sum. This makes it immediately understandable why such an evaluation of a person, or such an "attribute," never or very rarely shows a simple relationship with a certain behavior or any statistically calculable combination thereof.

Whether we want to or not, we constantly work with global attributes of this kind—whether we judge people directly, or have projective test material in front of us. This becomes dangerous only when we are unaware of the nature of these attributes and nonchalantly change them into scientific categories. As such they are worthless, and that is why they have been ignored in scientific psychology. But, perhaps, it has been a mistake not to use them as material for scientific study. Such descriptive personality attributes can have a degree of safety that is not inferior to that of test results. (In Holt's work[4] the judges indicated, on the basis of test data, how sympathetic applicants appeared. Rank order according to sympathy reactions corresponded better with the criterion than did attempts to judge aptitude.)

It is by no means impossible that certain personality attributes, in this phenomenological sense, provide a better foundation for comprehending the attributes of the inner personality structure than do preferred behavioral patterns. In character studies of infants,[9, 11] the use of a category which is neither a pure behavioral attribute nor a personality construct was most appropriate for observing further relationships. I believe that it may well be worthwhile to consider these purely descriptive personality attributes a little more in scientific work; proper description is one of the foundations of any scientific progress. This demand is not at all in contradiction to the previous emphasis on more exact analyses; rather, it is a necessary supplement.

In another respect, some expansion of our horizon, as apparent in the studies of Murphy [10] and the longitudinal concepts discussed in the chapter by Skard and her associates, appears desirable. Research in personality assessment was, understandably, long determined by projective methods; if not exclusively, certainly predominantly so. These techniques constituted a new, scientific approach to personality, but connected with them was some danger of narrowing the horizon.

There can be little doubt that personality theories also depend on the methods with which material is collected. When some investigators study the behavior of people at work, while others observe sports, and still others note relationships with the opposite sex, it may be expected that each will arrive at different personality categories. It is even more one-sided to derive basic variables solely from Rorschach responses, Szondi choices, or TAT stories. The importance of socio-economic determinants is particularly well demonstrated in the Shneidman and Farberow chapter on suicide.

Too much was expected from the principle, basic to all these techniques, that the total personality is mirrored in the reaction patterns of the most diverse kind. While the principle itself may be correct, the medium through which the personality then appears, is still noticeable. However, since we are above all supposed to perceive people relative to their daily life behavior, it is essential to pay more attention to this area. Methodologically, it is much more difficult to study daily life behavior than to work with tests; and questionnaires are hardly a dependable aid in overcoming these difficulties. But, experiments made on the basis of direct observations indicate that this method is more valuable than many tests.

SUMMARY

In this commentary, I have tried to review some central problems in personality research which deserve consideration in any discussion of investigative methods. Perhaps I have over-emphasized research in personality in general instead of focusing on methods. However, the chapters on "Personality" (Jensen) and "Theory and Technique of Assessments" (Kelly) in the 1958 *Annual Review of Psychology* [13] also have considerable content overlap. This is precisely what the past few years have taught us; namely, that the methods of personality assessment cannot progress unless our theoretical insights are more solidly grounded. Today this is (fortunately) almost commonplace. Still, Kelly's wish that we must discover more ideas appears justified.

"It would be far better," he writes, "to believe that all ideas are sheer fabrications and that it is only the palpable things that sit around waiting to be discovered. Such a view would help to advance creative thinking to its proper phase in the cycle of scientific reasoning." I have not "fabricated" any ideas in this commentary but have tried to loosen up a little some of the old ideas to facilitate the creation of new ones.

References

1. Burdock, E. J., Sutton, S., and Zubin, J. Persönlichkeit und Psychopathologie. *Schweiz Z. Psychol.*, 1958, 17, 258-284.

2. Fisher, S. Patterns of personality rigidity and some of their determinants. *Psychol. Monogr.*, 1950, No. 307.

3. Bialick, I. and Hamlin, R. M. The clinician as judge: detail of procedure in judging projective material. *J. consult. Psychol.*, 1954, 18, 239-247.

4. Holt, R. R. Clinical *and* statistical prediction: a reformulation of some new data. *J. abnorm. soc. Psychol.*, 1958, 56, 1-12.

5. Hörman, H. Zum Problem der psychischen Starrheit. *Z. exp. angew. Psychol.*, 1955-6, 3, 662-683.

6. Kornreich, M. Variations in the consistency of the behavioral meaning of personality test scores. *Genet. Psychol. Mongr.*, 1953, 47, 73-138.

7. Lesser, G. S. The relationship between overt and fantasy ag-

gression as a function of maternal response to aggression. *J. abnorm. soc. Psychol.*, 1957, 55, 218-221.

8. Meehl, P. E. *Clinical vs. statistical prediction*. Minneapolis: Univ. Minnesota Press, 1954.

9. Meili, R. *Anfänge der Charakterentwicklung*. Bern: Hans Huber Verlag, 1957.

10. Murphy, Lois B. *Personality in young children*. New York: Basic Books, 1956.

11. Pulver, U. Untersuchungen über Irritierbarkeit bei Säuglingen. *Schweiz. Z. Psychol.*, 1959, 18.

12. Shakow, D. Normalisierungstendenzen bei chronisch Schizophrenen. *Schweiz. Z. Psychol.*, 1958, 17, 285-299.

13. *Annual Review of Psychology*. Palo Alto, Cal., 1958.

XVIII

Beyond Provincialism:
A Note on the
International Congress

A NEW KIND OF PUBLICATION is finding its way into the field of psychology. Psychologists from many countries are invited to join in the preparation of a volume of papers stemming from selected contributions to the international congresses sponsored by the *International Union of Scientific Psychology*. The present volume is one of the fruitful results of the 15th International Congress of Psychology held at Brussels in the summer of 1957.

A meeting of 1256 participants from 47 different countries is a very rewarding but also a severely frustrating experience. Human capacity for assimilation and reaction is too limited to allow participants to profit fully from the heterogeneous display of approaches and viewpoints usually presented at an international congress. Time is far too short for fruitful discussion, and language barriers seriously limit the exchange of ideas and even the very understanding of the arguments proposed. The best an active participant can be expected to do is to register mentally a few data, approaches, or rationales striking his interest, in the hope that they may give him some new inspiration for his own work or that he may find time to consider them more carefully when back home.

Participants and readers from different countries need an opportunity to reflect on some of the data and methods presented at international meetings. Usually, even more time is required to assimilate and evaluate research results reported from other lands than in the case of papers from one's own country on current topics using familiar methods. The international congresses do not fully attain their purpose of establishing a personal sort of international scientific contact and exchange as long as their activity is limited to the organization of a series of sessions during a very few days. These sessions are only a starting point, stimulating scientific curiosity and opening some new perspectives. To have a lasting effect, the contact should be prolonged in a way that permits careful consideration of the points which stimulated interest during the days of the meeting. Publications, such as the present one, growing out of the Congress Program, should therefore be considered more and more an essential part of the activity of the International Congress of Psychology.

As a matter of fact, each of the 15 international congresses has published bound collections of abstracts of the papers read at the meetings. These 15 volumes of *Proceedings*—the first of which was published in Paris in 1890—make fascinating reading for the contemporary psychologist interested in the history of his field.* But, the *Proceedings* cannot fulfill the role just mentioned. A complete and even enlarged version of selected papers in some areas should be made available to achieve effective penetration of ideas on the international level.

It is to the great merit of the editors and publishers of *Perspectives in Personality Theory* that they took the initiative during the 14th International Congress, held in Montreal in 1954. Psychologists from nine countries collaborated in that volume. Following this example, the Program Committee of the 15th Congress made special efforts to promote the publication of still more material from its program.

Perspectives in Personality Research brings together work of psychologists from 11 countries and papers from such different Congress sections as *The Phenomenology of Behavior, Interper-*

---

* An interesting review of the previous international congresses of psychology was published by H. Piéron, Histoire succincte des congrès internationaux de psychologie. *Année Psychologique*, 1954, 54, 397-405.

sonal Perception, Dynamics of Perception, Longitudinal Study of Personality, Projective Techniques, and *Religious Psychology.*

Other sections of the Congress were also successful in achieving publication. Most of the material from the symposium on emotion, plus other symposia contributions made by French psychologists, were published in a special 1958 issue of *Psychologie Française.* The May 1958 issue of the *Journal of Social Psychology* carried the symposium on psychological research in Africa and related papers. Other publications are still in preparation, among them the symposium on psychological and social aspects of automation.

It is worthwhile to note that as a result of these publications, some papers originally prepared and read in English at the Congress are now available in French, while authors usually publishing in European or other languages have their contributions made available in English.

It seems unavoidable, and even acceptable, that volumes from international meetings, if they are to present a true picture of the variety of problems and approaches at work in a certain area, manifest a certain lack of unity and cohesion. If the exchange of ideas on an international scale is to be fostered in a field of research such as psychology, it will be necessary to overcome some of our prejudices on this point. This kind of publication has a special purpose to fulfill, one quite different from the aim of perfectly integrated chapters written by a team of co-workers or selected co-authors.

It might be suggested, as a possible remedy, that it would be preferable to plan the congress program so as to facilitate the publication of books. I am not at all sure that this would be the best thing to do. In my experience, international congresses such as those organized by the International Union of Scientific Psychology serve their specific purpose of international contact and exchange best by not doing too much advance "editing" in organizing the program, except of course with regard to level of presentation. It is important to provide an opportunity for a large number of relatively unknown research workers of all countries to communicate their problems, findings, and methods to an international audience. At the same time, most participants will agree that at least a certain degree of structure and inner cohesion should be maintained, even in the program of an International Congress of Psychology. It is not an easy task, therefore, to find the middle of the road in this striving towards both universal participation and a well-structured program.

To provide maximum opportunities for all psychologists, some previous international congresses simply issued a free call for papers, and the congress program then consisted of a succession of heterogeneous contributions. This formula did not seem the best possible to most participants. Other congresses in this international series then organized their programs under a single theme. More recently, in Montreal (1954), the approach used was that of a few symposia organized by the Program Committee in collaboration with a specialist in the field and a few invited contributors and discussants as panel members. Both types of structured programs greatly satisfied many participants. However, it was felt that, as one result of the limited invitations, a considerable number of research workers were frustrated, having to forego an opportunity to present their new data and/or fresh approaches to an international audience.

The Brussels Congress adopted a combination formula in which 26 specific topics were selected as "Themes of the Congress." This decision was reached after personal contacts with many groups and psychological research centers in the United States, Great Britain and Continental Europe, and also on the basis of occasional contacts with visitors from other continents during the two years of planning the program. Each of the Congress themes was treated in two ways. First, there was a symposium on each topic by invited members and discussants under the direction of an invited organizer. Secondly, announcements were sent to national psychological societies and members of university psychology departments, giving qualified psychologists the opportunity of contributing individual papers related to one of the Congress themes.

It is my impression that in organizing this type of international program much depends on the personal contacts established between members of the Program Committee and a large number of research centers in as many countries as possible, in

order to pinpoint "hot" topics and areas and to find men who
are willing and able to organize well-balanced symposia on each
theme.

It is not necessary to examine here the pros and cons of such
a program, but the very fact that the editors of several volumes
—published after the Congress—requested, in addition to the
material from several symposia, also a certain number of individual papers, seems to indicate that a combination of invited and
non-invited contributions enriches the program.

The international collaboration represented in this volume
gives only a partial view of the active participation of the different countries in the Congress Program as a whole. A few
more figures may complete this picture.

For the first time, the United States had the largest single
country representation in an international congress of psychology held in Europe.* Of the 356 American members of the
Congress, about 135 participated actively in the program. This
large attendance was facilitated, in part, by the assistance of the
Union, and the financial aid of foundations. Great Britain had
about 85 active participants. France followed with about 40;
Germany (plus Austria) and Italy, about 20 each. Several Western European countries, such as Switzerland, the Netherlands,
Scandinavian countries, and Belgium each had about 10 papers.
Eastern European countries had about 30 contributors (including 4 from USSR). There were 8 active participants from Canada, 5 from South America, 6 from Asia, 6 from Africa, and 1
from Australia.

The *Proceedings* of the Congress,† a volume of more than

---

* The International Congresses of Psychology started in 1889. Three of
them were held in France (Paris 1889, 1900, 1937) and three in Great
Britain (London 1892, Oxford 1923, Edinburgh 1948). One was held in
U.S.A. (Yale 1929) and one in Canada (Montreal 1954). The others took
place in the following European countries: Germany (Munich 1896), Italy
(Rome 1905), Switzerland (Geneva 1909), The Netherlands (Groningen
1926), Denmark (Copenhagen 1932), Sweden (Stockholm 1951), and
Belgium (Brussels 1957).

† *Proceedings of the 15th Congress of Psychology, Brussels, 1957*. Published by *Acta Psychologica – European Journal of Psychology*, Amsterdam:
North-Holland Publishing Company, 1958.

600 pages, published the more or less extensive abstracts of all symposia and individual papers read at the Congress, as well as the Presidential address (by Albert Michotte), the greetings and discourses of the opening session, and the three evening lectures delivered by Clyde Kluckhohn in English, by Wolfgang Köhler in German, and by Jean Piaget in French.

The Congress also successfully fostered international scientific exchanges in other ways. There were, for example, a few round-table conferences, organized by the Congress and attended by a small number of invited participants, on such specific topics as psychological terminology, theoretical and professional training of psychologists in different countries, etc. Following the round-table conference on psychological terminology, steps were taken by the Union to support the publication of an extensive lexicon of equivalent psychological terms in English, French, and German. This lexicon is to be published in the near future. Another small group was informally brought together to examine the possibility of preparing periodically an international yearbook of psychology in which outstanding journal articles published in several languages all over the world could be translated, for instance, into English or, from time to time, into another widely spoken language. This project is in progress at the moment. Suggestions for international research in the field of social psychology were also initiated and developed.

These few examples indicate how the concern with international affairs was actively and effectively pursued during the Brussels International Congress. More than ever, the Congress has an important role to accomplish. To attain its goals, the planning of the Congress program should grow from personal contacts between the organizers and as many research centers as possible all over the world. Its activity should then be prolonged, after the meetings, in the form of publications and other projects developed under the auspices of the *International Union of Scientific Psychology*.

Index

A

Abnormal motor development, 146-8; *see also* Voluntary action in children

Actual-genetic process, 259-301; *see also* Measurement techniques

Affective response mechanisms, 155-7; *see also* Psychotherapy
and drive mechanisms, 156
and the information processing system, 158

Allport, G. W., 3-13 *passim quoted*, 247, 249

American psychology
conceptual parasitism of, 7
contrasted with European psychology, 239
as functional and practical, 239
technical fecundity of, 7

Anglo-American personality theories, 4-13

Anxiety, 101-2; *see also* Denial; Religiosity

Anxiety potential, assessment of, 123-7; *see also* Behavior theory

Apperception processes, 32

Attitudinal studies, 322-3; *see also* Personality assessment

Autoerotism, as a step toward mature sexuality, 95

B

Basic character structure, 11

Behavior, the experience of, 162-3, 166-73

Gestalt factor in, 169

Behavior theory; *see also* Anxiety potential; Blacky pictures; Cannon-Bard theory of emotion; James-Lange theory of emotion; Stimulus-response sequence
approaches to, 107
electronic working model for study of, 110-3
description of, 113-9
strategy for developing, 109-10
suggested problem areas for research on, 119-21
summary of research program, 136-7

Behavioristic fallacy, the, 161-3

Behavioristic learning theory, 10

Blacky pictures, 121-6; *see also* Behavior theory
predicting recall of, 127-31

Blacky Test, 36

Brief projective methods; *see* Personality assessment

C

Cannon-Bard theory of emotion, 120; *see also Behavior theory*

Castration anxiety, 66

Cattell Manifest Anxiety Scale, 84

Children; *see* Voluntary action in children

Clinical screening devices, 319-22; *see also* Personality assessment

Cognition; *see* Person-cognition

Cognitive complexity, 205